ALLE · ZEIT · WACH · 1842 · SJ

Current Concepts of Infections in Orthopedic Surgery

Edited by Hans K. Uhthoff

Associate Editor Elvira Stahl

With 115 Figures

Springer-Verlag
Berlin Heidelberg New York Tokyo

Editor:
HANS K. UHTHOFF MD, FRCS(C)
Prof. and Head, Division of Orthopaedics
Faculty of Medicine of the University of Ottawa, Canada

Associate Editor:
ELVIRA STAHL, BA, FAAAS, FAMWA
2021 Atwater, Suite 1610
Montréal, Qué. H3H 2P2, Canada

ISBN-13:978-3-642-69835-4 e-ISBN-13:978-3-642-69833-0
DOI: 10.1007/978-3-642-69833-0

Library of Congress Cataloging in Publication Data:
Main entry under title: Current concepts of infections in orthopedic surgery.
Bibliography: 1. Orthopedic surgery–Complications and sequelae. 2. Surgical wound infections. I. Uhthoff, Hans K., 1925– . II. Stahl, Elvira. [DNLM: 1. Infection. 2. Orthopedics. WE 168 C975] RD732.C87 1985 617'.3 84-23672 ISBN-13:978-3-642-69835-4 (U.S.)

Softcover reprint of the hardcover 1st edition 1985

2124/3130-543210

Preface

"The philosophical investigation of Pasteur long since made me a convert to the germ theory and it was on the basis of this discovery that I founded the antiseptic treatment of wounds in surgery."

Joseph Lister
1875

"Knock out germs before they breed," Joseph Lister warned his colleagues, because 45% of his amputees were dying from tetanus, septicemia, and hospital gangrene.

Today, over 100 years later, infection following trauma or surgery is still the most dreaded complication facing orthopedic surgeons. Incapacitating illness, prolonged suffering, costly hospitalization, and permanent disability are the dire consequences.

The eleventh Annual Applied Basic Science Course INFECTION IN ORTHOPEDIC SURGERY held by University of Ottawa's Division of Orthopaedic Surgery in May, 1984 was a distinguished event for three important reasons. First, it focused on the absolute necessity for structured hospital infection control. Infection surveillance is now a recognized specialty, and for optimal results, the clinical microbiologist, the surgeon and infectious disease control physician have to work as a team.

Second, this meeting brought to us innovative European investigators who presented their concepts of preventive methods in total joint replacement procedures -- the method of using a biologic carrier for antibiotic therapy, such as the fibrin-antibiotic complex and the use of antibiotic-loaded acrylic cement.

The third important topic, and most widely discussed, was prophylaxis. Opinions still differ as to the best methods. Microbial transmission and transference can occur through direct or most tortuous indirect pathways. Transference by physical contact among patients, nursing staff, physicians, and surgeons will always remain a grave risk. Pre-, peri-, and postoperative antibiotic therapy was debated daily. When -- for how long -- which antibiotic -- and how much -- are still controversial issues and consensus could not be reached. Firm recommendations, however, were made by several authoritatives

In this era of high technologic air contamination control and hermetically sealed, sterile surgical garments, an ancient principle has remained as ever -- handwashing. Infection control specialists presented us valid data showing that the nosocomial wound infection rates can be markedly reduced by handwashing between patient contacts.

Sir William Osler once remarked that "soap, water and common sense are the best disinfectants." His dictum and that of another great man still prevail. It was a historic event in the annals of hospital infection control when, one day in 1847, Dr. Ignaz Philipp Semmelweiss put up a notice on the door of his Obstetric Clinic at Vienna's General Hospital: ". . . every doctor or student who comes from the dissecting room is required to wash his hands thoroughly in a basin of chlorine water."

I should like to express my special thanks to Mrs. Elvira Stahl, my faithful and patient associate editor, and her assistant, Mrs. Ruth Stocks. I am also most grateful to Springer-Verlag, Heidelberg, in particular to Mrs. Marianne Kalow, for their collaboration in the production and publication of these proceedings.

Hans-K. Uhthoff

List of Contributors

BEAUCHAMP, C.B.	Division of Orthopedic Surgery, Sunnybrook Medical Centre, 2075 Bayview Avenue, Toronto, Ontario M4N 3M5, Canada
BRAUN, A.	Department of Orthopaedic Surgery, University of Heidelberg, Heidelberg, West Germany
BRAUSE, B.D.	Hospital for Special Surgery, Cornell University Medical College, 535 East 70th Street, New York, New York 10021, USA
BUCHHOLZ, H.W.	Endo Klinik, Holstenstrasse, 2000 Hamburg 50, West Germany
CALLAGHAN, J.J.	Hospital for Special Surgery, Cornell University Medical College, 535 East 70th Street, New York, New York 10021, USA
CARRIÈRE, J.	Infection Control Laboratory, Department of Microbiology, Montreal General Hospital, 1650 Cedar Avenue, Montréal, Québec H3G 1A4, Canada
DAIGLE, G.-A.	Division of Orthopaedic Surgery, Department of Surgery, Hôtel-Dieu de Lévis, 143 rue Wolfe, Lévis, Québec G6V 3Z1, Canada
DINGELDEIN, E.	Department of Microbiology, E. Merck, Darmstadt, West Germany
ELSON, R.A.	Department of Orthopedic Surgery, Sheffield Health Authority, Northern General Hospital, Sheffield, England
FREEMAN, J.B.	Division of General Surgery, University of Ottawa, Ottawa General Hospital, 501 Smyth Road, Ottawa, Ontario K1H 8L6, Canada
GAESE, C.	Infection Control Unit, Department of Microbiology, Montreal General Hospital, 1650 Cedar Avenue, Montréal, Québec H3G 1A4, Canada
GAGNON, P.	Department of Microbiology, Hôtel-Dieu de Lévis, 143 rue Wolfe, Lévis, Québec G6V 3Z1, Canada

GALEY, J.P.	Department of Orthopaedic Surgery, University of Ottawa, Ottawa General Hospital, 501 Smyth Road, Ottawa, Ontario K1H 8L6, Canada
GÜSSBACHER, A.	Department of Orthopaedic Surgery, University of Heidelberg, Heidelberg, West Germany
GUSTILO, R.B.	Department of Orthopedics, Hennepin County Medical Centre, 701 Park Avenue South, Minneapolis, Minnesota 55415, USA
HÄRLE, A.	Orthopädische Klinik und Poliklinik der Westfälischen Wilhelms-Universität, Hüfferstrasse 27, D-4400 Münster, West Germany
HEINE, W.-D.	Department of Pathology, Leopoldina Hospital, Schweinfurt, West Germany
HUNTER, G.A.	Division of Orthopedic Surgery, Sunnybrook Medical Centre, 2075 Bayview Avenue, Toronto, Ontario M4N 3M5, Canada
KELLAM, J.F.	Division of Orthopedic Surgery, Sunnybrook Medical Centre, 2075 Bayview Avenue, Toronto, Ontario M4N 3M5, Canada
KEMPF, I.	Centre de Traumatologie et d'Orthopédie de Strasbourg, 10, avenue A.-Baumann, 67400 Illkirch-Graffenstaden, Strasbourg, France
KINNARD, P.	Department of Orthopaedic Surgery, University of Sherbrooke, Sherbrooke, Québec J1H 5N4, Canada
KLEIN, R.F.	The New York Hospital, Cornell University Medical College, 535 East 70th Street, New York, New York 10021, USA
KLEM, M.	Centre de Traumatologie et d'Orthopédie de Strasbourg, 10, avenue A.-Baumann, 67400 Illkirch-Graffenstaden, Strasbourg, France
KLOIBER, R.	Division of Nuclear Medicine, Foothills Hospital, 1403 - 29th Street N.W., Calgary, Alberta T2N 2T9, Canada
LAFLAMME, D.	Division of Orthopaedic Surgery, Department of Surgery, Hôtel-Dieu de Lévis, 143 rue Wolfe, Lévis, Québec G6V 3Z1, Canada
LECOCQ, L.	Centre de Traumatologie et d'Orthopédie de Strasbourg, 10, avenue A.-Baumann, 67400 Illkirch-Graffenstaden, Strasbourg, France
LETTS, R.M.	Division of Orthopaedic Surgery, University of Manitoba, Health Sciences Centre-Children's, 685 Bannatyne Avenue, Winnipeg, Manitoba R3E 0W1, Canada

LINDBERG, L. — Department of Orthopaedic Surgery, General Hospital, Kristiansted, Sweden

MACDONALD, N.E. — Departments of Pediatrics and Microbiology, University of Ottawa, Children's Hospital of Eastern Ontario, 401 Smyth Road, Ottawa, Ontario K1H 8L1, Canada

MACKENZIE, A.M.R. — Department of Microbiology and Immunology; Department of Pediatrics, University of Ottawa, Children's Hospital of Eastern Ontario, 401 Smyth Road, Ottawa, Ontario K1H 8L1, Canada

MAKAREWICZ, P.A. — Division of General Surgery, Ottawa General Hospital, University of Ottawa, 501 Smyth Road, Ottawa, Ontario K1H 8L6, Canada

MCELWAIN, J.P. — Division of Orthopedic Surgery, Sunnybrook Medical Centre, 2075 Bayview Avenue, Toronto, Ontario M4N 3M5, Canada

MCINTYRE, W.M. — Division of Orthopaedic Surgery, University of Ottawa, Children's Hospital of Eastern Ontario, 401 Smyth Road, Ottawa, Ontario K1H 8L1, Canada

MERCIER, D. — Division of Orthopaedic Surgery, Department of Surgery, Hôtel-Dieu de Lévis, 143 rue Wolfe, Lévis, Québec G6V 3Z1, Canada

MILLER, J.E. — Department of Orthopaedic Surgery, Montreal General Hospital, 1650 Cedar Avenue, Montréal, Québec H3G 1A4, Canada

MONTMINY, M. — Division of Orthopaedic Surgery, Department of Surgery, Hôtel-Dieu de Lévis, 143 rue Wolfe, Lévis, Québec G6V 3Z1 Canada

NOLIN, J. — Division of Orthopaedic Surgery, Department of Surgery, Hôtel-Dieu de Lévis, 143 rue Wolfe, Lévis, Québec G6V 3Z1, Canada

PAPINEAU, L.-J. — Division of Orthopaedic Surgery, Université de Montréal, Hôpital Notre-Dame, 1560, rue Sherbrooke est, Montréal, Québec H2L 4M1, Canada

PRENTIS, J.J. — Infection Control Laboratory, Department of Microbiology, Montreal General Hospital, 1650 Cedar Avenue, Montréal, Québec H3G 1A4, Canada

RICHARDS, G.K. — Department of Microbiology, Montreal General Hospital, 1650 Cedar Avenue, Montréal, Québec H3G 1A4, Canada

SALVATI, E.A. — Hip Clinic, Hospital for Special Surgery, Cornell University Medical College, 535 East 70th Street, New York, New York 10021, USA

SITTLER, M.A. — Centre de Traumatologie et d'Orthopédie de Strasbourg, 10, avenue A.-Baumann, 67400 Illkirch-Graffenstaden, Strasbourg, France

SMALL, R.D. — Hospital for Special Surgery, Cornell University Medical College, 535 East 70th Street, New York, New York 10021, USA

TILE, M. — Division of Orthopedic Surgery, Sunnybrook Medical Centre, 2075 Bayview Avenue, Toronto, Ontario M4N 3M5, Canada

TRAVERS, S. — Infection Control Laboratory, Department of Microbiology, Montreal General Hospital, 1650 Cedar Avenue, Montréal, Québec H3G 1A4, Canada

UHTHOFF, H.-K. — Division of Orthopaedic Surgery, University of Ottawa, Ottawa General Hospital, 501 Smyth Road, Ottawa, Ontario K1H 8L6, Canada

WESTWOOD, J.C.N. — Division of Microbiology, University of Ottawa, Ottawa General Hospital, 501 Smyth Road, Ottawa, Ontario K1H 8L6, Canada

WILEY, J.J. — Division of Orthopaedic Surgery, University of Ottawa, Children's Hospital of Eastern Ontario, 401 Smyth Road, Ottawa, Ontario K1H 8L1, Canada

WINK, I. — Infection Control Laboratory, Department of Microbiology, Montreal General Hospital, 1650 Cedar Avenue, Montréal, Québec H3G 1A4, Canada

Contents

Table I. Microbes of the normal flora of body surfaces

Body surface	Microbe
Respiratory	*Meningococcus* species *Pneumococcus* species *Haemophilus* species
Gut	*Escherichia coli* *Enterococci* species *Bacteroides* species
Skin	*Staphylococcus aureus** *Staphylococcus epidermidis* beta-hemolytic *Streptococcus** Diphtheroid bacilli *Candida*

* Note: If epidemic, then infection from without

The method that we use to identify which aerobic gram-negative microbes are likely to originate from the hospital environment consists of the analysis of urinary tract infections (UTI), which can be clearly defined, the causative microbes specified, and the location of the patient known. Two populations are defined: patients within the hospital and those remote from hospital contact. A further requirement is to exclude multiple reports from the same patient, since otherwise the data would be seriously biased.

This year we examined the data of 4,093 consecutive reports of urinary tract infections, excluding 1,328 (32%) on the basis of indeterminate location and 21% of the remainder for being multiples, giving an analyzable pool of 2,193 reports. Examination of the microbial species involved showed that some had a frequency of occurrence in a hospital five times or greater than that found in a domiciliary setting. This group (Table II) was clearly defined as "hospital-associated" (Table III).

Table II. UTI organisms distribution

Organism	Distribution		Ratio H/O)*
	Hospital	Outdoor	
Group A			
E. coli	42%	77%	0.5
Enterococci species	17%	6%	3
Proteus species	9%	4.5%	2
Klebsiella species	9%	8.5%	1
Group B			
Enterobacter species	5%	1%	5*
Pseudomonas aeruginosa	12.5%	2.5%	5*
Providencia species	1.5%	0.2%	8*
Serratia species	4.5%	0.5%	9*

* Ratio of 5-fold taken arbitrarily as significant

Epidemiology of Hospital Infection – The Role of the Microbiologist

G. K. RICHARDS, J. J. PRENTIS, and I. WINK

Introduction

If the source of infection could be identified and a correct procedure to eliminate the source be applied, then infection as a complication of surgery would disappear.

Epidemiology of hospital infection is a study to determine the sources of infection. It consists of three separate parts:

1) *The collection of data* concerning patients who have become infected.
2) *The analysis* of the data to determine the likely source of infection.
3) *Experimentation* to verify whether the analysis is correct and that appropriate procedures will reduce infection rates.

The source of infection can commonly be assigned either to the external microbial environment of the hospital (including staff and other patients) or to the internal microbial environment (normal flora of surfaces) of the individual patient.

The importance of this distinction lies in the fact that we can manipulate or exclude the external environment reasonably readily; therefore, infection identified with this source should theoretically be reducible to nil. Conversely, knowledge that particular types of infection are derived from the individual's normal flora permits concentration of preventive efforts (eg, antibiotic prophylaxis) in this area.

Epidemiologic Studies

The epidemiologic study begins with the collection of a minimally necessary amount of information [patient's name, location, site of infection, date of infection and causative organism(s)]. The key requirement for analysis is a guideline which permits sorting of these data into two groups: 1) infection associated with environment, and 2) infection associated with the patient's normal flora.

There is a general agreement concerning the microorganisms present in the normal flora of adults (Table I). The problem arises that the microbial environment of hospitals varies widely from institution to institution so that guidelines effective for one may not be relevant to another. It is here that the hospital microbiologist plays his role in defining his institution's guidelines.

Current Concepts of Infections in
Orthopaedic Surgery

Table I. Microbes of the normal flora of body surfaces

Body surface	Microbe
Respiratory	*Meningococcus* species *Pneumococcus* species *Haemophilus* species
Gut	*Escherichia coli* *Enterococci* species *Bacteroides* species
Skin	*Staphylococcus aureus** *Staphylococcus epidermidis* beta-hemolytic *Streptococcus** Diphtheroid bacilli *Candida*

* Note: If epidemic, then infection from without

The method that we use to identify which aerobic gram-negative microbes are likely to originate from the hospital environment consists of the analysis of urinary tract infections (UTI), which can be clearly defined, the causative microbes specified, and the location of the patient known. Two populations are defined: patients within the hospital and those remote from hospital contact. A further requirement is to exclude multiple reports from the same patient, since otherwise the data would be seriously biased.

This year we examined the data of 4,093 consecutive reports of urinary tract infections, excluding 1,328 (32%) on the basis of indeterminate location and 21% of the remainder for being multiples, giving an analyzable pool of 2,193 reports. Examination of the microbial species involved showed that some had a frequency of occurrence in a hospital five times or greater than that found in a domiciliary setting. This group (Table II) was clearly defined as "hospital-associated" (Table III).

Table II. UTI organisms distribution

Organism	Distribution		Ratio H/O)*
	Hospital	Outdoor	
Group A			
E. coli	42%	77%	0.5
Enterococci species	17%	6%	3
Proteus species	9%	4.5%	2
Klebsiella species	9%	8.5%	1
Group B			
Enterobacter species	5%	1%	5*
Pseudomonas aeruginosa	12.5%	2.5%	5*
Providencia species	1.5%	0.2%	8*
Serratia species	4.5%	0.5%	9*

* Ratio of 5-fold taken arbitrarily as significant

Table III. UTI organisms distribution

	Distribution Hospital	Outdoor	Ratio (H/O)
Group A	1028 (77%)	819 (96%)	0.8
Group B	308 (23.5%)	38 (4.2%)	5.1

Chisquare = 136; d.f. = 1; p = .00001

Table IV. Guideline summary

Suspect infection from environment
if due to:

a) *S. aureus* (when epidemic)*
b) *Streptococcus pyogenes* (when epidemic)*
c) *Pseudomonas aeruginosa*
d) *Serratia*
e) *Providencia*
f) *Enterobacter*

* 3 or more cases per unit

Therefore, for our hospital for the current year, guidelines (Table IV) can be used to indicate whether infection is likely to have been derived from the patient or from his environment.

Recommended procedure for epidemiologic studies

We recommend that the bacteriologic reports from all patients in a hospital unit be studied, selecting those naming an organism present in the guideline list as being likely environmentally acquired. The patient's name, the site of infection, the organisms and the date of infection are then written on a card or computer program. Once a week, the current week's data are added to that of the preceding three weeks. These are sorted into groups according to organism (Table V), and then resorted into groups according to site of infection (Table VI).

Analysis

Examination of data sorted into groups by microorganism may present a problem with infection acquired from the hospital environment. Table V shows results for a hypothetical unit where three patients are infected with *Providencia* sp, and three patients with *Serratia* sp. Clearly, this is not acceptable and demands further investigation.

Two patients are infected with *Pseudomonas aeruginosa*. This might be a suspicious finding, which would not necessarily trigger off a detailed investigation, but a trend to be examined in successive weeks.

Table V. Data sorted by microbes and patients' names*

Microbe	Patient		Site	Date of infection
Providencia sp.	White	F	Wound	18 June
Providencia sp.	White	F	Urine	14 June
Providencia sp.	Brooks	E	Urine	13 June
Providencia sp.	Green	P	Urine	9 June
Pseudomonas aeruginosa	Smith	J	Sputum	10 June
P. aeruginosa	Smith	J	Urine	14 June
P. aeruginosa	Smith	J	Wound	14 June
P. aeruginosa	Johnston	B	Sputum	12 June
Serratia sp.	Jackson	C	Blood	14 June
Serratia sp.	Brown	D	Blood	14 June
Serratia sp.	Black	E	Blood	14 June
Staphylococcus aureus	Page	R	Wound	13 June
S. aureus	Page	R	Sputum	16 June
S. aureus	Scott	J	Wound	13 June
S. aureus	Harrison	V	Urine	21 June
S. aureus	Harrison	V	Wound	13 June

* Evidence of infection from environment

Table VI. Data sorted by site, microbes and patients' names

Site	Microbe	Patient	Date of infection
Blood	*Serratia* sp.	Jackson	14 June
Blood	*Serratia* sp.	Black	14 June
Blood	*Serratia* sp.	Brown	14 June
Sputum	*Pseudomonas aeruginosa*	Johnson	12 June
Sputum	*P. aeruginosa*	Smith	10 June
Sputum	*Staphylococcus aureus*	Page	16 June
Urine	*S. aureus*	Harrison	21 June
Urine	*Providencia*	Brooks	13 June
Urine	*Providencia*	White	14 June
Urine	*Providencia*	Green	9 June
Urine	*P. aeruginosa*	Smith	14 June
Wound	*S. aureus*	Harrison	21 June
Wound	*S. aureus*	Page	21 June
Wound	*S. aureus*	Scott	21 June
Wound	*Providencia*	White	18 June
Wound	*P. aeruginosa*	Smith	14 June

Three patients may have *Staphylococcus aureus* infections. It could be argued that the infection was derived from the individual patients' own flora, but three or more patients in one short period is stretching coincidence and would suggest the necessity of further investigation -- eg, phage typing of isolates.

Examination of data sorted into groups by the site of infection may indicate the mode of transmission. Table VI indicates that three patients probably acquired *Serratia* infections by a route involving intravenous medication or equipment (transducers, i.v. lines, etc) particularly as the infections are recorded as identified on the same day.

Two patients had respiratory infections with *P. aeruginosa*. If both were on ventilator-assisted respiration or were having tracheal aspiration, this finding might well cause concern and require review of equipment and procedures (*P. aeruginosa* is spread by water, wet equipment and damp hands).

Three patients are noted to have urinary tract infections due to *Providencia*. If all three had indwelling catheters, then a serious defect in closed-catheter drainage care would be suspected.

Three patients had *S. aureus* wound infections, all noted to have started the same day. This might prompt a review of the members of the operating teams, and would certainly indicate the need for clarification by further investigation -- eg, phage typing.

The role of the hospital microbiologist is therefore seen, in practical terms, to be the provider of the necessary guidelines to permit the surgeon or his deputy, with the minimum effort, to identify possible major sources of infection within his own unit within a week of its onset, and to indicate possible steps for elimination.

The Role of the Infectious Disease Physician

N. E. MacDonald

In North America, infectious disease (ID) physicians are pediatricians, internists, and occasionally microbiologists who have taken further subspecialty training. As in other specialities, most ID physicians wear three heats: researcher, teacher, and clinician.

In clinical practice, ID physicians are concerned with four main areas: 1) the host; 2) the microbes; 3) the antimicrobial agents; and 4) the environment.

The Host

Patients with common, uncomplicated infections usually do not require the special expertise of an ID physician. However, they may be helpful in treating patients with compromised host defenses. For example, the management of the child with acute leukemia who also has *Staphylococcus aureus* septicemia and osteomyelitis is far more complicated than the therapy for the same infection in a normal patient (Carney et al, 1982; De Clerck et al 1978; Ladisch and Pizzo, 1978; Pizzo, 1981). Antibiotic therapy alone is often inadequate. Prolonged bactericidal antimicrobial therapy combined with surgery and granulocyte transfusions may be necessary to clear the infection. Signs of relapse may be subtle and treatment may be complicated by superinfections with fungi or other organisms (Sen et al, 1982). Other patient groups where infections are often difficult to treat include those with vascular insufficiency, sickle cell disease, chronic granulomatous disease, immune deficiency, malnutrition, and renal or hepatic failure as well as those who are very old or very young.

Another area of concern to ID physicians are patients without major underlying medical problems who do not respond in the expected manner during treatment of a common infection. For example, the child with *Haemophilus influenzae* B septic arthritis who initially responds well to joint aspiration and intravenous cefamandole may subsequently develop a secondary fever. This fever may be due to a nosocomial infection, such as a respiratory virus infection (Hall, 1981; Wenzel et al, 1977); failure of the cefamandole to adequately eradicate the *H. influenzae* B due to the inoculum effect (Azimi and Chase, 1981); or the partial treatment of unrecognized *H. influenzae* meningitis due to failure of cefamandole to attain adequate cerebrospinal fluid levels (Steinberg et al, 1978).

The Microbes

Isolation of an unusual or unexpected organism may be an indication for consultation with an ID physician, not only for discussion of the most

Current Concepts of Infections in
Orthopaedic Surgery

appropriate antimicrobial therapy but also for consideration of why the particular organism was involved. For example, *Serratia marcescens* is an unusual cause of osteomyelitis in childhood (Jackson and Nelson, 1982). These organisms are often multiple-resistant and difficult to treat (Marcowitz and Sibilla, 1980). More elaborate *in vitro* testing may be necessary to determine the best single or combination antimicrobial therapy. In addition, one would suspect that the child might have an underlying host defence problem such as chronic granulomatous disease with failure of the bactericidal action of the neutrophils (Tauber et al, 1983). This type of patient requires prolonged antimicrobial treatment and may then benefit from prophylactic therapy to decrease the incidence and severity of future bacterial infections.

Infection in an unusual site might also suggest the need for consultation with an ID physician. For example, frontal bone osteomyelitis is a rare but serious complication of sinusitis (Wald et al, 1981). It is imperative to prevent the spread of the infection to the epidural space. This is usually done with early surgery to debride the area and drain the sinus combined with aggressive antimicrobial treatment. Since the infection may be polymicrobial, including anaerobes as well as aerobes, appropriate cultures must be taken during the operation and the initial antibiotic coverage should be broad.

The Antimicrobial Agents

The myriad of antimicrobial agents currently marketed as well as the rapid proliferation of new agents often makes drug selection complicated. An ID physician can help in the selection of the most appropriate agent taking into account the type of infection, the offending organisms, the usual side effects of the antibiotic, drug interactions, and cost. This information may be particularly useful when dealing with a patient with a multiple resistant organism who also has major underlying medical problems, eg, the patient on renal dialysis with a methicillin-resistant staphylococcal osteomyelitis of the ribs secondary to an infected dialysis access shunt. Therapy might include surgical revision of the shunt, antibiotic therapy with vancomycin and rifampin, with careful monitoring of vancomycin serum levels to prevent ototoxicity. The dosage and timing of vancomycin must be modified significantly since the normal excretion route is renal and it is not easily removed by peritoneal lavage or hemodialysis (Bennett et al, 1980). This type of patient is best managed through coordinated efforts by the orthopedic and vascular surgeons, nephrologist, and ID physician.

The ID physician may also provide advice on the use of prophylactic antibiotics in orthopedic and severely traumatized patients (Caplan and Hoyt, 1981; Norden, 1983). These patients are at high risk for developing fatal infections, mostly directly related to an invasive procedure.

The Environment

Infectious disease physicians can offer expertise in the investigation, treatment and prevention of nosocomial infections. Over 300 of every 10,000 hospitalized patients develop nosocomial infections, predominantly surgical patients, patients under intensive care, and patients with burns (Allen et al, 1981). Physicians and other hospital personnel play major roles in spreading organisms from patient to patient (Albert and Condie, 1981; Maki et al, 1982). Infectious disease physicians are involved in revising and implementing infection control and isolation policies to reduce nosocomial infections and costs. This is particularly important with the emergence of multiple drug-resistant organisms as major causes of nosocomial infection (Weinstein and Kabins, 1981).

In summary, ID physicians can help orthopedic surgeons deal with complicated, unusual or difficult infections in their patients. They can provide liaison with the microbiology laboratories to facilitate specimen collection and culture techniques, and can help interpret culture results, resistance patterns, and antimicrobial drug concentrations. They can advise which antimicrobial agent is best suited for specific infections. They can coordinate infection control measures to reduce nosocomial infections. Together with the orthopedic surgeon, they can optimize the patient's care.

References

1. Albert, R.K., and Condie, F.: Hand-washing patterns in medical intensive care units. N. Engl. J. Med. 304,1465, 1981.
2. Allen, J.R., Hightower, A.W., Martin, S.M., and Dixon, R.E.: Secular trends in nosocomial infections: 1970-1979. Amer. J. Med. 70, 389, 1981.
3. Azimi, P.H., and Chase, P.A.: The role of cefamandole in the treatment of *Haemophilus influenzae* infections in infants and children. J. Pediatr. 98, 995, 1981.
4. Bennett, W.M., Muther, R.S., Parker, R.A., et al: Drug therapy in renal failure: Dosing guidelines for adults. Part I: Antimicrobial agents, analgesics. Ann. Intern. Med. 93, 62, 1980.
5. Caplan, E.S., and Hoyt, N.: Infection surveillance and control in the severely traumatized patient. Amer. J. Med. 70, 638, 1981.
6. Carney, D.N., Fossieck, B.E., Parker, R.H., and Minna, J.D.: Bacteremia due to *Staphylococcus aureus* in patients with cancer: Report on 45 cases in adults and review of the literature. Rev. Infect. Dis. 4, 1, 1982.
7. DeClerck, Y., DeClerck, D., Rivard, G.E., and Benoit, P.: Septicemia in children with leukemia. Canad. Med. Assoc. J. 118, 1523, 1978.
8. Hall, C.B.: Nosocomial viral respiratory infections: Perennial weeds on pediatric wards. Amer. J. Med. 70, 670, 1981.
9. Jackson, M.A., and Nelson, J.D.: Etiology and medical management of acute suppurative bone and joint infections in pediatric patients. J. Pediatr. Orthop. 2, 313, 1982.
10. Ladisch, S., and Pizzo, P.A.: *Staphylococcus aureus* sepsis in children with cancer. Pediatr. 61, 231, 1978.
11. Maki, D.G., Alvarado, C.J., Hassemer, C.A., and Zilz, M.A.: Relation of the inanimate hospital environment to endemic nosocomial infection. N. Engl. J. Med. 307, 1562, 1982.
12. Markowitz, S.M., and Sibilla, D.J.: Comparative susceptibilities of clinical isolates of *Serratia marcescens* to newer cephalosporins, alone and in combination with various aminoglycosides. Antimicrob. Agents Chemother. 18, 651, 1980.

13. Norden, C.W.: A critical review of antibiotic prophylaxis in orthopedic surgery. Rev. Infect. Dis. 5, 928, 1983.

14. Pizzo, P.A.: Infectious complications in the child with cancer. II. Management of specific infectious organisms. J. Pediatr. 98, 513, 1981.

15. Sen, P., Kapila, R., Chmel H., et al: Superinfection: Another look. Amer. J. Med. 73, 706, 1982.

16. Steinberg, E.A., Overturf, G.D., Wildins, J., et al: Failure of cefamandole in treatment of meningitis due to *Haemophilus influenzae* Type B. J. Infect. Dis. 137, S180, 1978.

17. Tauber, A.L., Borregaard, N., Simons, E., and Wright, J.: Chronic granulomatous disease: A syndrome of phagocyte oxidase deficiencies. Medicine 62, 286, 1983.

18. Wald, E.R., Pang, D., Milmoe, G.J., and Schramm, V.L.: Sinusitis and its complications in the pediatric patient. Pediatr. Clin. North Am. 28, 777, 1981.

19. Weinstein, R.A., and Kabins, S.A.: Strategies for prevention and control of multiple drug-resistant nosocomial infection. Amer. J. Med. 70, 449, 1981.

20. Wenzel, R.P., Chandler, E., and Hendley, J.O.: Hospital-acquired viral respiratory illness on a pediatric ward. Pediatr. 60, 367, 1977.

Diagnosis and Treatment of Malnutrition in the Traumatized Patient

P. A. MAKAREWICZ and J. B. FREEMAN

Introduction

Malnutrition is a commonly-recognized cause of intrahospital mortality and morbidity. Two main types of hospital malnutrition are observed. 1) Patients may develop nutritional deficiencies before or after admission. These patients may have coexisting diseases which can affect their metabolism (neoplastic disease and chemotherapy; diabetes mellitus; renal insufficiency). 2) Others suffer from diseases affecting intake, digestion and assimilation of nutrients (eg, ill-fitting dentures, strictures of the gastrointestinal tract, resection of intestine, fistulas, and malabsorption syndrome). Adverse social conditions (elderly and lonely persons) or poverty predispose to malnutrition. Some psychologic and psychiatric disorders may lead to a complete refusal to eat, as in anorexia nervosa, or lack of a balanced variegated diet (eg, living on toast, coffee, and cereal, etc).

To detect all possible forms of malnutrition in patients before elective surgery, the physician should assess the patient's nutritional status and correct any existing depletion before admission. It is also important to prevent iatrogenic malnutrition during hospitalization. Trauma and surgery can increase the basic metabolic expenditure by 10-20% after major, elective procedures, to as much as 30% following multiple fractures, and to 250% in extensive burns. Catabolism in traumatized patients has long been recognized and studied. In 1931, Sir David Cuthbertson showed an increase in the basal metabolic rate of animals with multiple fractures of long bones.

In emergency situations, physicians have to perform essential life-saving procedures and concentrate on acid-base and electrolyte equilibrium. Ordering 5% dextrose as a caloric supplement is common. These patients have much higher caloric and protein requirements and may develop profound nutritional depletion within a few days. This catabolic situation is frequently worsened by administration of corticoids.

Nutritional Assessment

A properly performed nutritional interview is important and can be crucial for the early detection of malnutrition. The history should include at least the following:

- recent weight change (significant if >10%);
- nausea, vomiting, or diarrhea;
- recent surgery or trauma;

Current Concepts of Infections in Orthopaedic Surgery

- presence of chronic illnesses (eg, neoplasm; diabetes mellitus; hyperlipidemia; renal, liver or heart failure; peptic ulcer);
- presence of digestive abnormalities (pancreatic disorders; milk intolerance; inflammatory bowel disease; fistula);
- abnormal social condition (elderly living alone; drug addiction);
- abnormal dietary habits (limited diet; loss of taste or smell; recent diet change);
- intake of drugs known to affect dietary absorption or food utilization (antacids; antibiotics; laxatives; diuretics; antineoplastics; contraceptives).

A complete physical examination with a careful search for signs of malnutrition is the next step in a nutritional assessment. Evidence of muscle and/or fat wasting is usually obvious but sometimes can be overlooked, especially when the patient is obese. In severe protein depletion, detection of muscle wasting in the temporal region and interosseal spaces of the hands may be helpful. Assessment of skin turgor, color, presence of any dermatologic changes, and hair loss may indicate specific vitamin deficiences. Baker et al (1982) showed that nutritional status assessments can be standardized and their validity has been repeatedly confirmed. If the presence of malnutrition has been determined or is suspected, confirmation and quantification should be obtained by anthropometric and laboratory studies.

The best and most reliable method is the assessment of body composition by measurement of radioisotope concentrations (Shizgal, 1981). This method requires highly specialized equipment; a specially designed laboratory with trained personnel is relatively expensive and not commonly available.

Simpler anthropometric measurements can be used for nutritional assessment: 1) body weight and its relation to the ideal body weight based on the patient's height and % weight loss; 2) skinfold thickness by measuring the alteration of patient's subcutaneous tissue. Measurements are taken from the posterior side of the nondominant arm and lower angle of the scapula, using a specially-designed skin caliper, such as the Lange and Harpender calipers. The triceps skinfold (TSF) combined with midarm circumference (MAC) allows calculating the arm muscle area (AMA) which is an indirect indicator of muscle body mass:

$$AMA = \frac{(MAC - Pi\ TSF)^2}{4\ Pi}$$

Most biochemical tests are based on the theory that protein malnutrition causes decrease in total body pool, affecting the serum protein levels. For nutritional purposes, the best tests are serum albumin and serum transferrin levels. Kaminski (1976) has shown that decrease in transferrin serum levels below 170 mg/L causes a 2.5-fold increase of mortality in postoperative patients.

Daily urinary nitrogen and creatinine excretion are also correlated with nutrition. Nitrogen excretion is closely related to its intake and utilization. Balancing nitrogen intake and excretion with respect to consumption versus inappropriate urinary and fecal losses is helpful in assessing the adequacy of nutritional support. Urinary creatinine excretion in humans is relatively constant unless there are major changes in creatine intake, muscle work or muscle mass. There is a constant relationship between creatinine excretion and height (the creatinine/height index). This index can be expressed as a percentage of normal indices taken from standard tables.

Malnutrition significantly alters the immunologic response manifested by a decrease in circulating lymphocytes and impaired cell-mediated immunity. The latter can be easily detected using four to six common antigens such as tetanus, diphtheria, streptococcus, trichophyton, or candida.

To quantify malnutrition, Buzby and Mullens (1980) combined several nutritional indices (age, weight, lymphocyte count and serum albumin) to create a numerical nutritional index. This mathematical formula is reputed to assess surgical risk in relation to the degree of malnutrition but it has recently come under serious criticism.

It is important to appreciate that each variable used to assess the degree of malnutrition can be affected by a number of other variables. For example, immunoresponse may also be reduced in patients with cancer, immunosuppression or zinc deficiency. There are many causes of albumin loss. Reductions in skin reactivity or serum albumin are generally not useful in specific patients or population groups. One cannot expect marked improvements in some measurements during nutritional repletion. Because of this lack of specificity, it is important to carry out a complex assessment of each patient consisting of a history, physical and biochemical examination (Grant et al, 1981). Following is a typical nutritional profile (Table I).

Table I. Nutritional profile: Patient _____

	Expected	Obtained	% Expected
Albumin	4.5 mg%	3.5 mg%	77.7
Weight	75 kg	62 kg	82.6
Creatinine/ height index	9.38	8.75	93.3
Skin test	7 +	2 +	RA*

* RA = relative anergy; anergy if patient has no response to any of the antigens - patient response to less than 3/7 antigens

Nutritional Support

1. *Correlating the composition of the diet* with the patient's requirements is the simplest and the most neglected method of correcting mild nutritional depletion in patients with intact gastrointestinal tracts, especially during periods of convalescence. A dietetic consultation in the presence of improper dietary habits may be helpful.

2. *Enteral feeding* is the most physiologic method of nutritional support. A staggering array of enteral formulas are available which differ in composition, concentration, osmolarity and degree of nutrient degradation. Blenderized formulas consist of whole food. Therefore, they contain all required nutrients and a high fiber content. The disadvantages of these

formulas are the necessity of having to use a large bore tube and the chance of bacterial contamination. Chemically defined formulas contain amino acids, simple sugars, essential fatty acids, vitamins and minerals. These formulas can be divided into two groups: elemental (all nutrients are in the simplest molecular form, usually with less than 2% fat content); and nonelemental, where sugars are more complex, protein is present as a hydrolysate rather than simple amino acids and fat content is higher. If the gastrointestinal tract is functioning, the nutritional values of these formulas do not differ. Because of the higher osmolarity of elemental formulas, however, nausea, vomiting and diarrhea are more frequent. Elemental formulas are ideal for patients in whom digestion and assimilation of nutrients are decreased (inflammatory bowel disease, pancreatitis, malabsorption, GI fistula, etc.) (Dubois et al, 1984). The selection of an enteral formula is primarily determined by the experience of the nutritional team and patient tolerance. Frequently, physicians turn to the elemental formulas prematurely. Evidence from our institution indicates that complications from these hyperosmolar elemental formulas may outweigh their theoretical benefits (Fairfull-Smith and Freeman, 1980).

Enteral feeding may be administered orally as a supplementary diet in patients with moderate or chronic depletion who are able to eat. Again, preference should be given to formulas which are isoosmotic and several varieties may have to be tried to find one which the patient tolerates. If elemental formulas are given orally, palatability is a problem because of the presence of the amino acids. There are flavored varieties but this increases osmolarity. Sometimes these formulas can be mixed with juice or frozen and then sucked like a popsicle. Alternatively, forced feeding using feeding tubes may be required in patients who are unable or unwilling to ingest food. When patients are eating but the quantity or quality of food consumed is in question, a three-day calorie and protein count should be made. An intake of less than 1000 Kcal and 50 g of protein daily is an indication for forced tube feeding.

Enteral feeding may be started immediately after major surgery even when the gastrointestinal tract is involved. Recent studies from our unit clearly show that patients can tolerate enteral feeding provided the stomach is bypassed after major abdominal procedures (Fairfull-Smith and Freeman, 1980). This can be accomplished by inserting a long tube transnasally, passing through the pylorus and into the duodenum or, alternatively, by inserting a jejunostomy tube during the operation. The latter is an essential maneuver in a multiple injured patient in whom oral intake will be delayed (eg, major pancreatic or duodenal injuries or head trauma). In this way, both parenteral nutrition and the necessity for prolonged nasogastric feeding are avoided.

Complications of enteral feeding may be caused by the tube used for administration of the formula. The risk of aspiration is greatest when nasogastric tubes are used because they permit free gastroesophageal reflux. Nasogastric feeding should ideally be done using fine bore (#8 French) silastic or teflon tubes with weighted mercury tips so that they will pass into the duodenum. All tubes should be carefully fixed to the external nares in such a way as to avoid ulceration. Other complications include cramping, abdominal distension, diarrhea and/or vomiting and are caused by hyperosmolarity or overload with formula. The latter complications can be avoided by gradually increasing the concentration and flow rate of the formula. We usually start with a half-strength solution at 25 to 50 mL/h, gradually increasing the rate and concentration to achieve full strength administration at 100 to 125 mL/h over 48 hours. However, each patient is different and the physician must individualize the procedure during this adaptation period. This emphasizes the importance of supplemental parenteral feeding since some patients require 7 days or more before they will accept this rate and concentration. Enteral feeding may be administered by continuous, 24-hour infusion or in larger boluses. The constant infusion technique has been recommended because it avoids diarrhea, and most enteral feeding progresses in this manner. However, some recent evidence indicates that bolus feeding over 12 to 18 hours per day may be more physiologic. Some surgeons give the entire day's requirements, with apparent success, in four equally divided bolus injections through a large nasogastric tube. This technique certainly saves time and money (no pumps required) but its safety, particularly with respect to aspiration, has not been documented. Also, the large volume of hyperosmolar formula will more frequently cause nausea, vomiting, cramps or diarrhea (Kaminski, 1976).

3. *Total parenteral nutrition (TPN)* is the most efficient form of support from a nutritional point of view because it assures that all required nutrients will be delivered and utilized. These nutrients are delivered via a catheter introduced into a large caliber vein such as subclavian or jugular. Since these nutrients are delivered directly into a large vein, immediately above the heart, dilution is instantaneous and there are few limitations with respect to solution concentration and osmolarity. Adaptation time is short (less than 72 hours) and repletion, although less physiologic, proceeds more rapidly than with enteral nutrition, at least in sick patients. The caloric source is 50% dextrose either alone or administered with a 10 or 20% lipid emulsion. The basic formula consists of 500 mL of 50% dextrose with 500 mL of an 8.5 to 10% amino acid solution. This results in a 25% dextrose-4.2 to 5.0% amino acid mixture. To this one must add all of the required fat- and water-soluble vitamins, now available in a single vial, and all required electrolytes and trace elements such as zinc, copper and chromium. Two 500 mL bottles of 10% lipid emulsion are given weekly to prevent essential fatty acid deficiency.

This technique is highly efficacious but the large concentrations of dextrose result in fatty infiltration of the liver and the excessive production of water and carbon dioxide may impair pulmonary function, especially in patients on ventilators. For these reasons, many have turned to the routine use of a more physiologic mixture using lower concentrations of dextrose while maintaining the caloric requirements with the simultaneous infusion of a lipid emulsion.

The normal resting energy requirements are approximately 30 Kcal/kg of ideal weight/day but these rise considerably in the presence of stress, sepsis, or trauma. Similarly, most patients will be adequately maintained with between 1 and 1.5 g of protein/kg ideal body weight. The total caloric requirements would normally be given either entirely as dextrose or in a 70:30% ratio to simulate normal oral intake. One liter of typical TPN solution (25% dextrose-5% amino acids) contains 250 g dextrose (1000 Kcal) and 50 g protein (8 g nitrogen). A liter of 10% lipid emulsion contains 50 g fat (450 Kcal) and 25 g glycerol (100 Kcal). Patients with high energy requirements or glucose intolerance require special attention and modification of the formula. Special consultation from the Nutritional Support Service is recommended for complicated cases.

The catheter is usually introduced into the superior vena cava via the subclavian or jugular vein. The introduction site should be covered with a transparent dressing (Op-Site), allowing for observation and early detection of infection. The metabolic status, catheter site and nutritional intake must be closely monitored, usually by a Nutrition Support Nurse and one or more physicians. Subclavian catheter insertion should not be approached lightly. We regard it as a highly skilled procedure carried out by experienced residents or members of the nutritional support team. It has been associated with many complications ranging from simple pneumothorax to hemothorax secondary to subclavian artery puncture, air and catheter embolism, myocardial perforation and death. Other complications related to the catheter or insertion site may develop later during TPN therapy and include sepsis (microbial or fungal), subclavian thrombosis and/or septic thrombophlebitis. The most common organisms responsible for sepsis are staphylococci and candida. Other complications during TPN are metabolic disturbances. They may include hyper- and hypoglycemia, hyperosmolar coma, acidosis/alkalosis and a number of electrolyte, vitamin, and macro and trace metal deficiencies (Burchett and Freeman, 1981).

4. *Peripheral parenteral nutrition (PPN)* is the delivery of calories and proteins via peripheral rather than large central veins, using 5% amino acids mixed with 5% rather than 25% dextrose. This reduction in calories (not protein) compared with TPN is due to the limited capacity of peripheral veins to tolerate hyperosmolar solutions. However, we have clearly shown that PPN improves nitrogen balance and is beneficial, particularly where the hospital personnel is unfamiliar with central vein catheter insertion techniques or the subsequent care of these catheters (Freeman, 1978). In addition, the indications for TPN are not always absolute; yet, one is reluctant to let the patient's malnutrition progress. In such instances, short 7 to 10-day periods of PPN are definitely justified until the patient can eat or clearly requires TPN. Such patients will obviously receive inadequate caloric intake. When the caloric requirements are higher, one can simultaneously infuse a fat emulsion. These emulsions are isotonic and nonirritating to peripheral veins, and are also valuable when fluid restriction or glucose intolerance are a problem. Since each 500 mL bottle of 10% lipid contains 550 calories (twice that amount in the 20% emulsion), insulin is not required for the metabolism of the fat. We have also shown improved PPN when glycerol rather than dextrose was added to the amino acid solution (Freeman et al, 1983).

The most frequent complication of PPN is peripheral phlebitis secondary to the hyperosmolarity of the amino acid component of the nutritional solution. This causes patient discomfort, necessitates frequent restarts, and may lead to a loss of peripheral veins. Each time phlebitis occurs, nutritional inflow is temporarily interrupted. Phlebitis may also cause fever which may prolong hospital stay, increase physician care, and result in increased costs as one has to diagnose the source of the fever. Recently, we have been able to prevent phlebitis during PPN by carrying out infusion of the nutritional solutions for a minimum of one week. In this double-blind, prospective study, considerable evidence suggests that a specially designed antiphlebitic mixture can significantly reduce the incidence of phlebitis (Bass et al, 1984; Makarewicz et al, 1984).

In summary, PPN is an ideal method for delivering calories and protein to the post-traumatic or postoperative malnourished patient provided the period of reduced food intake is expected to be short and the indication for TPN is not clear or the institution does not have the capabilities of administering TPN (Watters and Freeman, 1981).

HÔPITAL GÉNÉRAL D'OTTAWA
OTTAWA GENERAL HOSPITAL
501 CHEMIN SMYTH ROAD, OTTAWA K1H 8L6

ORDONNANCE DE NUTRITION PARENTÉRALE TOTALE
TOTAL PARENTERAL NUTRITION ORDER

LES ORDONNANCES DOIVENT ÊTRE REÇUES À LA PHARMACIE À **1200** HEURES. LES ORDONNANCES REÇUES APRÈS **1200** HEURES SERONT PRÊTES LE LENDEMAIN. CETTE ORDONNANCE EST VALIDE À PARTIR DE **1800** HEURES LE DATE ______	ORDERS MUST BE RECEIVED IN PHARMACY BY **1200** HRS. ORDERS RECEIVED AFTER **1200** NOON WILL BE PREPARED FOR THE FOLLOWING DAY. THIS ORDER WILL BE IN EFFECT STARTING AT **1800** HRS. ON DATE ______

A — SOLUTE FONDAMENTALE — BASIC SOLUTION

ACIDE AMINE / AMINO ACIDS / DEXTROSE

1. ☐ ACIDE AMINE 42.5g (4.25%) AMINO ACID — DEXTROSE 1250 mmol (25%) — TAUX/RATE ______ mL/hr — TOTAL ______ mL/24hr

OU/OR

2. ☐ ACIDE AMINE 42.5g (4.25%) AMINO ACID — DEXTROSE ____ mmol (____%) — TAUX/RATE ______ mL/hr — TOTAL ______ mL/24hr

LIPID

3. ☐ LIPID **10%** — TAUX/RATE ______ mL/hr — TOTAL ______ mL/24hr

OU/OR

4. ☐ LIPID **20%** — TAUX/RATE ______ mL/hr — TOTAL ______ mL/24hr

☐ QUOTIDIENNEMENT / DAILY
OU/OR
☐ LUNDI ET JEUDI POUR LE EFAD
MONDAY & THURSDAY FOR EFAD

NOTE: RÉSERVER AUX MALADES RESTRAINT AUX LIQUIDES SEULEMENT.
RESERVE FOR FLUID RESTRICTED PATIENTS ONLY.

B — ADDITIFS — ADDITIVES

1. ELECTROLYTES
AU **1000** ml PER **1000** ml

	☐ STANDARD	OU/OR ☐ SPÉCIAL SPECIAL
SODIUM	35 mmol	mmol
POTASSIUM	30 mmol	mmol
CHLORURE-CHLORIDE	35 mmol	mmol
CALCIUM	2.25 mmol	mmol
MAGNESIUM	2.5 mmol	mmol
PHOSPHATE	15 mmol	mmol
ACETATE	68 mmol	26 mmol
GLUCONATE	mmol	mmol

2. OLIGO ÉLÉMENTS / TRACE ELEMENTS ☐
(Ajouter à **1** unité par jour/Add to **1** unit per day)

CHROMIUM	0.2 µmol
CUIVRE-COPPER	15 µmol
MANGANESE	9 µmol
ZINC	60 µmol

3. VITAMINES / VITAMINS ☐
(Ajouter à **1** unité par jour/Add to **1** unit per day)
MVI-12 10 mL

À L'USAGE DE LA PHARMACIE - PHARMACY USE ONLY

CALORIES / 24 hr. CHO ______ K cal
Lipid ______ K cal
TOTAL ______ K cal

PROTÉINE
PROTEIN / 24 hr. ______ g
INGÈRE EN NITROGÈNE
NITROGEN INTAKE 24 hr. ______ g

PROPORTION DE CALORIES SANS PROTÉINE (grammes utilisable N) (proportion idéale 150 cal/gm N) ______
RATIO NON-PROTEIN CALORIES (grams utilizable N) (ideal ratio 150 cal/gm N)

VALEURS DU LABORATOIRE - LABORATORY VALUES:

DATE:						
Na						mm/l
K						mm/l
Cl						mm/l
Ca						mm/l
PO_4						mm/l
Mg						mm/l
Zn						mm/l
TCO_2						mm/l
GLU						mg/dl
BUN						mg/dl
CR						mg/dl
Alb.						g/dl
Poids WEIGHT						kg

ORDONNÉE PAR: ORDERED BY:	COMITE DE NUTRITION NUTRITION COMMITTEE CONSULTANT	DATE

66-59 (08-82) CAT: 413295

Fig. 1. Total parenteral nutrition order form

Nutrition support team. To coordinate and supervise nutritional support in our institution, a Nutrition Committee was formed. Representatives from medicine, surgery, pharmacy, nursing, and dietetics are members of this Committee. Guidelines for nutritional assessment and support (both intravenous and enteral) protocols for individual procedures have been developed and a consultative service organized to assure the delivery of safe and cost-effective nutritional support. An order form for the delivery of nutritional support has been designed which greatly simplifies the ordering of solutions and encourages participation by the individual physician (Fig. 1). This nutrition support team, after performing an initial assessment, recommends a particular method of nutrition, the calorie-protein requirements, duration of support, and follows the patient during the entire period of nutritional support.

References

1. Baker, J.P., et al: A comparison of clinical judgement and objective measurements. N. Engl. J. Med. 306, 969, 1982.
2. Bass, J., Freeman, J.B., et al: Prevention of phlebitis in surgical patients. A double blinded prospective study. 8th Clinical Congress, Aspen. 1984.
3. Burchett, H., and Freeman, J.B.: Current concepts of total parenteral nutrition. J. Can. Hosp. Assoc. 58, 14, 1981.
4. Buzby, G.P., and Mullen, J.L.: Prognostic nutritional index in gastrointestinal surgery. Am. J. Surg. 139, 160, 1980.
5. Dubois, P., Fairfull-Smith, R.J., and Freeman, J.B.: A comparison of elemental and nonelemental diets in postoperative enteral feeding. Cont. Surg. 24, 65, 1984.
6. Fairfull-Smith, R.J., and Freeman, J.B.: Immediate postoperative enteral nutrition with nonelemental diet. J. Surg. Res. 29, 236, 1980.
7. Freeman, G.B., Fairfull-Smith, R.J., et al: Safety and efficacy of a new peripheral intravenously administered amino acid solution containing glycerol and electrolytes. Surg. Gynecol. Obstet. 156, 625, 1983.
8. Freeman, J.B.: Peripheral parenteral nutrition. Can. J. Surg. 21, 489 1978.
9. Grant, J.P., Custer, P.B., and Thurlow, J.: Current techniques of nutritional assessment. Surg. Clin. North Am. 61, 437, 1981.
10. Kaminski, M.: Enteral hyperalimentation, Surg. Gynecol. Obstet. 143. 1976.
11. Makarewicz, P.A., Freeman, J.B., et al: Prevention of phlebitis during peripheral parenteral nutrition (In preparation).
12. Shizgal, H.M.: Body composition and nutritional support. Surg. Clin. North Am. 61, 729, 1981.
13. Watters, J.M., and Freeman, J.B.: Parenteral nutrition by peripheral vein, Surg. Clin. North Am. 61, 593, 1981.

Recommended Reading

Fisher, J.E.: Surgical Nutrition. Little, Brown & Co. 1983.

Kirkpatrick, J.R.: Nutrition and Metabolism in the Surgical Practice. Futura Publications Co. 1983.

Skin Bacterial Populations - Contamination or Infection?

G. K. RICHARDS, J. E. MILLER, and J. CARRIÈRE

The bacterial causes of deep wound infection after total joint replacement are well known. Review of 17,170 infected total hip replacements (THR) procedures (Franco and Ennekin, 1979) implicated *Staphylococcus aureus* in 50%, *Staphylococcus epidermidis* in 29%, and gram-negative rods in 14% of patients.

Infection originating at the time of surgery could theoretically be derived from the bacterial flora of the patient's skin, be blood-borne, or derived from the external microbial environment either directly at the time of surgery or indirectly by prior colonization of the patient.

The air in a modern operating room equipped with microfiltration and properly engineered laminar flow air-delivery systems is known to be free of large numbers of organisms. It can therefore be reasonably discounted as a major source of these organisms. The desirable current practice of operating with the minimum duration of prior hospital stay diminishes the chance of significant colonization from the environment.

The two probable sources, therefore, are the patient's skin flora (known to include staphylococci and, possibly, gram-negative rods) and bacteremias, for which the likeliest origin is colonization or infection of the urinary tract (primarily gram-negative rods).

To clarify this problem, a bacteriologic screening procedure was designed to evaluate the bacterial skin and urinary tract flora of patients before carrying out total joint arthroplasty.

The screening took place approximately three weeks before the date booked for surgery and consisted of four parts:

1) A questionnaire for high risk factors, covering the preceding 12 months, including a history of respiratory tract infection (middle ear, sinuses, teeth, gums, bronchitis and pneumonia), skin infection ("spots", pustules, boils, eczema, psoriasis), urinary tract infection (symptoms and surgery), and the use of antibiotics. Previous surgical procedures and associated infections, the use of steroids and known antibiotic allergy were also noted.

2) A clean-catch midstream specimen of urine was collected for microscopic examination and culturing.

3) Cultures were taken as a minimum from the nostrils, the hairline of the forehead, both arms and hands (particularly from the fingers), the

Current Concepts of Infections in
Orthopaedic Surgery

lateral aspects of both hips, thighs and lower legs, plus three overlapping cultures of the proposed area for incision.

A preliminary trial examined various sampling techniques including high volume slit-sampling of air close to the patient, clothes and skin; a variety of contact plates; and swabs using adhesive solutions. The most effective practical method was found to be the use of swabs, previously immersed in a tube of 5 mL of peptone water, streaking the skin firmly in a standardized manner (eg, 12 strokes to cover an area of approximately 18 x 10 cm). The tubes containing the swabs were directly subcultured, incubated for a further 18 hours and then replated. (More nutritious primary culture media were found to increase technical problems by the overgrowth of dubiously pathogenic organisms, eg, diphtheroids).

4) The isolates of *S. epidermidis* obtained from the planned operating sites were pooled and tested against a number of antibiotics, including cloxacillin, cefazolin, cefamandole, and tobramycin to determine their ability not only to inhibit but to kill completely the inoculum at appropriate concentrations.

Coagulase-negative staphylococci (*S. epidermidis* and *Staphylococcus albus* in routine laboratories) are now known to be separable into 14 species of varying pathogenic potential (Kloos, 1982). *S. epidermidis* is associated with infections of prostheses and i.v. catheters, and *Staphylococcus saprophyticus* with urinary tract infections. The remaining 12 species are of dubious or rare pathogenicity (Kloos, 1982; Lowy et al, 1983). Of particular relevance is the description of mucoid strains of *S. epidermidis* of enhanced pathogenicity in experimental models (Christensen et al, 1983). Our data do not distinguish among these species, but groups them as *S. epidermidis*.

The *S. aureus* carriage status was recorded as: negative; nasal only; passive contact (occasional isolates commonly of mixed phage types); and dispersers, which appear to be covered head to foot in *S. aureus*, a state associated with spread of organisms (Richards, 1973) and a high risk of self-infection.

Results

To date, 212 patients have been surveyed, comprising 152 hip, 54 knee total arthroplasties, and six other procedures.

A. *Urine cultures* of 106 patients revealed six (7%) clinically unsuspected bacteriurias or urinary tract infections by gram-negative rods (coliforms/enterobacteriaceae).

B. *S. aureus screening* of 212 patients showed 121 (57%) negative; 21 (10%) nasal carriage only; and a surprising 70 (33%) were positive at the proposed surgical site (25% dispersers, 8% passive contacts). This high incidence parallels the high incidence in THR sepsis (Table I). Awareness of this finding allowed elimination by hexachlorophene shampoos and baths in good time for the booked procedure.

C. *Skin survey* results are given in Table II. All patients carried *S. epidermidis* (the second most frequent cause of THR sepsis). Six patients

Table I. Bacteriology of deep wound infections in THR*
n = 17,170 procedures

	Early	Late	Total
S. aureus	58%	39%	50%
S. epidermidis	21%	41%	29%
Gram-negative rods	17%	10%	14%
Others	4%	5%	7%

* Franco, J.A. and Enneking, W.F., 1979

(3%) carried hemolytic streptococci (Lancefield groups A, B), of high destructive potential, at the operating site.

It would have been reasonable to assume that hips would be more likely to be colonized by fecal organisms (coliforms, enterococci) than knees, but this was not found. Perhaps this is a drawback of the modern flush-toilet, a producer of major aerosols.

Colonization with *S. epidermidis* alone was found in only 12%, an unsuspected finding.

Table II. Preoperative skin flora

	Hips n = 152		Knees n = 54		Totals n = 206	
S. epidermidis	152	100%	54	100%	206	100%
S. aureus	45	30%	23	43%	68	33%
Hemolytic streptococci	4	3%	2	4%	6	3%
Streptococcus viridans	26	17%	16	30%	42	20%
Bacillus subtilis	49	32%	28	52%	77	37%
Enterococci	40	26%	17	32%	57	28%
Coliforms	43	28%	14	26%	57	28%
Pseudomonas aeruginosa	1	0.7%	1	2%	2	1%
Alkaligenes	14	9%	13	24%	27	13%
Acinetobacter	51	34%	24	44%	75	36%
S. epidermidis only	22	15%	2	4%	24	12%

D. *Antibiotic sensitivity* results are summarized in Table III. Routine antibiotic sensitivity testing requires generally pure isolates (the predominant strain), and use methods (disc, agar and broth dilutions) to determine whether the isolates are inhibited by the antibiotic. For prophylaxis of skeletal prosthetic implantation procedures, it is evidently preferable to use an antibiotic known to be bactericidal, ie, that does not merely inhibit but kills the entire test population of microorganisms (which in our test is pooled).

Table III. Summary of antibiotic tests of pooled *S. epidermidis*

		Bacteriostatic (sensitive)	Bactericidal
Cloxacillin	n = 177	86%	24%
Cefazolin	n = 177	98%	96%
Cefamandole	n = 156	99%	74%
Tobramycin	n = 167	96%	68%

Tests for inhibition alone (Table III) would indicate that cloxacillin (86%) was a reasonable prophylactic choice, cefazolin was better (98%), and cefamandole (98.6%), with only one resistant pool in 156 tested, would be preferred overall.

Tests for bactericidal activity give a different picture. Cloxacillin is no longer desirable, and cefazolin (96%) is preferred over cefamandole (74%) as the desirable prophylactic antibiotic on the basis of this test procedure. This is a significant finding.

The advantages of preoperative screening (skin and urine) before THR surgery are summarized in Table IV. Our results indicate that this is a worthwhile procedure, particularly the reassurance for the surgeon that the antibiotic chosen for prophylaxis has not failed laboratory testing for bactericidal efficacy. Should infection occur, even several months later, the earlier findings may indicate likely pathogens, and reviving the stored frozen pooled cultures would enable the use of advanced typing techniques to confirm or disprove the identity of the skin strains with those found on investigative surgery.

Skin bacterial populations are apparently sufficiently large to be the main source of infection complicating prosthetic surgery (with possible contri-

Table IV. Advantages of preoperative screening

Excludes unsuspected bacteriuria or UTI
Excludes the presence of *S. aureus* at the surgical site (if present can be removed in time)
Maps the individual skin flora
Confirms the choice of an appropriate prophylactic antibiotic
Baseline should infection occur later: a) Suggests possible pathogens b) If culture obtained, may indicate if infection from patient or environment
Permits epidemiologic studies
Security

butions from the urinary tract). Further study, incorporating newly available subspeciation and typing procedures, is necessary to confirm this identity beyond any reasonable doubt.

References

1. Christensen, G.D., Simpson, W.A., Bisno, A.L., and Beachey, E.H.: Experimental foreign body infections in mice challenged with slime-producing *Staphylococcus epidermidis*. Infection and Immunity 407, 1983.

2. Franco, J.W. and Enneking, W.F.: Infections of skeletal prostheses. In, Bennett, J.V., and Brachman, P.S. (Eds.): Hospital Infections. Little, Brown, 1979. p. 323.

3. Kloos, W.E.: Coagulase-negative staphylococci. Clin. Microbiol. Newsletter 4, 75, 1982.

4. Lowy, F.D. and Hammer, S.M.: *Staphylococcus epidermidis* infections. Ann. Int. Med. 99, 834, 1983.

5. Richards, G.K.: The epidemiology of sepsis. Clin. Orthop. 96, 5, 1973.

Infections in Orthopedics: Patient Preparation and Skin Scrub

J. C. N. Westwood

Introduction

With the introduction of antiseptic surgery by Lister at the end of the last century, sterilization of the hands of the operating team became a cardinal requirement. The first antiseptic chosen for the purpose was phenol -- a substance which was anything but kind to the surgeons' hands. At a later date, mercurials replaced phenol. Although the mercurials were found eventually to be inefficient degerming agents since they are bacteriostatic but not bactericidal, they made a most vital, albeit accidental, contribution to surgical antisepsis by leading to the development of the surgical rubber glove. Originally produced to protect the hands of Halsted's operating room nurse from the antiseptic to which she became sensitized, these gloves were not used as a deliberate barrier against contamination of the surgical site.

Despite its humble start, however, the rubber glove opened the door to the entirely new concept of aseptic surgery which was to depend not on the chemical destruction but on the total exclusion of all microbial contamination. This concept, coupled with prior sterilization of all materials in contact with the wound, produced a miraculous change in the entire application of surgery. Eventually, it made possible the reconstructive techniques that are now commonplace and a major accomplishment in orthopedic surgery.

In theory, the interpolation of the sterile impermeable barrier supposedly provided by the operating room clothing should eliminate the necessity for sterilization of the surgeons' hands and should also provide complete protection from the entire body flora of the operating team. Unfortunately, this ideal has never been achieved. The failure of the barrier in practice will become abundantly clear from the presentations of other speakers and has necessitated the introduction of elaborate space-age measures to reduce wound infections in critical procedures. Rubber gloves, on the other hand, are both sterilizable and impermeable and should therefore have eliminated the need for special measures as far as the surgeons' hands are concerned. Even this measure, however, has not been successful since it has been repeatedly shown that some 30% of gloves are punctured by the end of an operation. By then, the untreated hand is bathed in a soup of sweat and microbes that are squirted into the wound with every hand movement. Double- and even triple-gloving cannot entirely eliminate this danger. Work has therefore continued towards the goal of attaining total hand degerming with maintenance of sterility for the many hours needed for elaborate surgical procedures. This research has been extensive, and I will present only the conclusions together with a few illustrative highlights.

Current Concepts of Infections in
Orthopaedic Surgery

Requirements

Degerming of the skin, whether for "scrub" preparation of the hands of the surgical team or for preoperative preparation of the patient's skin, makes special demands on the antiseptic chosen, the requirements being:

1. A wide spectrum of activity.
2. Rapid action.
3. Bactericidal, not merely bacteriostatic, action.
4. It must be nonirritant, nonsensitizing, and nontoxic to skin and deep tissues.
5. It must not be absorbed from the wound into the general circulation with toxic consequences.
6. It should not react with or be inactivated by soaps, detergents, or other antiseptics with which it may be combined.

Only a few antiseptics meet these requirements:

Alcohol

Ethyl alcohol was one of the earliest substances used for rapid degerming and also one of the most successful. It acts rapidly, has a wide spectrum of activity, and is bactericidal. Its main disadvantages are that it is effective only in a restricted range of concentrations, between 70 and 95%, and may thus become quickly diluted to inffectiveness when incorporated into a surgical scrub procedure, especially when it is used at or near its lower limit of bactericidal activity. This is usually the case for financial reasons since it is expensive. It is also potable in pure form and so must be adulterated or it becomes subject to pilfering. An important characteristic of ethyl alcohol is that it is synergistic with a number of other antiseptics; this will be discussed further below.

The problems of cost and required adulteration have been overcome by the substitution of *isopropyl* for ethyl alcohol. *Isopropanol* is as effective and has the additional advantage that its bactericidal activity does not decline at concentrations below 90%. It is synergistic with other antiseptics but is a strong fat solvent so that its repeated use requires the incorporation of an emollient to prevent excessive dryness of the skin. This is not, however, essential for single applications such as for preoperative skin preparation.

Hexachlorophene

Hexachlorophene, a bisphenol, is a slow-acting disinfectant, relatively ineffective against gram-negative microbes, especially *Pseudomonas aeruginosa*, but has the great advantages that it is bland, is not inactivated by soap or detergents, and has a marked cumulative action which is useful to reduce the load of microbial skin flora to a low level by repeated use for about one week. The original microbial load will be restored in about three days after it is discontinued. The slow antimicrobial action of hexachlorophene greatly reduces its value as a surgical degerming agent, even in combination with an efficient detergent, and makes it unsuitable for preoperative preparation of patients' skin. There is also a danger of gram-negative colonization of dilute solutions of the chemical. These disadvantages are largely overcome, however, if hexachlorophene is used at concentrations of 0.1% or more in 70% ethyl or isopropyl alcohol. Rapid degerming can then be achieved in combination with long-term effect.

Iodine

Iodine is one of the oldest germicides used for skin disinfection. It has a wide spectrum of activity and is more strongly sporicidal than the other antiseptics available for degerming. It acts fast, especially as an alcoholic tincture, and its staining action is useful since it delineates clearly the treated skin area. Unfortunately, iodine may provoke severe skin reactions in some patients and others may be systemically hypersensitive to it. There is also the danger that the concentration of the iodine may increase progressively through evaporation of the alcohol, leading to skin burns. Elemental iodine has therefore been almost abandoned as a skin disinfectant and the application of iodine is carried out by the use of the more recently introduced *iodophors* in which the element is organically bound with a detergent carrier. These substances release free iodine slowly, retaining most of the bactericidal properties of the element without irritant or toxic side effects. They have, however, a slower bactericidal action and are less sporicidal. Again, combination with alcohol greatly increases their speed of action and degerming effectiveness.

Quaternary ammonium compounds (QUATS)

A wide range of these compounds is available -- cationic, anionic, and nonionic. Of these, the cationic group possesses the widest and strongest antimicrobial activity while the nonionics are almost inactive but all quats are more active against gram-positive than against gram-negative organisms and some of the latter, particularly *Pseudomonas aeruginosa*, are resistant to their action. These substances are active against sensitive organisms at high dilutions, are almost totally bland and nontoxic. In addition, they possess detergent activity so that they can be used as skin cleansing agents as well as for antisepsis. They do, however, have two serious disadvantages limiting their use in the surgical field. First, they are incompatible with a variety of substances and are inactivated by soap to such an extent that even traces of soap left on the skin may render them ineffective. Second, on the skin they tend to be bacteriostatic rather than bactericidal, so that microbes may regain their activity after entry into a surgical wound. At the present time, only cetrimide is extensively used, usually combined with 70% alcohol, for preoperative skin preparation. None is commonly used as a preoperative surgical scrub.

Chlorhexidine

This substance, a biguanidine, was introduced as a skin disinfectant in the early 1960s and has been extensively studied in Europe, especially in Britain. Like hexachlorophene, to which it is chemically unrelated, its action is predominantly on gram-positive flora, but it acts much faster and its degerming activity is more powerful. Combined with ethyl or isopropyl alcohol, it appears to be the most effective skin antiseptic for surgeons' hands and for patients' skin.

Soap

Soap is not an antiseptic and possesses no bactericidal properties in its own right. For many years it formed the basis for the surgical scrub, contributing mainly as a simple cleansing agent but also being capable by this action of removing a large part of the contaminating microbes which form the so-called transient flora. It has no action, however, on the resident skin flora. Its main value lies in its ability to combine effectively with hexachlorophene to produce an antibacterial soap which is socially acceptable and can make use of the cumulative action of hexachlorophene either to reduce the flora on the hands of the operating team or on the patient's skin. Its use even for this purpose, however, has been largely taken over by synthetic detergents.

Fuller descriptions of these groups of disinfectants may be found in Price (1967) and Block (1983).

Experimental Studies

Blank et al (1950), building on the fundamental studies of Price (1938a; 1938b), demonstrated the value of alcohol as a degerming agent and their conclusions have been repeatedly confirmed. Table I has been derived from the data published in their thorough study and clearly shows the effectiveness of isopropyl alcohol in enhancing the antimicrobial activity of hexachlorophene and as a degerming agent in its own right. It also shows another important point -- that the alcohol should not be removed from the skin with a towel but should be allowed to dry by evaporation.

Table I. Percentage recoveries of microbial flora of the hand after various scrub procedures (derived from Blank et al, 1950)

Scrub procedure	Recoveries		
	Before	After	Percent
2-5 min with soap and 2% hexachlorophene	5.5×10^6	1.1×10^7	200
10 min with soap 15 sec isopropyl alcohol Towel dry	1.4×10^7	6.5×10^6	46
2 min with soap 2 min isopropyl alcohol Dried by evaporation	3.8×10^6	6.5×10^5	16
2 min with soap 2 min hexachlorophene .1% in 70% isopropyl alcohol with 2% cetyl alcohol Dried by evaporation	1.12×10^7	1.4×10^5	1.3

Lowbury (1965) fully confirmed the importance of alcohol, especially in combination with other chemical agents. The figures in Table II are taken from his studies.

A further development of this work (Lowbury et al, 1974) demonstrated not only the synergistic action of both ethyl and isopropyl alcohols with chlorhexidine but also showed that their antimicrobial action continued for at least three hours provided the hand was covered with a rubber surgical glove (Table III). They also showed that the process of washing the hands was not essential to the degerming activity. The application of two successive doses of 5 mL of 0.5% chlorhexidine in 95% alcohol, each applica-

Table II. Percentage reduction in skin flora recoverable from the hand after two minute scrub with various antiseptics (from Lowbury, 1965)

Antiseptic	% Reduction in viable count
70% alcohol	68.6
Alcoholic iodine	80.7
Lugol's iodine	67.4
Aqueous chlorhexidine	60.7
Alcoholic chlorhexidine (0.5%)	81.3
Aqueous iodophor	62.3

Table III. Effect of gloving for three hours after various scrubs

Scrub technique	% Reduction in viable count	
	Immediate	After 3 hours wearing gloves
Chlorhexidine 0.5% in 70% ethyl alcohol	81.5	96.2
70% ethyl alcohol	73.6	90.7
Chlorhexidine 0.5% in 70% isopropyl alcohol	89.3	96.9
Chlorhexidine 0.5% in water	60.7	94.2
Aqueous iodophor	62.3	89.4

Table IV. Effect of alcoholic chlorhexidine alone without prior washing

Scrub technique	% Reduction in viable count	
	After first application	After sixth application
Chlorhexidine 0.5% in 95% ethyl alcohol *	97.9	99.9
Chlorhexidine 0.5% in distilled water	65.1	91.8
4% chlorhexidine detergent	86.7	99.2

* Two applications of 5 mL rubbed on the hands and wrists until dry.

tion being rubbed into the skin of the hand until it was dry, was as effective as scrubbing in the conventional manner with 4% chlorhexidine in a detergent mixture (Table IV).

Finally, Lowbury and Lilly (1975) tested for microbial growth, washings taken from over 600 surgical gloves worn by surgeons and nurses for various operations. The results are presented in Table V. It is apparent that either of the last two degerming techniques may achieve apparent sterility of the operating teams' gloved hands in a significant number of surgical procedures.

Table V. Effect of scrub technique in reducing release of microorganisms into the glove during surgical procedures

Scrub technique	Count/mL of handwashing after scrub	Number of gloves tested	Percent giving no growth
5 min soap scrub + alcohol swab	20.8	274	1.1
2 min scrub with 3% hexachlorophene detergent	3.6	250	22
2 min scrub with 4% chlorhexidine detergent	2.1	101	70
2 x 5 mL chlorhexidine in 95% ethyl alcohol + 1% glycerol	0.6	80	66

Conclusions

The surgical scrub

From results obtained by different workers over the last 35 years, the value of alcohol in skin degerming may be accepted with confidence. Either ethyl or isopropyl alcohol may be used with equal effect but the latter is less costly and its concentration is less critical. Its repeated use for the hands requires the incorporation of an emollient to prevent excessive dryness, but either 1% glycerine or 2% cetyl alcohol solve this problem effectively. Ethyl or isopropyl alcohol may be used in concentrations from 70 to 95%; and by the incorporation of one of the antimicrobial chemicals discussed above immediate degerming to the extent of 90% may be achieved. This will increase to about 97% within three hours. Under these conditions, about 70% of gloves worn by the surgical team can be expected to yield no microbial growth from washings taken at the end of the surgical procedure.

Lowbury et al (1974) consider that, of the options available, two applications of alcoholic chlorhexidine with 1% glycerine as emollient gives the best results and obviates the need for the classical "scrub" procedure using soap or a detergent-based antimicrobial mixture. They advocate the latter only for the first degerming of the day to remove social dirt. This initial scrub should be followed by two applications of the alcoholic chlorhexidine formulation. For subsequent operations, only the latter is then required. They state that this procedure has been standard practice in Germany for a number of years.

Preparation of the patient's skin

For optimal preoperative preparation of the patient's skin, the same procedure may be followed using 0.5% alcoholic chlorhexidine. The solution should be rubbed on the skin until dry, using a gloved hand since this is a more effective degerming technique than a gauze swab held in an applicator (Lowbury and Lilly, 1975).

If desired, advantage may be taken of the cumulative effect of chlorhexidine by instructing the patient to use a chlorhexidine soap for bathing on each of the three or four days before surgery. This could be carried out at home.

Shaving preparation. Shaving of the skin of the operation site increases both the microbial flora of the shaved area (Price, 1967) and the infection rate following clean surgery (Cruse, 1970; Seropian et al, 1971). Seropian recommended the use of a depilatory to avoid superficial abrasions caused by shaving and demonstrated a reduction in the subsequent infection rate. It is therefore logical that shaving be carried out as close to the time of operation as possible, preferably in the operating room, to avoid the danger of microbial colonization in nicks or abrasions produced in the surgical site.

Recommendations

The work quoted above permits selection of the most effective procedures for preoperative treatment of the surgical team's hands and the patient's skin using the same reagents for both purposes.

Surgical scrub

For the first operation of the day

1. Wash with gentle scrubbing for 2 minutes using detergent-based solution of 4% chlorhexidine.
2. Dry hands on sterile towel.
3. Apply 5 mL of 0.5% chlorhexidine in 70% isopropyl alchohol (or 95% ethyl alcohol) containing 2% cetyl alcohol or 1% glycerine. Rub hands together until dry by evaporation.
4. Apply second measure of 5 mL of alcoholic chlorhexidine and again rub hands until dry by evaporation.
5. Glove.

For subsequent operations

1. Apply two successive measures of 5 mL of alcoholic chlorhexidine to hands and rub dry by evaporation as in #3 and 4 above.
2. Glove.

Preparation of the patient's skin

1. When necessary, shave surgical site and immediate surrounding skin using a disposable safety razor.
2. Wash for 2 minutes with detergent-based solution of 4% chlorhexidine.
3. Dry with sterile towel.
4. Apply 5 mL of 0.5% chlorhexidine in 70% isopropyl alcohol. Rub firmly over surgical site, using gloved hand, until the skin is dry.
5. Repeat #3.

References

1. Blank, I.H., Coolidge, M.H., Soutter, L., and Rodkey, G.V.: A study of the surgical scrub. Surg. Gynecol. Bostet. 91, 577, 1950.
2. Block, S.S.: Disinfection, Sterilization, and Preservation. Lea & Febiger, Philadelphia, 1983. p. 157.
3. Cruse, P.J.E.: Surgical wound sepsis. Can. Med. Assoc. J. 102, 251 1970.
4. Lowbury, E.J.L.: Removal of bacteria from the operation site. In, Maibach, H.I. and Hildick-Smith, G. (Eds): Skin Bacteria and Their Role in Infection. McGraw-Hill, 1965. pp 263-275.
5. Lowbury, E.J.L. and Lilly, H.A.: Gloved hand as applicator of antiseptic to operation site. Lancet 2, 153, 1975.
6. Lowbury, E.J.L., Lilly, H.A., and Ayliffe, G.A.J.: Preoperative disinfection of surgeons hands: Use of alcoholic solutions and effects of gloves on skin flora. Brit. med. J. 4, 369, 1974.
7. Price, P.B.: The bacteriology of the normal skin. J. Infect. Dis. 63, 301, 1938b.
8. Price, P.B.: New studies in surgical bacteriology and surgical technique. J.A.M.A. 111, 1983, 1938b.
9. Price, P.B.: Surgical scrubs and preoperative skin preparation, J. Hosp. Res. 5, 7, 1967.
10. Seropian, R., and Reynolds, B.M.: Wound infections after preoperative depilatory versus razor shave. Am. J. Surg. 121, 251, 1971.

Clean Air Operating Environment and Superficial Infection

R. A. Elson

It is redundant to affirm that for orthopedic operations, especially total joint replacements, clean air is a mandatory requirement. The problem of wound pollution, however, has not yet been solved. I remember conversations with Sir John Charnley in which he expressed optimism that one day we would be able to pursue long surgical procedures with complete confidence that infection would never occur. However, even in one of his early papers (Charnley and Dandy, 1974) it was clear that despite a marked fall in the incidence of deep infection to 0.5%, superficial infection continued to occur in 7% of patients -- a serious and worrisome problem. At that time, many bacteriologists and surgeons remained sceptical as to the need for clean air and to the contention that so-called "nonpathogenic" organisms were significant; the succeeding ten years have amply substantiated both points. The problem of superficial infection remains, however, with its potential to cause more serious deep infection. As bacteriologists have become more aware of the pathogenicity of low grade organisms, we are in a better position to take the final steps of overcoming the problem.

Superficial infection may be defined as an inflammation of the skin and subcutaneous tissues which does not extend to the implant or its adnexae (wires, cement, etc.). It usually occurs during the first three postoperative weeks, and any later manifestations are more likely to relate to emerging deep infection (except for the occasional "stitch abscess"). Frequently, it is a highly subjective diagnosis by the surgeon, but if the normal course of wound healing is accepted as one of dryness after 24 hours and progressive uninterrupted subsidence of edema in the subcutaneous fat, comparison with this process is objectively possible.

Such comparisons were attempted in the recent Medical Research Council investigation conducted in Great Britain and Scandinavia, presented in what I regard as classical papers by Lidwell et al (1978, 1982, 1983a, 1983b) and another paper awaiting publication. My hospital made a small contribution to this investigation, and I therefore have some insight into the ancillary aspects of the study which prove so interesting. In this study, good correlation was shown between the incidence of proven deep infections requiring reoperation and the degree of air cleanliness (Table I). Furthermore, the efficacy of prophylactic antibiotics was substantiated. The combined benefits of these two measures were not mutually exclusive.

Superficial infection was graded as: major, minor, and possible wound sepsis. These grades were chosen by the individual surgeons and their criteria were recorded; the correlation of objective factors differed markedly (eg, redness, wound discharge and its contents, ESR, pain, etc.), but an approximate grading was nevertheless possible and useful for comparison.

Current Concepts of Infections in
Orthopaedic Surgery

Table I. Effect of air cleanliness on the incidence of deep infection requiring reoperation

Operating environment	Incidence of proven deep infection	
	Without antibiotics	With antibiotics
Conventional	3.4%	0.8%
Ultraclean air	1.2%	0.3%

Charnley and Dandy (1974) recorded an unsatisfactory superficial healing of 8.5%, but none of these led to known deep infection. In an earlier study, however, the authors reported that, based on photographic recording of wounds in 3,627 patients, imperfect healing led to a 3.8% deep infection rate while perfect healing was associated with a subsequent 0.25% deep infection rate; this discrepancy is not explained.

Salient conclusions made in the MRC trial are presented in Table II.

Table II. Effect of air cleanliness on incidence of wound sepsis*

Type of wound sepsis	OR environment	Incidence	
		Without antibiotics	With antibiotics
Major	Conventional	2.3%	0.7%
	Clean air	0.7%	0.6%
Minor	Conventional	5.1%	5.2%
	Clean air	5.2%	3.7%

* wound sepsis = superficial infection

Thus, the major wound sepsis incidence is affected by clean air and antibiotics whereas minor wound sepsis is reduced significantly only be antibiotics.

The relationship between deep infection and a preceding superficial wound sepsis is also reported in Table III.

The final analysis supporting these figures has to await full publication but the implications are obviously of great import. A recognized aggressive pathogen, *Staphylococcus aureus*, causing or colonizing a superficial wound infection was, if followed by deep infection, more commonly found in the latter as the same organism.

Thus, the Charnley and Dandy finding (1974) that superficial infection did not predispose to deep infection is not substantiated in the MRC trial, especially when the former is graded into major and minor.

Table III. Relationship between deep infection and preceding wound sepsis

	No. of cases	Resulting deep infection rate
Wound sepsis		
Major	64	30%
Suspected	565	3%
Normal healing	7423	0.7%

Surin et al (1983), in a review of 803 total hip arthroplasties, found strong correlations between superficial wound discharge, especially when containing microorganisms, and deep infection developing later. Again, the notable efficacy of prophylactic antibiotics was evident in both groups. Furthermore, other factors such as postoperative complication, previous surgery, or remote infections compounded the risks when present at the same time. These workers stressed that each problem should be attacked; I agree, and at the present time use clean air, systemic antibiotics, and antibiotic-loaded cement.

With regard to the prophylactic benefits of ALAC, we have to note the same differences between superficial and deep infection. Thus, in a prospective comparison of gentamicin-loaded acrylic cement (ALAC) and systemically administered antibiotics, Josefsson, Lindberg and Wiklander (1980) showed a statistically significant better effect for ALAC in deep infections but a reversed preference for systemic antibiotics in superficial infections (6.0% incidence for systemic antibiotic and 8.6% for ALAC). The authors had the same problems of subjective diagnosis and do not mention the incidence of deep infection following superficial infection. Their explanation was that ALAC is unlikely to produce high levels of gentamicin in the superficial tissue comparable with those obtained in the deeper layers. However, suction drainage aspirates yield, for a short 24-36 hours, gentamicin levels of <27 mμ (Elson et al, 1981).

The four references cited above all offer the same message -- superficial infections comprise a mixed group, at risk of developing deep infections. It is difficult to know what other prophylactic measures can be taken and certainly its incidence can be evaluated only in large centres. It is most unfortunate that Charnley did not complete a further study related to the method of wound closure. We had discussed the possibility of a controlled study, using a method of wound closure where no fat suture (buried or otherwise) would be used and coaptation of the fat maintained only by vacuum drainage. The earlier methods used by Charnley ranged from catgut to polythene tension sutures on foam plastic cushions. Buchholz and his team in Hamburg convinced me in 1977 that no fat suture was necessary but the technique is a little more sophisticated than that commonly employed: first, the drains must be copious, two or more depending upon the adiposity of the patient; second, they must be withdrawn a little every 12 hours, thereby unblocking the perforations; in this manner they are being removed progressively. Even with this care, occasional hematomas occur associated with anticoagulant prophylaxis.

The matter of wound closure is cogent because any strangulation of fat or irritation from buried resorbing suture material causes inflammation or local necrosis in a wound which is nearly always contaminated. Antibiotics do not reach strangulated tissue so easily. Not one of the series related to superficial infection describes the presence, absence or nature of a subcutaneous suture except Charnley's. If the information could be obtained, it might resolve another uncertainty. Comparisons with other types of surgery are not valid.

With regard to management, when major superficial wound inflammation occurs, it is reasonable to fear its spread (especially if suppuration occurs) either deeply or superficially towards vulnerable suture lines in the deep fascia or skin respectively. Any sign of inflammation or tension should induce the surgeon to open the wound early to decompress outwardly. I suggest that one should not fear secondary infection as much from outside compared with build-up of tension and spread inwardly. I am sure that two fulminating early postoperative deep infections I encountered began as inadequately treated superficial infections. Superficial hematoma demands release when it is obviously localized adjacent to the suture line; but the more patchy diffuse type, more commonly seen associated with warfarin prophylaxis and presenting as a brownish staining and thickening, is not as likely to produce necrosis and secondary infection.

In principle, I suggest that most supperficial infections are secondary to inflammation from tissue necrosis, tension, suture material reaction, and contaminating organisms implanted at the time of operation, or which may spread hematogenously. Avoiding fat sutures may reduce the incidence of infection, a suggestion that still requires evaluation.

Acknowledgement

I am most grateful to Dr. Owen Lidwell and his colleagues for permission to quote some results from the MRC Trial which awaits publication.

References

1. Charnley, J. and Dandy, F.: Wound infection after total hip replacement performed in clean air operating room. Internal Publication No. 45. Wrightington Hospital, 1974.

2. Elson, R.A., Jephcott, A.E., McGechie, D.B., and Verettas, D.: Antibiotic-loaded acrylic cement. J. Bone Joint Surg. 59B, 200, 1977.

3. Josefsson, G., Lindberg, L., and Wiklander, B.: Systemic antibiotics and gentamicin-containing bone cement in the prophylaxis of postoperative infections in total hip arthroplasty. Clin. Orthop. 159, 194, 1981.

4. Lidwell, O.M., Lowbury, E.J., Whyte, W., Blowers, R., Stanley, S.J., and Lowe, D.: Effect of ultraclean air in operating rooms in deep sepsis in the joint after total hip or total knee replacement: a randomized study. Brit.med.J. 285, 10, 1982.

5. Lidwell, O.M., Lowbury, E.J.L., Whyte, W., Blowers, R., Stanley, S.J., and Lowe, D.: Bacteria isolated from deep joint sepsis after operation for total hip or knee replacements and the sources of infection with *Staph. aureus*. J. Hosp. Infect. 4, 19, 1983a.

6. Lidwell, O.M., Lowbury, E.J.L., Whyte, W., Blowers, R., Stanley, S.J., and Lowe, D.: Airborne contamination of wounds in joint replacement operations: the relationship to sepsis rates. J. Hosp. Infect. 4, 111, 1983b.

7. Surin, V.V., Sundholm, K., and Backmann, L.: Infection after total hip replacement. J. Bone Joint Surg. 65B, 412, 1983.

Specific Measures to Reduce Operating Room Infections

R. M. LETTS

Surgical Wound Contamination

The primary sources of surgical wound contamination are a) contact, b) endogenous, and c) airborne.

The introduction of microorganisms directly into the wound by contact with instruments, surgeons, and operating room personnel can be reduced by good barrier systems encompassing both surgeon and patient. Endogenous infections are basically contamination from the patients own microflora that invade the wound. Airborne contamination of the wound results from microorganisms invading the wound, usually from debris contaminated by the surgical staff. It has been demonstrated that particulate matter in the operating theatre can be reduced by clean air control systems (Charnley, 1973; Charnley and Eftkar, 1969). Controversy exists, however, whether or not this on its own is responsible for a decrease in wound infections. At the present time it is debatable whether the most important factor is clean room technology or an efficient microbial barrier system demarcating the surgical personnel.

Factors Decreasing Contamination of the Surgical Wound

1. Preoperative wound site preparation.
2. Efficacy of the surgical garb: a) mask, b) hood, c) gown, and d) gloves.
3. Clean air system.
4. Wound irrigation.
5. Surgical procedure: a) length of operation, b) wound irrigation, c) patient barrier systems, and d) temperature of the operating theatre.

Operating Room Architecture

It has been shown that the design of the operating room will have a direct effect on the efficiency of the surgical team as well as those providing diagnostic and supportive services (Laufman, 1973). Design primarily aims to prevent outside contamination and provide sufficient space for material handling and equipment. Commonly recommended designs are the central core concept, the central corridor design, the cluster pattern, and the peripheral corridor design. All help to reduce the risk of operating room (OR) contamination.

Current Concepts of Infections in
Orthopaedic Surgery

Changes in materials have also decreased particulate matter entering the operating theatre. The use of harder and less porous walls and ceilings are an example and also assist in cleansing by wet vacuum methods.

Control of Foot Borne Contamination

A weak link in the operating room decontamination system involves the stretchers and personnel who enter the operating room from other parts of the nonsterile operating suite.

The methods to control such contamination have traditionally been a) use of OR overboots, b) antiseptic impregnated rugs at the entrance to the operating theatre, c) disposable sticky mats, and d) Dycem screens.

It appears from a practical aspect that the OR boots combined with a decontamination control screen at the entrance to the operating theatre provide the best method to decrease contamination from feet and wheels of OR stretchers. This also serves to decrease the contamination from the operating theatre out into the remainder of the operating suite and hospital. Meddick (1977) has demonstrated that contamination control mats decrease particle contamination of the operating theatre and that Dycem mats are highly efficient in removing particles from wheeled vehicles and shoes. These mats are easily cleaned and assist in reducing particle contamination of the operating theatres.

Traffic Flow in the Operating Room

Since microbial contamination in 80% of instances arises from surgical and support personnel within the operating environs (Hill et al, 1974), it is logical to try to decrease the number of persons who enter the operating theatre. This can be accomplished by decreasing access to the operating theatre and having a control system to limit unnecessary visitors and personnel.

We have studied the degree of microbial air contamination in an orthopedic operating theatre by air slit samplers (Letts and Doermer, 1983) (Fig. 1). This sampler, combined with agar plates placed throughout the operating theatre, and combined with traffic flow diagrams of the circulating nurses, indicate increased air counts and cultures associated with increased activity in the operating theatre (Fig. 2). We found a significant increase in gram-positive cocci and bacilli counts related to occupation and activity of the operating theatre (Fig. 3). The highest counts obtained were in high traffic areas.

Airborne contamination of the operating theatre is decreased by decreasing the number and activity of personnel within the operating theatre.

Video Camera Systems

Furthermore, outfitting the operating room with audiovisual equipment so that consultation services, teaching and communication can be handled in a much more efficient way without individuals having to enter the operating theatre constantly to observe the lesion, the incision or the problem. Cameras can now be attached directly to the operating lights and through a video hookup provide a much better view than if the individual were actu-

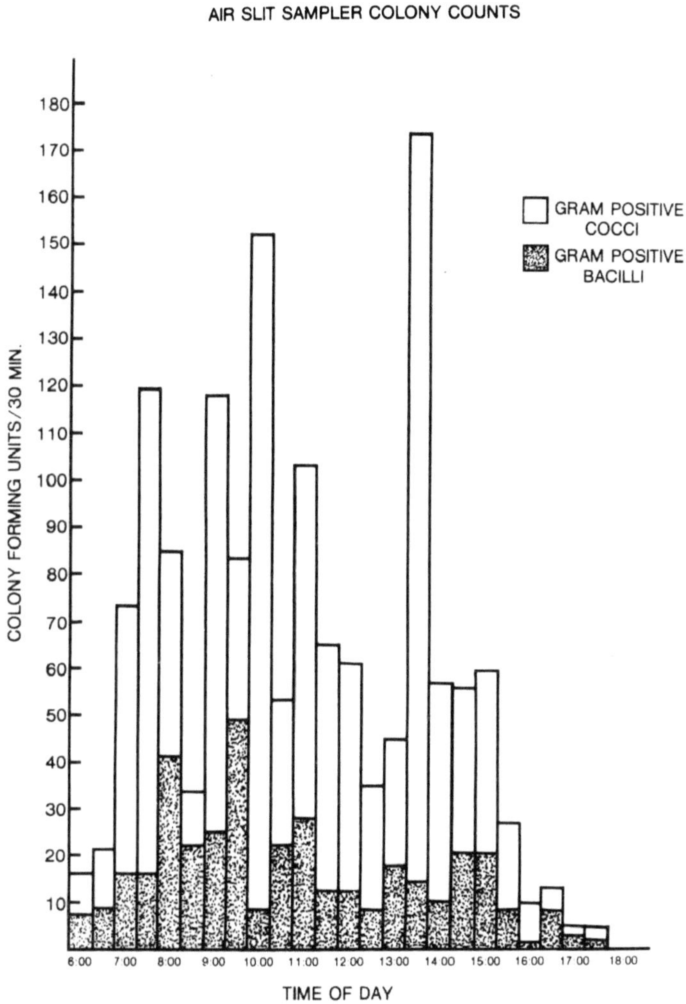

Fig. 1. Air slit sampler counts over a 12-hour period in a busy orthopedic operating room used 0700 h to 1530 h. (From J. Bone Joint Surg. 65A, 357, 1983 - with permission.)

ally in the operating theatre. Teaching is thus greatly enhanced and the patient made safer from contamination.

Operating Room Air

Particle counts in the average operating theatres have been found to contain 20,000 to 30,000 particles of 0.5 μ or larger per cubic ft per min. Microbes in the operating theatre air are attached to particles and most emanate from the surgical OR staff (Charnley, 1973). Microbes range in size from 0.3 μ to 10 μ, the most common organism being the *Staphylococcus*, measuring approximately 0.75 μ. The particles carrying microbes are usually

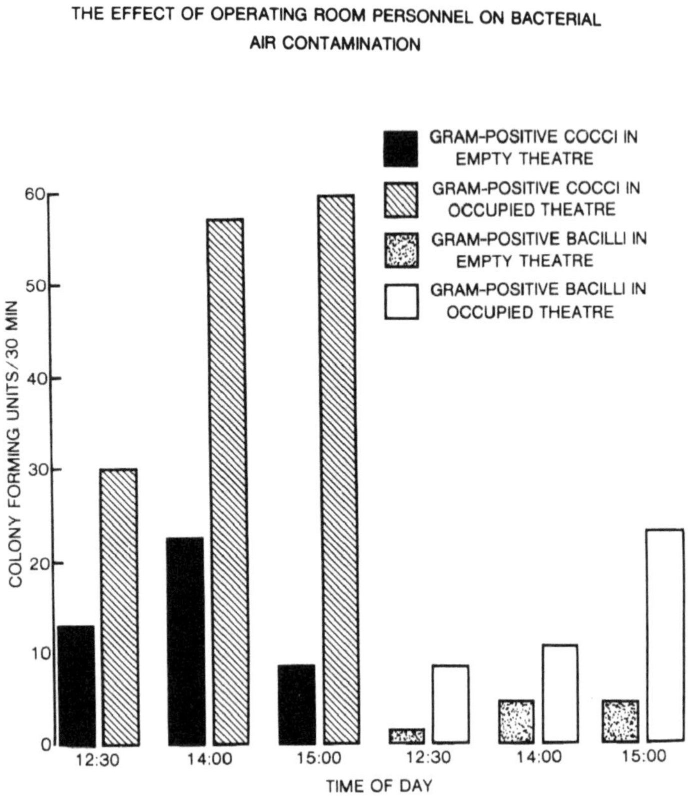

Fig. 2. Occupied theatres consistently show increased colony forming units when compared to dormant OR theatres. (From J. Bone Joint Surg. 65A, 357, 1983 - with permission.)

in the 8 to 14 μ diameter range. It seems reasonable to assume that decreasing particulate matter in the operating theatre can assist in decreasing wound contamination.

Surgical Gowns

The barrier effects of surgical gowns are important in preventing particle and microbial contamination of the operating room air. Standard cotton OR apparellel has a pore size of approximately 100 μ. This is insufficient to prevent the 8 to 14 μ particles laden with microbes from entering the OR environment. It has even been demonstrated that an individual in a surgical apparel actually sheds more microbes in the environment than if the individual were naked (Ulrich, 1966). The increased particle contamination when cotton suits are worn is simply due to the "cheese grater" effect of the material scraping off epithelial cells that pass through the large apertures of the cloth. In a study by Charnley and Eftekar (1969), it was found that the surface area of the surgical gowns was contaminated in 50% of surgeons at the conclusion of total hip arthroplasty. This may increase depending on the activity of the occupant; the more active the surgeon is,

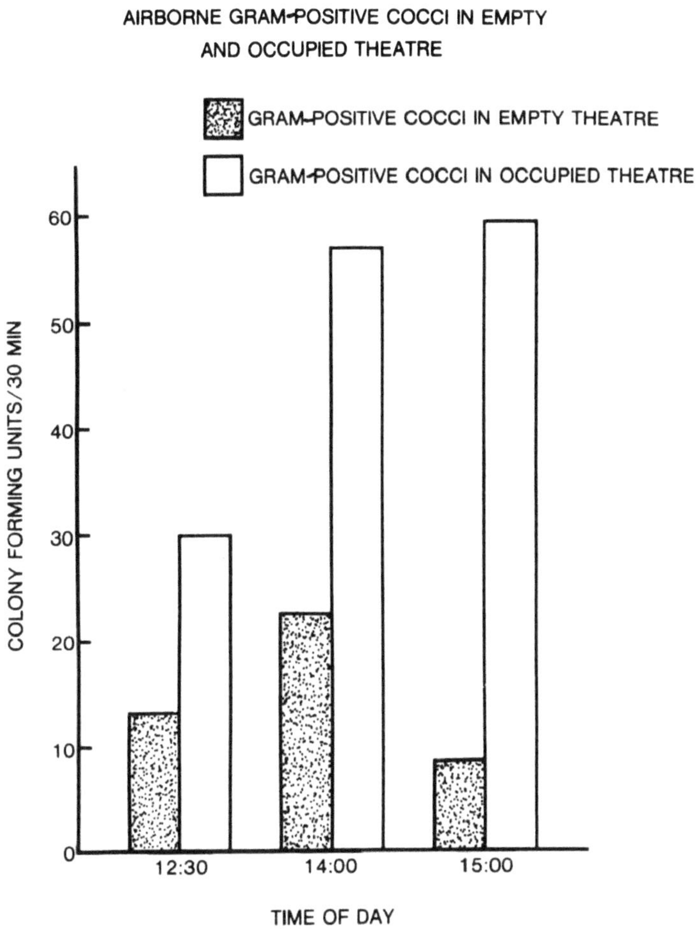

Fig. 3. Gram-positive cocci consistently elevated in the occupied theatres. (From J.Bone Joint Surg. 65A, 357, 1983 - with permission.)

the more shedding will occur. This is accentuated during activity because of a "bellows action" of the material which actually forces the cells out through available apertures. In a warm environment sweating also increases contamination of the external surgical garb since fluids pass by capillary action and microbes follow along with it (Alfred et al, 1973; Moylan and Kennedy, 1980).

Gown material

To prevent and reduce contamination of the external surfaces of surgical gowns, closer weave materials such as paper, close weave cotton, and plastics are important but have the added disadvantage of being warm. Muslin cotton has a thread count of 140 whereas newer cloth products have a thread count of 280. Disposable Tyvek gown and drape barrier systems are more efficient than cotton in providing a barrier to the surgeon. Isolator suits are the ultimate and have been shown to decrease the shedding from 70 colonies per cu ft to 7 colonies per cu ft in the operating theater. It has been demonstrated by Hamilton et al (1979) that the greater the pore size the greater the contamination of the external surface of the gown. Even the ventile material with 10 μ pore size will still, with time and increased temperature, result in contamination of the external surface of the gown. The closer the weave of surgical gown material the higher rises the temperature surrounding the surgeons and the greater the tendency to contamination of the external surface of the gown -- the Wick phenomenon. This can be reduced, as shown by Hamilton, by using a body exhaust system.

Using radioactive-labelled human albumin microspheres, Ha'eri and Wiley (1981) were able to demonstrate penetration of woven gowns and drapes by the microspheres. Wound contamination was noted in patients whose skin covered by the drapes was sprayed with the human albumin microspheres. Contamination of the wound by microspheres was noted whenever woven drapes were used. Similarly, the chest and shoulder region of surgeons were also sprayed with the microspheres and contamination of the wound was noted only when woven material was used in the surgical garb. It was not detected when nonwoven material was worn. Human albumin microspheres, particle size 10-35 μ in diameter, were found to pass through the woven gown in greater numbers when the gowns had been washed repeatedly or were wet.

Surgical Gloves

Carbolic acid was first used to prepare the skin at the surgical site as well as the surgeon's hands. It has been reported that the gross irritative properties of this solution led William S. Halstead to invent latex rubber gloves, thus protecting the delicate skin of the scrub nurse who later became his wife (Sharpe and Geelhoud, 1983).

The hands have one of the highest concentrations of staphylococci. The type of gloves used in the operating theatre is therefore of most importance. Virtually 100% of operating personnel tested during a surgical procedure will grow *Staphylococcus aureus* from the hands, even after standard surgical scrub. A needle hole in the glove will result in as many as 18,000 staphylococci passing through during a 20-minute period (Sharpe and Geelhoud, 1983). Holes in gloves are extremely common in orthopedic procedures and double gloving for procedures such as total joint replacement is insurance against this.

Double gloving

A review by McCue et al (1981), testing the efficacy of double gloving as a barrier to microbial contamination during total joint arthroplasty, revealed little evidence that the actual double gloving decreased microbial contamination. It was, however, shown that the double gloving technique was useful during draping since gloves are often contaminated during this procedure. The outer gloves were frequently holed with the surgeon having the thumb and index finger ruptured, most commonly the assistant having a rupture rate of about half as much. Following the draping, however, most colonies grew from the index and thumb although the gloves had no holes at this time.

Glove cuff junction

The glove cuff junction is a weak area of protection, and since the hands and wrists are highly contaminated areas this is a weak link in the surgeon's garb. Hamilton and coworkers (1979) have recommended a "mitt cuff" to provide better coverage and to prevent the sleeve from sliding up the arm. These authors found that positive cultures were obtained from the external surface of the standard stocking net cuffs in 36% of OR personnel whereas only 17% of the mitt cuffs demonstrated positive cultures. It appears that the mitt cuffs do provide an improved barrier to microbial contamination at this site in the OR gown.

Surgeons gloves and polymethylmethacrylate

Since polymethylmethacrylate is frequently used by orthopedic surgeons, its effect on glove viability is of great import not only to prevent the egress of organisms on the surgeons hands but also to prevent sensitization of the surgeon using the cement. Waegemaker et al (1983) have observed that the permeability of surgeons' glove material to polymethylmethacrylate is a function of time and increases with increasing temperature. It has also been shown that the permeability of the glove materials increases after exposure to polymethylmethacrylate to other fluids such as water. To date, no rubber glove on the market protects adequately against the permeability of polymethylmethacrylate.

Surgical Site Preparation

The standard preparation of the surgical site has not changed over the last few decades. Preoperative cleansing with scrubs, paints and sprays have shown considerable effectiveness. Isolation of the wound from the rest of the patient is essential, and barrier drapes plus plastic draping has decreased wound contamination from the patient.

Skin preparation of the surgical site

The antiseptic solution.

The antiseptic solution used on the patient's skin has three basic functions: a) dilution of the inoculum on the skin, b) defatting the skin surface and c) antimicrobial activity after application.

The preoperative solution which, of course, is mostly water, disperses the flora on the skin surface and when combined with a scrubbing action dislodges debris and microbes. All skin has a surface of secretions including perspiration, oils, and desquamated epithelium. The emolient added to the scrubbing solution dissolves the material, the most efficient being isopropyl alcohol. This also has an antiseptic action. Water, alcohol and iodoform are the most commonly used preoperative scrub solutions (Ritter et al, 1980).

Methods of skin preparation

a) Spray produces defatting and an antimicrobial effect but has little ablution or mechanical debriding action.

b) Scrubbing is the most obvious method of skin preparation.

c) The painting wipe technique is used for alcohol and iodoform paint. This takes little time and does not disturb the patient.

d) Film-incision drapes can be impregnated with a long-lasting antiseptic solution that is slowly released. This is a new technique, the antimicrobial film being applied to the skin and remaining during the operation.

The comfortable polymeric film adheres to the skin at the surgical site and slowly releases active iodine during the procedure. The film has been shown to be at least equivalent to other skin preparations (Sharpe and Geelhoud, 1983).

Surgical Masks

Masks are used in the operating theatre to prevent the transfer of pathogens from the nasopharynx of the operating team to the open wound of the surgical patient. Many shapes, sizes, and filtering efficiency masks are currently in use.

Basically, two types of surgical face masks exist: a) the nonfiltering or reflecting mask and b) the filtering mask. Unless an exhaust system is used, the filtering masks are usually preferred because of comfort. Synthetic face masks are extremely efficient against large particle leakage, ie, 8 to 15 µ and about 75 to 80% efficient against particles smaller than 1 µ (Dineen, 1971; Madsen and Madsen, 1967). Mask wiggle is also reduced when soft synthetic masks are used (Schweizer, 1976).

Ha'eri and Wiley (1980) first used tracer particles of human albumin microspheres 10 - 35 µ in diameter to test the efficiency of masks. These investigators found little transmission through the mask but noted some transmission around the mask. Letts and Doermer (1983) carried this a step further, measured the leakage of microspheres around the mask and correlated it with talking during surgery. They found that when the hood did not encompass the edge of the mask, there was a direct correlation between increased talking and increased retrieval of microspheres in the surgical wound. The hood, therefore, becomes an essential component of the surgical garb to ensure minimal leakage around the edge of the mask from a bellows effect accentuated by conversation. The importance of face masks is emphasized in a study by Ford (Ford and Peterson, 1963; Ford et al, 1967) in which the same spectrum of microorganisms was found in the nasopharynx of operating room personnel and in exudates taken from wound infections.

It seems logical that airborne organisms can cause wound infection and that masks will prevent the escape of most large nasopharyngeal droplets and organisms. If this is not simply a redirection outside of the masks and the organisms are kept contained within the surgical garb by completely covering hoods, contamination of operating room air from this source can be greatly reduced.

Conversation in the operating theatre as a source of airborn contamination

Using a technique developed by Ha'eri and Wiley, human albumin microspheres were applied to the face in the area covered by the mask. The human albumin microspheres are spherical aggregates of albumin ranging from 10 to 35 µ in diameter, used to simulate particles carrying microbes. Face mask testing was done on Johnson and Johnson "Surgine" face masks. A dose containing approximately 300,000 human albumin microspheres was sprayed onto the subject's face with a syringe over an area covered by the face mask and some was sprayed into each nostril. The face was allowed to dry and the mask was then applied. A control series was then set up by having the subject's face 12 inches above a water bath, 11.6 x 9.2 cm, simulating a wound. One of the following sets of two words was said every 30 seconds: scalpel please, sponge please, clamp please, or hemostat please. Trials were done for 5, 10, 20, 30, 40, 50 and 60 minutes. Following each trial, the distilled water from the wound simulator was collected and several drops of crystal violet were added to the water to stain the contaminating human albumin microspheres. The mixture was then passed through polycarbonate microfilter membranes with perforations of either 5 or 8 micra. The membrane was scanned under 10 X on the light microscope and human albumin microspheres and their size were noted.

To determine the effect of talking on the efficiency of face masks, the above experiments were carried out under identical conditions except that the subject read out loud for the entire time. The microspheres were collected and processed as before (Fig. 4).

The effect of wearing the face mask underneath the hood rather than over it was measured by comparing the results of human albumin microspheres dropout over 30 min with a talking control (2 words every 30 sec) where the face mask was worn over the hood.

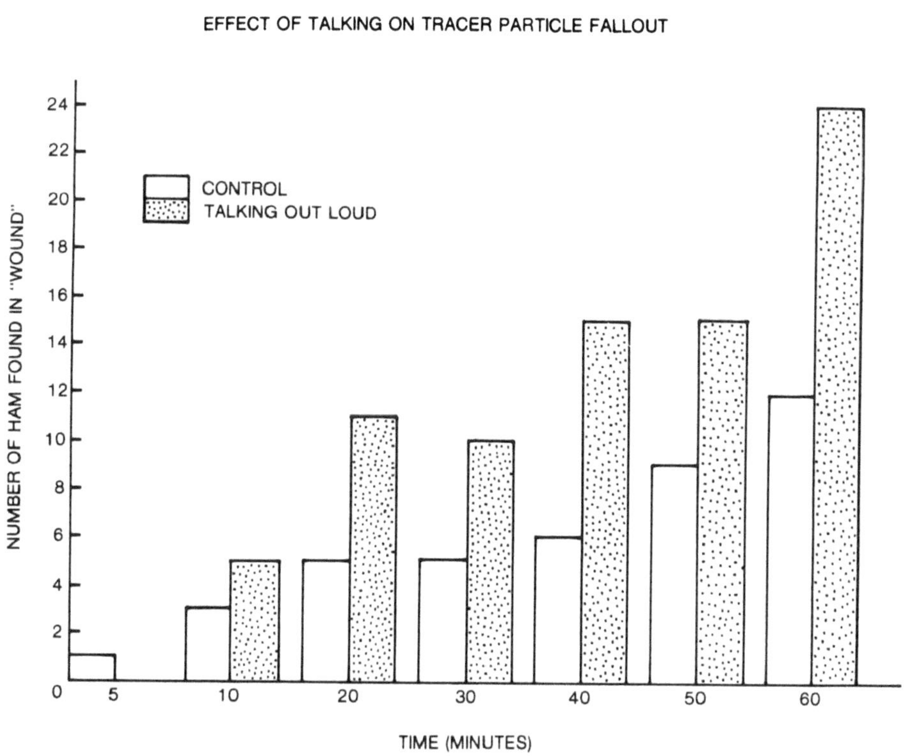

Fig. 4. The effects of conversation on wound contamination with passage of time. (From J. Bone Joint Surg. 65A, 357, 1983 - with permission)

The longer the masks were worn the more human albumin microspheres were found in the "wound." The same was true of the talking study except that the absolute number of human albumin microspheres was larger. By analysis of variance both the effect of time and talking on producing an increased human albumin microspheres count was found to be significant to the $.01<p<.05$ level. When the mask was worn under the hood, a reduced human albumin microspheres' count was noted.

From the results of the face mask control it was apparent that the longer the mask was worn the greater number of human albumin microspheres found in the "wound." As the duration of surgery is one of the factors involved in rendering the wound more suceptible to infection, it can be contended that microbes from behind the mask, in increasing numbers as time goes by, are a source of infection. Dineen has shown that moistening the mask and testing it for up to 8 hours does not adversely affect the filtration efficiency of modern masks. It follows, then, that the human albumin microspheres found in the "wound" fell out of the sides and/or bottom of the mask.

Although often suspected by some surgeons, it has now been proved that one of the ways to cut down the route of infection from behind the mask is to decrease the amount of conversation in the operating room.

Another way of eliminating this route of infection is to wear the mask under a hood which completely overlaps the sides and the bottom of the mask. This would prevent any particles from escaping out the sides and bottom (Fig. 5).

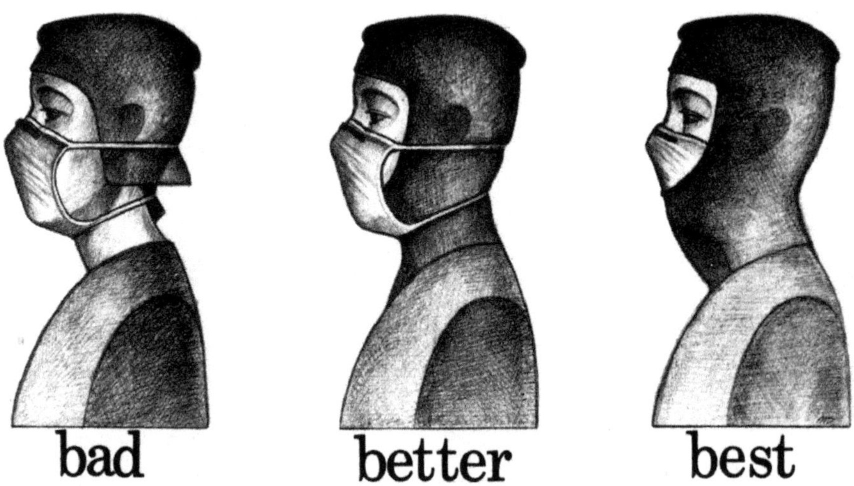

Fig. 5. The hood should cover the edges of the mask to prevent particle spill from the sides. (From J. Bone Joint Surg. 65A, 357, 1983 - with permission.)

References

1. Alfred, H.M., Ritter, M., French, M., and Hait, J.: The operating room gown as a barrier to bacterial shedding. Amer. J. Surg. 125, 589, 1973.

2. Charnley, J.: Clean air in the operating room. Cleveland Clin. Quart. 40, 99, 1973.

3. Charnley, J. and Eftkar, N.: Penetration of gown material by organisms from the surgeon's body. Lancet 1, 172, 1969.

4. Dineen, P.: Microbial filtration by surgical mask. Surg. Gynec. Obstet. 133, 812, 1971.

5. Ford, C.R. and Peterson, D.E.: The efficiency of surgical face masks. Amer. J. Surg. 106, 954, 1963.

6. Ford, C.R., Peterson, D.E., and Mitchell, C.R.: An appraisal of the role of surgical face masks. Amer. J. Surg. 113, 787, 1967.

7. Ha'eri, G.B. and Wiley, A.M.: The efficacy of standard surgical face masks: An investigation using tracer particles. Clin. Orthop. 148, 160, 1980.

8. Ha'eri, G.B. and Wiley, A.M.: Wound contamination through drapes and gowns. Clin. Orthop. Rel. Res. 154, 182, 1981.

9. Hamilton, H.W., Booth, A.D., Lone, F.J., and Clark, N.: Penetration of gown material by organisms from the surgical team. Clin. Orthop. Rel. Res. 141, 237, 1979.

10. Hill, J., Howell, A., and Blowers, R.: Effect of clothing on dispersal of *Staphylococcus aureus* by males and females. Lancet 4:1131, 1974.

11. Laufman, H.: Surgical hazard control: Effect of architecture and engineering. Arch. Surg. 107, 552, 1973.

12. Letts, R.M. and Doermer, E.: Conversation in the operating theatre as a cause of airborne bacterial contamination. J. Bone Joint Surg. 65A, 357, 1983.

13. McCue, S.F., Berg, E.W., and Saunder, E.A.: Efficacy of double gloving as a barrier to microbial contamination during total joint arthroplasty. J. Bone Joint Surg. 63A, 811, 1981.

14. Madsen, P.O. and Madsen, R.E.: A study of disposable surgical masks. Amer. J. Surg. 114, 431, 1967.

15. Meddick, H.M.: Bacterial contamination control mats - a comparative study. J. Hyg. 79, 133, 1977.

16. Moylan, A. and Kennedy, B.V.: The importance of gown and drape barriers in the prevention of wound infection. Surg. Gynec. Obstet. 151, 465, 1980.

17. Ritter, M.A., French, L.V., Eitzen, H.E., and Gio, T.E.: The antimicrobial effects of operative site preparative agents. J. Bone Joint Surg. 62A, 826, 1980.

18. Schweizer, R.T.: Mask wiggling as a potential cause of wound contamination. Lancet 2:1129, 1976

19. Sharpe, K., and Geelhoud, G.W.: The rational and ritual of pre-operative skin preparation. Contemp. Orthop. 7, 29, 1983.

20. Ulrich, J.A.: Skin carriage of bacteria in the human. Space Craft Sterilization and Technology. National Aeronautics and Space Administration Publication, NASA sp. 108, 87, 1966.

21. Waegemaker, T.H.J.M., Seutter, E., Den Arend, J.A.C.J., and Maltern, K.E.: Permeability of surgeons gloves to methylmethacrylate. Acta Orthop. Scand. 54, 790, 1983.

Clean Wound Surveillance

G. K. Richards, C. Gaese, and S. Travers

Clean wound surveillance is regarded by some as the study of bacteriologic cultures taken from clean incised tissue at the time of surgery. Others apply this term to the surveillance of patients having undergone clean surgical procedures to measure the rate of postoperative wound sepsis.

The culturing of incised tissue at the time of clean surgery to predict the likelihood and nature of postoperative sepsis has been the subject of extensive study. The results are clear-cut. With reference to the National Research Council - US Public Health study of 11,690 clean elective procedures, there is a somewhat puzzling lack of correlation between the identity of organisms cultured from wounds at the time of closure and those later cultured from wound infection (Altemeier, 1979). In a series of 658 total hip replacements (THR), intraoperative cultures were positive in 195 (30%). Of the seven patients who developed deep wound infection, only four had positive intraoperative cultures, and in three of these the findings were irrelevant (Fitzgerald et al, 1973). In another series of 740 THR, joint capsule cultures were positive in 233 (31%), and fascia lata cultures were positive in 22/272 (8%). Of the 12 patients who developed a deep infection, eight had negative intraoperative cultures, and two of the four positive cultures were irrelevant. According to Murray (1973), "There was no correlation between the recovery of bacteria from the hip joint capsule and the incidence or onset of postoperative infection." The routine intraoperative culture of clean wounds without clinical indication is seen to be neither predictive nor diagnostic.

The alternative concept that clean wound surveillance is an epidemiologic study of postoperative infection, is of great practical value. This form of study can conveniently be divided into three steps (Brachman, 1979):

1) *Description* - the collection of data concerning wound infections to establish an average infection rate which can be used for comparisons (eg, institution to institution) and to detect unexpected deviations.

2) *Retrospective analysis* of the descriptive data to arrive at theories of the possible causes of infection or of unexpected variations.

3) *Prospective experiment and modification* based upon the analysis to reduce infection rates, using descriptive data as a guide.

The ultimate purpose of clean wound surveillance is the reduction or elimination of postoperative infection (the third step), and it is obvious that this cannot come about without the previous steps of data collection and analysis conducted consecutively. Since modifications of surgical methods

Current Concepts of Infections in
Orthopaedic Surgery

and patient care cannot be introduced without the consent and active cooperation of the surgeon, it would be senseless to conduct any such study without his full involvement. In the ideal situation it is the surgeon who has full responsibility for patient care and who initiates and coordinates the entire process.

It is most surprising when visiting some institutions to find that descriptive data are obsessively collected but filed away without analysis. Others do analyses and write reports which are then filed without consideration of further action or change. Equally surprising is the institution where wide-sweeping (and expensive) changes are made with no attempt to collect prior or follow-up data to determine whether a problem existed beforehand or whether it had been resolved. Some institutions have systems which do not involve surgeons; or individual surgeons refuse to cooperate since their patients (unlike others) never get infection! Regrettably, only the minority of institutions implement all three steps as a coordinated routine with the full involvement of the surgical teams, thereby bringing about impressive and prompt reductions in infection rates as a result of investigation, experiment and change.

Collection of Data

There are several ways in which data collection can be organized.

Surveillance of all clean wounds, hospital wide, all year round. This is comprehensive, but requires considerable manpower and organization, with centralization usually in an Infection Control Unit.

Surveillance of all clean wounds, one unit, all year round. This is an excellent choice. It requires surprisingly little manpower, and no centralization. The surgeons conduct their own study on their own patients.

Surveillance of all clean wounds, one unit, periodically. This is periodic surveillance, which in practice occurs when someone remembers or has spare time (!), or when an outbreak occurs too great to be ignored. Such a system is not recommended.

Analysis of Data

The purpose of analysis is to find causes for events. The data are reviewed periodically (eg, weekly) to check whether an epidemic of infection is present (multiple infections of the same type originating from outside the patient), or whether the rate of infection has increased (multiple infections not of the same type, but above the normal rate).

Can causes of any increased or epidemic rate be found? In the presence of an acceptable low rate, can infections be divided into those which originate from the environment, and into those which arise from the patient's own microbial flora, using guidelines provided for this purpose by the hospital microbiologist? (Richards, 1984) If this division can be made then it halves the number of variables (Tables I and II) that need to be considered or investigated to arrive at the cause of concern.

Table I. Analysis: Infection derived from the environment

Important considerations
Efficacy of handwashing
Glove punctures
Air supplies to OR (sterility, positive pressure, effective exhaust, rate of change)
Air sterility at operating site (filtration, turbulence)
Sterility of instruments and prostheses
Sterility of solutions and materials (sutures, swabs)
Break in sterile techniques
Staphylococcus aureus disperser in OR team
Streptococcus pyogenes carrier (perineal) in OR team
Prolonged hospital stay before surgery

Table II. Infections derived from the patient

Important considerations	Prophylaxis
Skin shaving	Selection of bactericidal antibiotic
Skin disinfection	Dosage regimen
Surgical technique	Timing
Excess trauma	Length of treatment
Hematoma formation	Monitoring of serum levels
Duration of surgery	Monitoring adequate tissue distribution
Bacteremias	
UTI and catheterization	
Impaired immune status	

Planned Experiment and Change: An Example

An increase in postoperative clean wound sepsis rates was noted, and *Staphylococcus aureus* was found in 40%, suggesting origins in the hospital environment. At that time there was uncertainty how the *S. aureus* spread and how best to investigate such a situation effectively, promptly and economically. An experimental model was devised, using the newborn nursery.

Neonates are ideal subjects for the study of *S. aureus* transfer, since they are born virtually germ-free, have a standardized wound (the umbilical stump), a large surface of sterile skin, a built-in air sampler (the nostrils), and are skin colonized by staphylococci (sometimes by *S. aureus)* within the first few days of life.

Daily cultures were taken from the babies, from nostrils, umbilicus and groin. During the same period, twice-weekly cultures were taken from nostrils, clothing and hands of all 71 attendant nurses. The mean time for colonization by *S. aureus* of nine neonates was 1.9 days for the umbilicus, 2.8 days for the groin and, surprisingly, 3.1 days for the nostrils, suggesting spread by contact rather than by air. Of the 71 nurses, 58 (82%) were negative, 15 (21%) had passive contamination of hands or clothing, and only eight (11%) were *S. aureus* dispersers, covered head to foot with *S. aureus* of a single phage type contaminating their hair, hands, and clothing. Five phage groups were involved. These eight nurses could be directly related to the nine colonized babies in their care, with corresponding phage types. The provisional conclusion of this model was that *S. aureus* was spread by contact rather than by air, and the origin was from a *S. aureus* disperser, a state easy to identify.

Application

Three neurosurgical patients, operated on during the same session, developed severe wound infection with *S. aureus* of a distinctive antibiotic sensitivity pattern and phage type 84/85. *S. aureus* dispersers of this strain were sought amongst the 97 ward and OR staff. Only two were found, a nurse with a discharging ear (not present at the time of surgery) and a surgical resident, member of the OR team, who had a discharging abscess of the thumb, which he claimed could not be the source, since it had been covered by a glove, and the germs would drop inside! This discounted the fact that his body was covered in the organism, contaminating clothing and disseminating into the air. The conclusion from this study was that in the event of further *S. aureus* outbreaks related to single OR sessions, investigation would be limited only to looking for dispersers in those members of the OR team having direct contact with the surgical field. Subsequent investigations have confirmed the utility of this approach. The disperser state can be abolished readily by hexachlorophene shampoo and bath, preferably confirmed by overnight culture before returning to full duty.

Another experiment

The clean wound infection rate in one surgical team had risen to a disturbing level, without obvious cause on repeated investigation. An experiment to determine the rates of clearance of airborne microbes in an empty OR room demonstrated a defect in the air exhaust system and that the OR suite used by that team was under negative pressure. Cleaning of the exhaust system throughout the hospital for the first time in 25 years, due to a design error, corrected the situation.

Conclusions

Clean wound surveillance is a sensitive biologic indicator of environmentally acquired infection. It is a simple essential tool for any surgeon wishing to monitor or prevent postoperative wound sepsis or to investigate the basic causes. It is most strongly recommended.

References

1. Altemeier, W.A.: Surgical infections: incisional wounds. In, Bennett, J.V. and Brachman, P.S. (Eds.): Hospital Infections. Little, Brown, 1979, p. 296.

2. Brachman, P.S.: Epidemiology of nosocomial infections. In, Bennett, J.V. and Brachman, P.S. (Eds): Hospital Infections. Little, Brown, 1979, pp 13-17.

3. Fitzgerald, R.H., Peterson, L.F.A., Washington, J.A., Van Scoy, R.E., and Coventry, M.B.: Bacterial colonization of wounds and sepsis in total hip arthroplasty. J. Bone Joint Surg. 55A, 1242, 1973.

4. Murray, W.R.: Results in patients with total hip arthroplasty. Clin. Orthop. 95, 80, 1973.

5. Richards, G.K.: Epidemiology of hospital infections: the role of the microbiologist. Companion paper in this publication.

Microbial Study of Surgical Drain Cultures

M. MONTMINY, G.-A. DAIGLE, P. GAGNON, D. LAFLAMME, J. NOLIN, and D. MERCIER

A prospective study was undertaken at the Hôtel - Dieu de Lévis Hospital, covering a period of eight years, to assess the predictability of orthopedic surgical infections before the appearance of clinical signs and symptoms. We used surgical drain cultures for our investigation.

We postulated that if an infection were detected without delay, it would be possible to initiate appropriate therapy at once and thereby reduce not only morbidity, but also the high costs of prolonged hospitalization.

Materials and Methods

Drains were inserted into all surgical wounds, clean or contaminated, including open noninfected fractures. The wound was then covered with sterile dressing. After several days a member of the nursing staff removed the drain, cut off about 2 cm at the tip of the drain and sent it to the microbiology laboratory for culturing.

We have used several types of drains in this investigation: Penrose® and Hemovac® suction drains and a "feeding" drain, ie, a small nasogastric tube without suction.

The original surgical dressing was not changed before the first drain sample was taken for culturing.

Specimens were tested for aerobic and anaerobic isolates. By this method we investigated 900 wounds, of which 784 were included in this study as conforming to our test criteria. In all, we evaluated 52 variables for each documentation. The most important of these were the type and number of drains used, the length of time the drain had remained in the wound, antibiotic therapy before and/or after removal of the drain, and the identification of the infecting organisms (Tables I-IV).

Table I. Types of drains used in this study

Drain	No. of cases	%
Feeding	426	54
Hemovac	238	30
Penrose	59	7.5
(Unknown)	66	8.4

Current Concepts of Infections in
Orthopaedic Surgery

Table II. Surgical procedures

Procedure	No. of cases	%
Osteoarticular	490	62.1
Soft tissue	249	31.6
Total hip replacement	50	6.3

Table III. Number of drains used per wound

No. of drains	No. of cases	%
One	626	79.3
Two	163	20.7

Table IV. Duration drains left in wounds

Days	No. of cases	%
Less than two	29	3.7
Two	368	46.6
More than two	389	49.3

We then tried to correlate these variables. We particularly tried to correlate the isolated organisms, the type of wound infections, and the pathogenic organisms isolated from the wounds with the organisms cultured from the drains. All findings were then computerized and analyzed by qualified statisticians.

Almost one-half of the patients had received antibiotics. The number of patients receiving antibiotic treatment before removal of the drain almost equalled the number who received antibiotics after removal of the drain (Fig. 1).

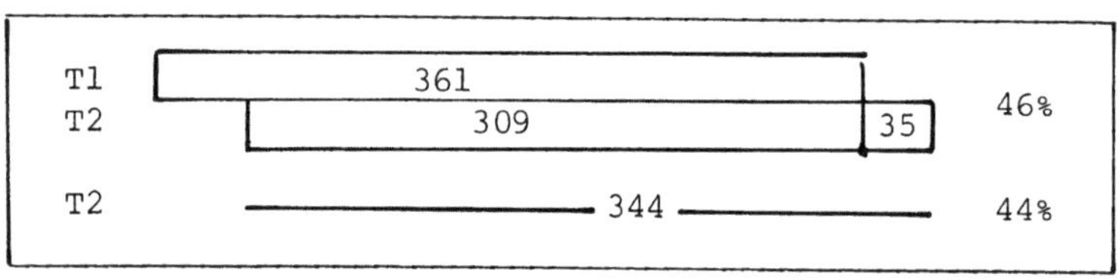

Fig. 1. T1 = Antibiotic treatment before drain removal
T2 = Antibiotic treatment after drain removal

Table V shows the follow-up periods except for infected wounds. Total hip replacement cases are being followed up for two postoperative years and longer.

Table V. Postoperative follow-up periods

Days	No. of patients	%
0 - 14	38	4.8
15 - 29	45	5.7
30 - 179	251	31.8
180 - 359	165	20.9
More than 360	289	36.6

Results

The results of the drain cultures and the status of the wounds were analyzed to determine correlations between the cultured microbes and the condition of the wounds (Fig. 2).

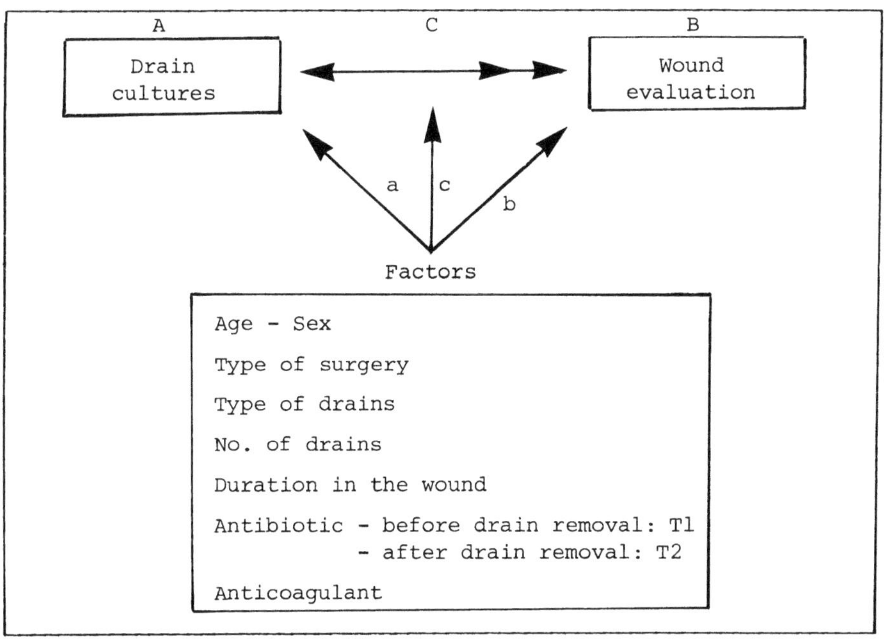

Fig. 2. Correlation between drain culture and wound status

Drain cultures

1. Approximately 33% of the drain cultures were positive. When excluding coagulase-negative staphylococci, however (justified because these were found in this study to be contaminants)11% of the cultures were positive (Table VI).

Table VI. Number of drain cultures isolated

	No. of patients	%
+ drains	254	32.4
- drains	530	67.6
Excluding coagulase-negative staphylococci		11

2. Penrose drains appeared to develop positive cultures more frequently tha than the other types of drains (Table VII).

Table VII. No. of cultures isolated per drain

Type of drain	No. of isolates	%
Feeding	145/424	34.2
Hemovac	50/237	21.1
Penrose	32/58	55.2

3. The number of drains per wound had minimal or no effect on the rate of positive cultures except with the Hemovac drain (Table VIII).

Table VIII. No. of drains per wound related to the rate of positive cultures

Type of drain	No. per wound		
	1	2	1 or 2
Feeding	33%	36%	34.2%
Hemovac	12%	28%	21%
Penrose	50%	60%	55%

4. Antibiotic therapy tended to invalidate culturing of drain specimens (Fig. 3).

	T1 +	T1 -
+ Drains	25	38.5

Drains: T1 +	T2 -
36%	50%

Fig. 3. Effect of antibiotic therapy on drain cultures.
T1 + = Antibiotic treatment before drain culturing
T2 - = Antibiotic treatment after drain culturing

5. The most commonly isolated microorganisms were coagulase-negative staphylococci (Table IX).

Table IX. Identification and percentage of microbes isolated from drain cultures

Microbes	No. of patients	%
Coagulase- staphylococci	189	67
Coagulase+ staphylococci	25	8.8
Mixed flora	21	8.1
Escherichia coli	14	5.3
Streptococcus faecalis	11	4.2
Streptococcus viridans	4	1.7
Enterobacter sp.	5	1.7
Pseudomonas aeruginosa	3	1.0
Proteus sp.	2	0.6
Alginobacter sp.	3	1.0
Flavobacterium sp.	2	
Candida albicans	1	

Wound infections

1. A deep wound infection was observed in 3.5% of patients. We did not include superficial infections since they are not associated with any morbidity (Table X).

Table X. Incidence of deep wound and superficial infections

	No. of patients	(%)		
Deep			Manifestations:	
Cultured	26	(3.5)	Swelling	+
Noncultured	2		Symptoms	+
			Systemic signs	+
			Antibiotic need	+
			Apprehension	+
			Fear of complications	+
Superficial	15	(1.9)	Causes:	
			Stitches	-
			Blisters	-
			Tape irritation	-
			Pressure points	-
			Drain holes	-
			Skin necrosis	-
			Wound dehiscence	
Total	43	(5.4)		

+ =
- =

2. The microorganism causing deep infection was identical in 93% to that present in drains. In no instance was a different organism isolated (Table XI).

Table XI. No. of drain cultures correlating with deep wound infections

	Deep culture	Superficial wound
Positive drain(s) same agent	93%	0%
Negative drain(s)	7%	84%
Positive drain(s)	0%	16%

3. The incidence of infection in the presence of Penrose drains was higher than with any other drain (Table XII).

Table XII. Incidence of infection related to type of drain

	Infection	
Type of drain	Deep	Superficial
Feeding	2.6%	0.9%
Hemovac	2.5%	3 %
Penrose	10.3%	1.7%

4. The incidence of infection rises significantly when the drains remain in situ longer than two days (Table XIII).

Table XIII. Incidence of infection relative to duration of drain in situ

	Infection	
Duration	Deep	Superficial
Two days	2.5%	-
More than two days	4.7%	1.6%

5. Most deep infections occurred early after surgery (Table XIV).

Table XIV. Occurrence of infection following surgery

Days after surgery	Infection	
	Deep	Superficial
0 - 14	25/28	8/16
15 - 29	2/28	6/16
30 - 179	1/28	1/16
179 - 359	0	1/16

Correlation of drain cultures with wounds

1. The incidence of microorganisms found in drains and in deep wound infections, as well as the percentage of correlation, was 10% overall. However, when eliminating the coagulase-negative staphylococci, which is justified in view of the low percentage of correlation compared with the overall infection rate, the correlation rate is 22% (Table XV).

Table XV. Percentage of drain culture and deep wound infection correlation

Microbes	Positive cultures		W/D %
	Drains (D)	Wounds (W)	
Coagulase - staphylococci	189	6	3.2*
Coagulase + staphylococci	25	7	28
Mixed flora	21	3	13
Escherichia coli	14	3	20
Streptococcus faecalis	11	3	25
Streptococcus viridans	4	1	20
Enterobacter sp.	5	2	40
Pseudomonas sp.	3	1	33
Proteus sp.	2	0	0
Alginobacter sp.	3	0	0

* Coagulase-negative staphylococci excluded : 22

2. Only 0.4% of patients who had a negative drain culture later developed a deep infection (Fig. 4).

3. Antibiotic therapy either before swabbing the drain (T1) or after sampling (T2), the number of drains inserted, and the duration of drains in situ do not seem to change significantly the drain-wound correlation, established at 22% for a positive and at 0.4% for a negative correlation (Table XVI).

DRAINS CULTURES +/-

WOUND INFECTIONS +/-

		WOUND INFECTONS -	WOUND INFECTONS +
DRAIN CULTURES	+	88%	11.8%
	-	97.5%	2.5%

TYPE OF WOUND INFECTION

	-	+ DEEP	+ SUP.
+	88%	10.2	1.6
-	97.3%	0.4	2.3

DEEP WOUNDS INFECTIONS

		DEEP -	DEEP +
DRAIN CULTURES	+	89.8%	10.2%
	–	99.6%	0.4%

DRAIN CULTURES +

DEEP WOUND INFECTIONS +/-

SAME AGENT(S)

INCLUDING COAGULASE - STAPHYLOCOCCI

	WOUNDS INFECTIONS -	WOUNDS INFECTIONS +
DRAINS CULTURES +	89.8%	10.2%

EXCLUDING COAGULASE - STAPHYLOCOCCI

	WOUNDS INFECTIONS -	WOUNDS INFECTIONS +
DRAINS CULTURES +	79.5%	22%

Fig. 4. Deep wound infections developing despite negative drain cultures

Table XVI. Effects of antibiotic therapy and drain sampling on drain culture-wound correlation*

	Positive drains n = 254			Negative drains n = 530		
T1						
+		8	77		173	2
-		14	147		265	
+/- %		46	34		37	
Infection	Sup.	Deep	No	Sup.	No	Deep
No	4	26	224	12	515	2
%		10.2	88.2	2.3	97.2	0.4
T2						
+	2	11	78		240	
-		15	246		272	
+/- %		42	34		47	
One drain	4	18			412	
Two drains		8			103	
1/2 %		70			80	
More than 2	4	16			225	
Two days		9			266	
Less than 2		3			21	
+ 2/2-2 %		54			45	

* Type of drain or surgical procedures also did not affect correlation rates

Discussion

1. The culturing of drains is a simple procedure which permits early detection of deep infection in 22% of all wounds. Coagulase-negative staphylococci were considered contaminants and consequently eliminated from further analysis.

2. Since only 0.4% of negative drain cultures later developed deep infection, an early identification of wounds not at risk is recommended.

3. Early detection of wounds at risk not only alerts surgeons to a possible complication but also to initiation of aggressive therapy to prevent or at least limit the infection. We suggest the treatment plan shown in Figure 5.

4. Since the cost of a postoperative infection is five to ten times higher than the cost of the original operation ($16,000 to $37,000 for an infected total hip replacement), it is evident that the cost for microbiologic testing of drains is comparatively negligible.

5. Penrose drains seem to be a direct cause of infection and their use is not recommended.

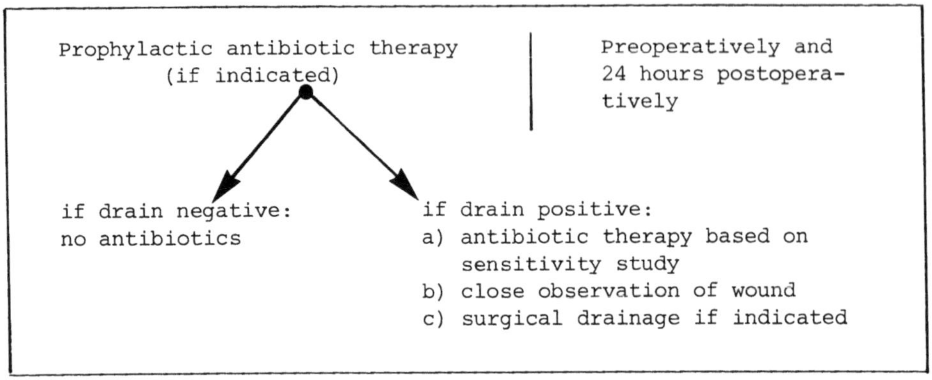

Fig. 5. Suggested treatment plan

6. Surgical drains should not remain in wounds longer than two days, since later removal will significantly increase the risk of infection.

7. Many questions await further clarification, in particular the incidence of coagulase-negative staphylococci, and the fact that three out of four patients with positive cultures from drains did not develop a subsequent infection.

The following techniques should be assessed and explored further:

a) The position of the drain and the length of its subcutaneous route.

b) The importance of suction on the drain, its force and its duration in situ.

c) The importance of manipulations while emptying the suction container.

d) Possible contamination of drains by the skin.

e) Determination of the rate of microbial growth at the distal end of the drain could predict more precisely the risk of infection. At the same time, it would augment the diagnostic value of the drain cultures.

The Microcomputer for Operating Room Infection Surveillance

R. M. LETTS

The operating room is most amenable to computerization from several points of view. The statistics generated in the operating theatre are immense and are necessary for health care workers at many levels (Johnson, 1983). In the operating room a computer can be used to

a) provide information regarding surgical procedures to members of the health care team -- ie, residents, surgeons and nursing staff;

b) monitor infections and personnel within the operating theatre;

c) establish a system to control inventory, equipment maintenance and staff scheduling;

d) ensure rapid, accurate records for annual reports, hospital certification committees and Royal College accreditation committees;

e) improve operating room scheduling and distribution of O.R. slating;

f) assist administration personnel in budget planning and forecasting; and

g) assist in billing.

Software is now available or can be produced for individual operating theatres to compile the above data and produce documentation and statistics required by administrative and medical management staff of the hospital (Edmunds, 1984; McGuire, 1984).

Computerizing the operating theatre requires a computer terminal in each theatre. The circulating nurse records all of the patient data on the computer instead of the operation sheet. Basic information that can be recorded includes virtually all hand-recorded material that is currently documented and later collated. For example, basic patient information can be recorded together with the operation performed as well as the names of the attending resident and surgical staff. This would enable residents, for instance, to have a printout immediately of all surgical procedures in which they have participated.

Furthermore, starting times can easily be recorded together with anesthetic starting times, intubation times, finishing times, types of skin preparation, types of anesthesia, etc. Data concerning the surgical procedure can also be recorded such as drains used, types of equipment used, type of

Current Concepts of Infections in
Orthopaedic Surgery

transfusions, implants, etc. Specimens, complications, type of operations and roentgenographic data are other items that can be programmed to record and analyze.

The Microcomputer and Infection Monitoring

We have designed a software package for monitoring operating room and postoperative infections using the Apple II computer (Letts and McQueen, 1981). Each member of the operating room staff is assigned a number and data are collected on all patients as to preoperative infections, operating room complications, and postoperative infective microorganisms. The data can then be readily analyzed by the computer. For example, it can be ascertained how often each individual member of the operating staff was involved in an infected case over a period of one year. Various combinations and permutations of staff can also be studied together with the incidence of infection that occurs with that combination. Data can also be collected regarding types of antibiotics administered, including preoperative and postoperative antibiotic treatment. The computer is ideally suited for compiling and analyzing the numerous variables always encountered in patients with infections.

References

1. Edmunds, L.: Computers in patient care. AORN Journal 39, 176, 1984.
2. Johnson, R.L.: Hospital computer trends for the 1980's. Computers in Health Care 2, 36, 1983.
3. Letts, R.M., and McQueen, D.: The Microcomputer, an essential component of a busy department of orthopaedic surgery. Orthopaed. Rev. 10, 49, 1981.
4. McGuire, H.P.: Computerizing in O.R. AORN Journal 39, 184, 1984.

Diagnosis of Acute Bone Infection

P. KINNARD

Prompt diagnosis of acute bone infection is essential and cannot be overemphasized. Failure to identify the causative microorganisms and to begin appropriate antimicrobial therapy lead to further bone destruction and increased morbidity (Septimus and Musher, 1979). Excellent three-dimensional visualization of the osteomyelitis may now be obtained by sophisticated diagnostic techniques, enabling the physician to identify the cause and to start the appropriate treatment without undue delay.

It is advisable to consider the age of the patient because differential diagnosis, prognosis and management may vary when facing acute bone infection in neonates and infants, in children, in adults and in elderly persons. In each group, the osteomyelitis may have a hematogenous origin due to a bacteremia from an identifiable or nonidentifiable source or it may be secondary to a contiguous focus of infection which may be post-traumatic or iatrogenic ie, following surgery or investigative procedures (Weinstein et al., 1983).

Neonates and Infants

Lack of clinical signs and fever of undetermined origin may delay the diagnosis and treatment in neonates and infants who not uncommonly have a fever of unknown origin. Careful examination is therefore necessary to reach the diagnosis.

The origin is usually hematogenous, caused by a *Staphylococcus aureus*, although a recent shift to the group A beta-hemolytic *Streptococcus* has been described (Fox and Sprunt, 1978) but may also be due to contiguous septic focus (Canale and Manugian, 1981).

Several reports indicate the increased role of diagnostic procedures as a cause of infection, such as umbilical catheterization, fetal monitoring, femoral puncture or heel puncture (Canale and Manugian, 1981; Edwards et al, 1978; Lilien et al, 1976; Overturf and Balfour, 1975). The patient may have a septicemia or only swelling with localized tenderness and inability to move a leg freely (Weissberg, et al., 1974). Multiple infected sites are common, the femur being most frequently involved (Fox and Sprunt, 1978), with a high incidence of septic arthritis due to the free connection between metaphyseal and epiphyseal vessels (Septimus and Musher, 1979). After the clinical examination, the first step is to obtain appropriate blood culture. Infants and neonates have a bacteremia with a high order of magnitude; the sensitivity of a single 1 mL blood culture is around 85% while three separate blood cultures within a 24-hour period have a sensitivity of nearly 100% (Mandell et al, 1979; Reller et al, 1982).

Current Concepts of Infections in
Orthopaedic Surgery

Other laboratory data are of little help; the white blood count is unreliable (Fox and Sprunt, 1978; Morrey et al, 1975); erythrocyte sedimentation rate (ESR), however, is almost consistently elevated (Fox and Sprunt, 1978). Appropriate radiologic examination is the second step. Neonatal osteomyelitis is fulminant (Bonakdar-Pour and Gaines, 1983; Waldvogel and Vasey, 1980; Weissberg et al, 1974) demonstrating early radiologic signs of soft tissue swelling adjacent to the involved bones, obliteration of tissue planes or early lytic lesions (Resnick and Niwayama, 1982). Within the first three days after the onset of the disease, in most cases the other procedures can be bypassed. An immediate microscopic examination may be made following a direct needle aspiration or, if necessary, an open incision and drainage (Peterson, 1983). This permits a diagnosis within a few hours after examination (Morrisy, 1982).

Radionuclide scans may delay the diagnosis and should not be prescribed routinely (Morrisy, 1982). Technetium bone scan is often difficult to interpret in neonates. Normal scintigraphy does not exclude osteomyelitis; cold spots may be obtained when the microcirculation of bone is compromised by an abscess (Green, 1983; Jones and Cady, 1981; Kirchner and Simon, 1981) but it may also become positive within hours after onset of an infection (Kirchner and Simon, 1981; Resnick and Niwayama, 1982); it may be particularly helpful when one suspects multiple sites of infection (Morrisy, 1982) and infantile vertebral osteomyelitis (Eismont et al, 1982). Gallium scanning takes up to 24 hours and is of no value in the early diagnosis of acute infantile osteomyelitis (Green, 1983).

Children

As the child grows older, the growth plate becomes a barrier and the metaphysis becomes a frequent site of infection (Septimus and Musher, 1979). Hematogenous spread is most common with localization in tibia and femur in 70% of the patients (Morrey and Peterson, 1975), *S. aureus* being the pathogenic organism in 80 to 90% of patients (Resnick and Niwayama, 1982). Contiguous infection from a septic focus becomes more common in open fracture surgical procedures or in traumatic puncture wounds of the foot (Fitzgerald and Cowan, 1975) where gram-negative organisms predominate. The diagnosis should be made within 72 hours of the onset of symptoms. Immediate appropriate treatment prevents serious complications (Morrisy, 1982).

History and physical examination will usually detect the site of infection, ie, increased warmth, tenderness, swelling, and pseudoparalysis with a sudden onset of fever or toxic state (Resnick and Niwayama, 1982). Diagnosis may become more difficult: 1) in spine infections because of the absence of back pain (Boston et al, 1975; Wenger et al, 1978); 2) in iliac osteomyelitis (Beaupre and Carroll, 1979; Resnick and Niwayama, 1982) which may cause gluteal, abdominal or back pain; 3) in patients having received antibiotic therapy; or 4) when the infection is primarily epiphyseal (Green et al, 1981). Appropriate blood cultures must be ordered, and because a bacteremia in children has a low order of magnitude, three separately collected blood cultures must be taken (Mandell et al, 1979; Reller et al, 1982) which will yield the organisms in about 30 to 50% of the cases (Norden, 1979; Petersen, 1983; Smith, 1979; Waldvogel and Vasey, 1980; Wenger et al, 1978).

Routine laboratory data may not be helpful (Boston et al, 1975; Mollan and Piggot, 1977; Morrey and Peterson, 1975; Morrey et al, 1975; Peterson, 1983) although the ESR is almost always elevated.

Radiologic examination can demonstrate early changes in soft tissues with displacement of fat lines and obliteration of tissue planes around the bone in the first three days following the onset of the disease (Bonakdar-Pour and Gaines, 1983; Resnick and Niwayama, 1982). It will not, however, demonstrate bony changes in the early phase of infection because alteration in the bone architecture may take from 7 to 14 days (Peterson, 1983; Resnick and Niwayama, 1982) after destruction of at least 40% of the infected bone (Resnick and Niwayama, 1982; Septimus and Musher, 1979; Waldvogel and Vasey, 1980).

Bony changes in the spine and flat bones may also be difficult to detect, indicating a need for other more sensitive modalities. Most often, clinical examination, plain roentgenograms with or without tomograms, and laboratory data will localize the site allowing to undertake a biopsy or aspiration without too much delay.

In difficult cases, a radionuclide scan is the procedure of choice to localize the site of infection (Beaupre and Carroll, 1979; Peterson, 1983; Wenger et al, 1978).

Technetium bone scanning may be positive within 24 hours after the onset of the infection (Kirchner and Simon, 1981) and 10 to 14 days before any radiologic changes (Alazraki, 1982; Septimus and Musher, 1979) are observed. False positive or negative images, however, may occur (Peterson, 1983). A normal technetium bone scan does not exclude osteomyelitis (Green, 1983). It may show cold spots due to an interruption of the blood supply by the abscess, or may demonstrate multiple hot spots not progressing to osteomyelitis. Moreover, a positive scan cannot always differentiate infection from trauma and tumor, although cellulitis and arthritis can be distinguished from osteomyelitis by doing a radionuclide angiogram (Alazraki, 1982).

Gallium scanning may take up to 24 hours to detect infection and is not indicated in acute cases (Green, 1983) but is very helpful in difficult sites and when a technetium bone scan is doubtful, revealing infection in nearly all cases (Alazraki, 1982).

The final diagnostic procedure is to obtain a specimen for Gram stain and cultures which must routinely be done for aerobic and anaerobic organisms, mycobacteria and fungi (Septimus and Musher, 1979).

Routine exploration, drainage and culture are integral parts of the correct management of acute osteomyelitis (Mollan and Piggot, 1977), to confirm the inflammatory nature of the lesion, to identify the organism, and to determine the treatment (Morrisy, 1982).

Needle aspiration of bone is positive in only 69% of the patients (Norden, 1979), while the culture of surgical biopsy is positive in nearly 100% of the scans. It must be remembered that a negative aspiration is of no significance but indicates a need for more material; furthermore, the value of the bacterial culture report is only as good as the care with which the specimen was obtained (Kind and Williams, 1982) and transported to the laboratory (Morrisy, 1982).

Adults

The clinical picture of adult osteomyelitis differs from children by an increased incidence of infection secondary to a contiguous septic process, by the localization of the hematogenous osteomyelitis and by an insidious clinical course.

Hematogenous osteomyelitis is typically located in the axial skeleton (Kelly, 1975; 1977; Resnick and Niwayama, 1982; Septimus and Musher, 1979) although other sites may be affected. The spreading will occur through the Batson plexus or, more commonly, through the nutrient branches of the posterior spinal arteries (Septimus and Musher, 1979).

Predisposing factors are skin, urinary and postpartum infections, urologic and gynecologic diagnostic or surgical procedures (Rosenthal et al, 1982; Stauffer, 1975), gastrointestinal diseases (Resnick and Niwayama, 1982) or systemic diseases in a patient with a compromised immune system.

The spine will be the main site with *S. aureus* being the offending organism in 90% of the patients (Stauffer, 1975). Other sites include sacroiliac and manubriosternal joints in drug abusers due to gram-negative organisms (Kelly, 1975; 1977; Resnick and Niwayama, 1982; Waldvogel and Vasey, 1980) and the symphysis pubis after urologic or gynecologic procedures (Rosenthal et al, 1982).

Systemic signs with back pain can be present, marked with only low grade fever (Stauffer, 1975). Blood culture may be positive in 10 to 60% of acute untreated cases (Mandell et al, 1979; Waldvogel and Vasey, 1980); however, three 10 to 20 mL samples may have to be taken by separate venipunctures because the bacteremia is of a low order of magnitude (Mandell et al, 1979; Reller et al, 1982).

Laboratory data may be unreliable but the ESR is almost always elevated Mandell et al, 1979; Septimus and Musher, 1979; Stauffer, 1975).

Radiologic examination is not positive before 10 to 14 days following the onset of infection (Waldvogel and Vasey, 1980) and demonstrates progressive narrowing of the disk space and blurring of the subchondral bony plate before more obvious changes occur. It is not therefore of much help for an early diagnosis (Stauffer, 1975). Radionuclide scanning with technetium and gallium are essential in the diagnosis, allowing early detection of the infected area and offering a chance to look at the bone in a dynamic fashion (Deutsch et al, 1981; Hogues, 1980).

The infected site will be located quickly allowing early biopsy and culture (Waldvogel and Vasey, 1980). Technetium bone scan may be positive as early as 24 hours after the onset of symptoms (Alazraki, 1982) but is related to vascularity and may also be positive in the presence of a tumor and trauma. Gallium scanning takes up to 48 hours but, being more specific, reveals the infection in almost all patients (Alazraki, 1982).

In more severe conditions, computed tomography will be useful in localizing the site for a biopsy, and in assessing the spine and its contents demonstrating adjacent paravertebral abscess (Genant, 1982; Schumaker et al, 1978). The last procedure is the biopsy. The need for an exact bacteriologic diagnosis cannot be overemphasized (Septimus and Muscher, 1979). Bacterial proof is important because the organisms may be unusual and empiric antimicrobial therapy could be inappropriate (Kelly, 1975). Specimens may be retrieved through needle biopsy (Resnick and Niwayama, 1982) under roentgenographic or CT-Scan control (Genant, 1982; Schumaker et al, 1978), but the biopsy may be unrewarding in up to one-third of the patients (Septimus and Musher, 1979; Waldvogel and Vasey, 1980), necessitating an open biopsy.

The specimens must be sent for histologic examination (Pritchard, 1975; Washington, 1975) to rule out a granulomatous lesion (Pritchard, 1975) and for microbiologic studies including aerobic and anaerobic cultures as well as mycobacteria and fungi.

Osteomyelitis secondary to a contiguous septic focus may be post-traumatic: open fractures, infected wounds or iatrogenic infections after surgical or investigative procedures.

Post-traumatic osteomyelitis may be caused by penetrating injuries, human bites, puncture wounds, irradiation and burns. Open fractures are contaminated wounds and, if left untreated over an eight-hour period, will probably become infected (Kind and Williams, 1982).

Early closure may precipitate infection in 73% of patients while closure after the fourth day may cause infection in only 4% (Septimus and Musher, 1979). Although *S. aureus* accounts for 50% of the organisms, almost any pathogen may be responsible (Resnick and Niwayama, 1982). Contamination by gram-negative organisms and anaerobes is frequent (Sim, 1975).

The first step in the diagnosis is at the time of initial debridement: Gram staining and culture must then be done (Fitzgerald, 1979). It will be found that the cultured organisms are the causes in 65 to 70% of the cases (Kind and Williams, 1982). Contiguous osteomyelitis behaves insidiously, with increasing wound drainage and sinus formation as the sole manifestations but, at times, systemic signs may be severe as in anaerobic infections (Sim, 1975). Blood cultures are usually negative (Mandell et al, 1979). The soft tissue infection will show radiologic changes such as periostitis, cortical erosion and bone lysis (Resnick and Niwayama, 1982) but late in the course of the infection. The technetium scan is not reliable because it shows abnormalities during the repair process following a fracture, whereas the gallium scan may be more specific, although its role has not yet been fully established (Kirchner and Simon, 1981).

The specificity of both scans may be increased by first using transit blood pool imaging (Kirchner and Simon, 1981), allowing differentiation between cellulitis and osteomyelitis (Alazraki, 1982).

The definitive procedure to reflect the state of affairs in the deeper tissues is needle aspiration of bone biopsy (Kind and Williams, 1982).

Iatrogenic osteomyelitis. Infection may occur after elective surgery in 1 to 7.4% of the cases (Fitzgerald, 1979) or after investigative procedures, such as discography or myelography.

The diagnostic workup may be similar to the one following post-trauma osteitis but may not be easy in the case of spinal involvement. Iatrogenic spinal infection may be suspected by a persistant back pain and if the ESR has not decreased three months after the procedure (Stauffer, 1975). Blood cultures are negative and the technetium scan is usually elevated in surgical trauma. In this event, a gallium scan may add useful information (Kirchner and Simon, 1981) and a CT-scan will be helpful to confirm the presence of a prevertebral abscess and to determine the site for a biopsy (Resnick and Niwayama, 1982; Schumaker et al, 1978).

Infected arthroplasties present a particularly difficult problem for diagnosis. Arthroplasties may become infected in 1% of patients (Hunter, 1982) due to surgical contamination (Resnick and Niwayama, 1982) or late hematogenous infection (Cruess et al, 1975; Stinchfield et al, 1980). Early detection is important for a successful outcome but the diagnostic process is different in acute infections (1-4 weeks) and delayed sepsis (after 1 year).

Early acute arthroplasty infection may be difficult to differentiate from inflammation (Gristina and Kolkin, 1983). The cardinal clinical sign is pain (Eftekhar, 1977) while fever may or may not be present.

Radiologic examination is useless because bony changes will not be demonstrable in the first six weeks (Eftekhar, 1977; Gristina and Kolkin, 1983). Radionuclide scans are not helpful because they are positive for three to six months postoperatively (Gristina and Kolkin, 1983) and are therefore not specific in acute infections (Goergen, 1982) although the gallium scan appears promising (Goergen, 1982; Reing et al, 1979).

The diagnostic procedure of choice is aspiration of the joint (Eftekhar, 1977) followed by injection of saline and reaspiration if indicated (Gristina and Kolkin, 1983). Gram stains and cellular morphology may be diagnostic in the presence of increased neutrophils and a decrease of cytoplasmic granules in the neutrophils (Efteknar, 1977; Gristina and Kolkin, 1983). The offending organism is *S. aureus* in 50% of the cases (Gristina and Kolkin, 1983); it must be remembered, however, that no organisms are demonstrated in seven to 15% of documented infections because, in part, the organisms in contact with biomaterials may be surrounded by a polysaccharide membrane called the glycocalyx (Gristina and Kolkin, 1983) and, if antibiotics were already given, L forms may be present which will show up only if the culture is continued for at least five days (Gristina and Kolkin, 1983). In doubtful cases, an open biopsy will be the last diagnostic procedure.

Forty-two to 76% of the late arthroplasty infections become clinically evident within the first postoperative year.

Pain is again the cardinal sign (Eftekhar, 1977; Hunter, 1982). It is gradual, persistent at night while, in aseptic loosening, the pain is more sudden and increases with walking (Gristina and Kolkin, 1983). Laboratory data are not helpful but the ESR is often elevated (Eftekhar, 1977; Gristina and Kolkin, 1983).

Radiologic changes may become evident if periodic films are available for comparison (Eftekhar, 1977). Increasing lucency between bone cement or prosthesis cement interfaces, change in the position of the prosthetic components, and cement fracture may all be signs of septic or aseptic loosening (Eftekhar, 1977).

Radionuclide scans although nonspecific are more informative; however, one must remember that they may remain abnormal up to one year postoperatively (Gristina and Kolkin, 1973). Negative scans essentially rule out the presence of significant loosening or infection (Weissman, 1983). A positive focal uptake of technetium is more suggestive of loosening while a diffuse intense uptake is more likely due to infection (Weissman, 1983).

A gallium scan is indicated in all patients with positive technetium uptake (Reishton et al, 1982), and suggestive of infection if the gallium uptake is intense or incongruent with the technetium uptake (Weissman, 1983). Both scans have a specificity and sensitivity of 75% (Reing et al, 1979) and must be part of the routine assessment of suspected arthroplasty loosening.

The final diagnostic procedure will be the aspiration biopsy which may be done during arthrography (Eftekhar, 1977; Insall, 1982; Murray, 1982). Arthrography of the hip may demonstrate the extension of contrast materials into the bone cement or metal cement interface, and have a true positive rate of 78% for loosening (Weissman, 1983). In established infections, it may demonstrate the extent of soft tissue lesions with fistulae and para-articular cavities (Weissman, 1983) but is usually not helpful in the diagnosis of infection per se and could be misleading as to the presence of loosening (Eftekhar, 1977). If the aspiration biopsy fails to yield the organism and other data suggest infection, then an open surgical biopsy will have to be done.

Elderly

The clinical picture may be, as in the neonates, subtle with a lack of systemic symptoms and fever (Stauffer, 1975) and a high index of vigilance will be needed to make the diagnosis.

Hematogenous osteomyelitis may induce vertebral osteomyelitis (Septimus and Musher, 1979; Stauffer, 1975) and late hematogenous infection of total arthroplasties. Because of an impaired immune mechanism, systemic diseases such as diabetes, atherosclerosis, rheumatoid arthritis, neoplasms, or in patients on chronic hemodialysis or corticotherapy (Norden, 1979), there is an increased risk of hematogenous seeding from infection elsewhere in the body (Cruess et al, 1975; Stinchfield et al, 1980) due to dental work, poor oral hygiene, pneumonia, cellulitis or medicosurgical procedures (Kelly, 1977). As to suspected spinal infections, the diagnostic workup was discussed in the adult section. In late hematogenous infection of total arthroplasties, the pain may appear suddenly, years after asymptomatic arthroplasty (Fitzgerald and Cowan, 1975). The assessment is similar to the one discussed for adults.

Osteomyelitis contiguous to a septic focus becomes more common in the elderly who suffer from diabetes and atherosclerosis.

Infected decubitus ulcers and infected ulcerated callosities or toenails may lead to osteomyelitis. It commonly affects the feet but pain may not be present in cases of diabetic neuropathy (Selvapandian, 1982; Wagner, 1981).

The determination of the true pathogen may be difficult and mixed flora with both aerobes and anaerobes is always present (Wagner, 1981; Weinstein, 1982). Radiologic examination may be difficult to interpret and magnification radiography may be helpful (Resnick and Niwayama, 1982) in detecting bone erosion. Radionuclide scanning may confirm the infection and surgical biopsy may yield the organisms.

Conclusions

Delay in diagnosis is the single most important factor determining the prog nosis of acute osteomyelitis. It is the physician's prime responsibility to identify without delay the cause of the infection and to start appropriate treatment.

Sophisticated techniques are indicated only to detect and confirm the nature of the lesion but should not delay identification of the causative organisms.

Acknowledgements

The author is grateful to Drs. J. Basora, G. Lamoureux, R. Levesque, R. Duperval and J.A. Marcoux for their useful comments and criticisms.

References

1. Alazraki, N.: Bone imaging by radionuclide techniques. In, Resnick and Niwayama: Diagnosis of Bone and Joint Disorders, Saunders, 1982. pp. 639-677.
2. Beaupre, A. and Carroll, N.: The three syndromes of iliac osteomyelitis in children. J. Bone Joint Surg. 61A, 1087, 1979.
3. Bonakdar-Pour, A. and Gaines, V.: The radiology of osteomyelitis. Orthop.Clin. North Am. 14, 21, 1983.
4. Boston, H., Bianco, A., and Hable-Rhodes, K.: Disk space infections in children. Orthop. Clin. North Am. 6, 953, 1975.
5. Canale, S. and Manugian, A.: Neonatal osteomyelitis of the os calcis. Clin. Orthop. 156, 178, 1981.
6. Cruess, R., Bickel, W.S., and Von Kessler, K.: Infections in total hips secondary to a primary focus elsewhere. Clin. Orthop. 106, 99, 1975.
7. Deutsch, S., Gandsman, E., and Spraragen, S.: Quantitative regional blood flow analysis and its clinical application during bone scanning. J. Bone Joint Surg. 63A, 295, 1981.
8. Edwards, M., Baker, C., Wagner, M., Taber, L., and Barrett, F.: An etiologic shift in infantile osteomyelitis: The emergence of the group B streptococcus. J. Pediat. 93, 578, 1978.
9. Eftekhar, N.: The infected total hip. Instr. Course Lecture 26, 66, 1977.
10. Eismont, F., Bohlman, H., Soni, P., Goldberg, V., and Freehafer, A.: Vertebral osteomyelitis in infants. J. Bone Joint Surg. 64B, 32, 1982.
11. Fitzgerald, R.: Laboratory diagnosis of postoperative sepsis of the musculoskeletal system. Orthop. Clin. North Am. 10, 361, 1979.
12. Fitzgerald, R. and Cowan, J.D.: Puncture wounds of the foot. Orthop. Clin. North Am. 6, 965, 1975.
13. Fox, L. and Sprunt, K.: Neonatal osteomyelitis. Pediat. 62, 535, 1978.
14. Genant, H.K.: Computed tomography. In, Resnick and Niwayama: Diagnosis of Bone and Joint Disorders, Saunders, 1982. pp 380-408.

15. Goergen, T.: Radiographic evaluation of the postoperative patient. In, Resnick and Niwayama: Diagnosis of Bone and Joint Disorders, Saunders, 1982, pp 814-845.

16. Green, N.: The use of bone scans for the detection of osteomyelitis. Instr. Course Lecture 32, 40, 1983.

17. Green, N., Beauchamp, R., and Griffin, P.: Primary subacute epiphyseal osteomyelitis. J. Bone Joint Surg. 63A, 107, 1981.

18. Gristina, A., and Kolkin, J.: Current concepts review: total joint replacement and sepsis. J. Bone Joint Surg. 65A, 128, 1983.

19. Hugues, S.: Radionuclides in orthopedic surgery. J. Bone Joint Surg. 62B, 141, 1980.

20. Hunter, G.: The natural history of the patient with an infected total hip replacement. Instr. Course Lecture 31, 38, 1982.

21. Insall, J.: Infection in total knee arthroplasty. Instr. Course Lecture 31, 42, 1982.

22. Jones, D., and Cady, R.: Cold bone scans in acute osteomyelitis. J. Bone Joint Surg. 63B, 376, 1981.

23. Kelly, P.: Osteomyelitis of the adult. Orthop. Clin. North Am. 6, 983, 1975.

24. Kelly, P.: Infections of bones and joints in adult patients. Instr. Course Lecture 26, 3, 1977.

25. Kind, A. and Williams, D.: Antibiotics in open fractures. In, Gustilo: Management of open fractures and their complications, Saunders, 1982. pp. 59-69.

26. Kirchner, P., and Simon, M.A.: Current concepts review: Radio-isotopic evaluation of skeletal disease. J. Bone Joint Surg. 63A, 673, 1981.

27. Lilien, L., Harris, V., Ramamurthy, R., and Pilder, R.: Neonatal osteomyelitis of the calcaneus, complications of heel puncture. J. Pediat. 88, 478, 1976.

28. Mandell, G., Douglas, G., and Bennet, J.: Infectious Diseases. Wiley, 1979, pp 145-146.

29. Mollan, R., and Piggot, J.: Acute osteomyelitis in children. J. Bone Joint Surg. 59B, 2, 1977.

30. Morrey, B., Bianco, A., and Rhodes, K.: Septic arthritis in children. Orthop. Clin. North Am. 6, 923, 1975.

31. Morrey, B., and Peterson, H.: Hematogenous pyogenic osteomyelitis in children. Orthop. Clin. North Am. 6, 935, 1975.

32. Morrisy, R.: Bone and joint sepsis in children. Instr. Course Lecture 31, 49, 1982.

33. Murray, W.: Treatment of the established deep wound infection after total hip arthroplasty. In, Leach, Hoaglund and Riseborough: Controversies in Orthopedic Surgery. Saunders, 1982, pp 382-398.

34. Norden, C.W.: Osteomyelitis. In, Mandell: Infectious Diseases. Wiley, 1979. pp 946-956.

35. Overturf, G. and Balfour, G.: Osteomyelitis and sepsis: severe complications of fetal monitoring. Pediat. 55, 244, 1975.

36. Peterson, H.: Musculoskeletal infections in children. Instr. Course Lecture 32, 33, 1983.

37. Pritchard, D.: Granulomatous infections of bones and joints. Orthop. Clin. North Am. 6, 1029, 1975.

38. Reller, L., Murray, P., and McLowry, J. In, Cumitech, I.A., Am. Soc. for Microbiology. 1982.

39. Reing, M., Richin, P., and Kenmore, P.: Differential bone scanning in the evaluation of painful total joint replacement. J. Bone Joint Surg 61A, 933, 1979.

40. Reishton, N., Coakley, A., Tudor, J., and Wraight, E.: The value of technetium and gallium scanning in assessing pain after total hip replacement. J. Bone Joint Surg. 64B, 313, 1982.

41. Resnick, D. and Niwayama: Osteomyelitis, septic arthritis and soft tissue infection. In, Resnick and Niwayama: Diagnosis of Bone and Joint Disorders. Saunders, 1982. pp 2042-2236.

42. Rosenthal, R., Spickard, W., Markham, R., and Rhamy, R.: Osteomyelitis of the symphysis pubis. J. Bone Joint Surg. 64A, 123, 1982.

43. Schumaker, T., Genant, H., Korobkin, M., and Bovill, E.: Computed tomography: its use in space occupying lesions of the musculoskeletal system. J. Bone Joint Surg. 60A, 600, 1978.

44. Selvapandian, A.: Infections of the foot. In, Jahss: Disorders of the Foot. Saunders, 1982. pp 1398-1428.

45. Septimus, E. and Musher, D.: Osteomyelitis: recent clinical and laboratory aspects. Orthop. Clin. North Am. 10, 347, 1979.

46. Sim, F.: Anaerobic infections. Orthop. Clin. North Am. 6, 1049, 1975.

47. Smith, J.: Bone and joint infections. In, Mandell: Infectious Diseases Wiley, 1979.

48. Stauffer, R.: Pyogenic vertebral osteomyelitis. Orthop. Clin. North Am 6, 1015, 1975.

49. Stinchfield, F., Bigliani, L., Nev, H., Goss, T., and Foster, C.: Late hematogenous infection of total joint replacement. J. Bone Joint Surg. 62A, 1345, 1980.

50. Waldvogel, F., and Vasey, H.: Osteomyelitis: the past decade. N. Engl. J. Med. 303, 360, 1980.

51. Wagner, W.J.: The dysvascular foot. Foot-Ankle 2, 64, 1981.

52. Washington, J.: The microbiology of musculoskeletal infection. Orthop. Clin. North Am. 6, 1115, 1975.

53. Weinstein, A.: Selection of antimicrobial therapy. Instr. Course Lecture 31, 14, 1982.

54. Weinstein, A.: Classification of adult osteomyelitis and antibiotic therapy. In, Evarts Surgery of the Musculoskeletal System 10, 5. Churchill Livingston, 1983.

55. Weissberg, E., Smith, A., and Smith, D.: Clinical features of neonatal osteomyelitis. Pediat. 53, 505, 1974.

56. Weissman, B.: The radiology of total hip replacement. Orthop. Clin. North Am. 14, 171, 1983.

57. Wenger, D., Bobechko, W., and Gilday, D.: The spectrum of intervertebral disk space infection in children. J. Bone J. Surg. 60A, 100, 1978.

The Role of Radionuclide Studies in the Diagnosis of Infections in Orthopedic Surgery

R. KLOIBER

Introduction

The sensitivity of technitium phosphate imaging in the detection of reparative bone reaction, local alteration of blood flow, and inflammation make such procedures valuable in the assessment of infections of the musculoskeletal system. In acute osteomyelitis, scintigraphic abnormalities precede plain radiographic evidence by ten to 14 days and are also useful in differentiating soft tissue and joint involvement. With secondary infection following surgery or trauma and in chronic osteomyelitis, the ability to detect the inflammatory response directly with gallium or indium-labelled leukocyte imaging can assist in diagnosing active disease in situations with complex radiographic appearance.

The localization of the technetium phosphate compounds depends on the number of accessible binding sites on metabolically-active bone mineral or matrix as well as the rate of delivery or blood flow. The amount of uptake does not depend on total mineral content but on the rate of turnover which is increased in reparative bone. Studies with these compounds, therefore, indicate the normal bone response to injury. They are sensitive, obtain good resolution and anatomic detail but are very low in specificity. Gallium and indium-labelled leukocytes show the pathologic process directly and offer greater specificity. Nevertheless, in the case of gallium, inflammation and certain neoplasms cannot be differentiated and neither gallium nor indium leukocyte imaging can distinguish septic from nonseptic inflammation. When radionuclide studies are used in combination and correlated with clinical findings and other imaging techniques, maximum sensitivity and specificity can be achieved.

Radiophosphate Compounds in Uncomplicated Disease

The clinical diagnosis of osteomyelitis can be difficult, particularly in children. Differentiation of cellulitis, septic arthritis, and osteomyelitis can have a significant effect on duration of therapy and prognosis. In the early stage, radiographs unfortunately show little more than nonspecific edema in most cases. The spine, carpals, tarsals and pelvis are particularly difficult to assess radiographically. Moreover, up to 45% of radiographs of osteomyelitis may remain normal with early antibiotic therapy (Duszynski et al, 1975).

In osteomyelitis, delayed technetium phosphate images characteristically show a well defined focus of increased activity in the bone (Fig. 1). This is often accompanied by diffuse regional hyperconcentration due to hyperemia. In septic arthritis, the periarticular bone shares in the synovial

Current Concepts of Infections in
Orthopaedic Surgery

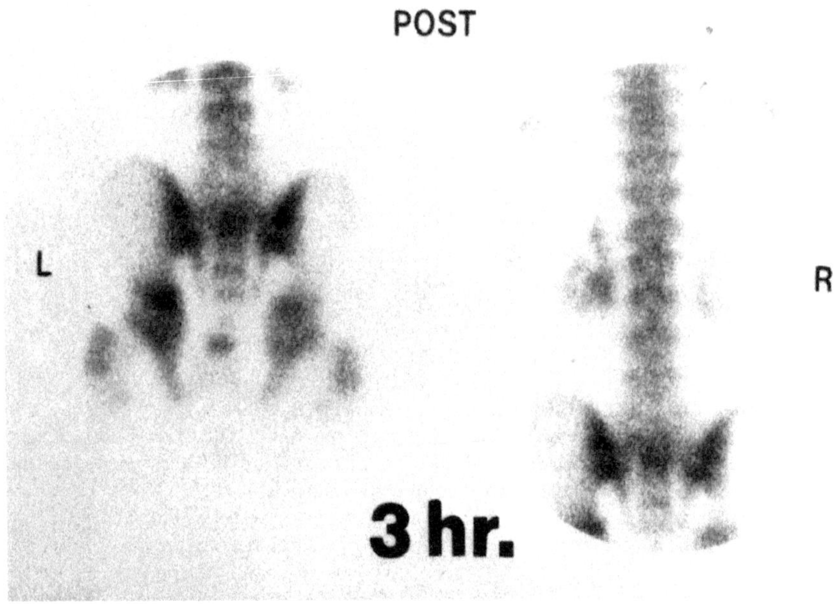

Fig. 1. Osteomyelitis: delayed technetium phosphate bone images showing focal increased activity in the left acetabulum due to acute osteomyelitis

hyperemia and results in diffuse increased periarticular uptake (Fig. 2). This is symmetrical about the joint and lacks the focal increased activity that signifies direct bone involvement. In cellulitis, images may be normal or show diffuse hyperemia of the entire limb. Addition of blood flow and blood pool images immediately after injection of the radiotracer allows direct visualization of the hyperperfusion not only in the soft tissues or synovium, but can also define the most active area in acute or chronic osteomyelitis and guide aspiration or surgical biopsy. Areas of decreased activity on blood pool images may signify areas of ischemia or the presence of joint effusions displacing vascular structures.

In acute hematogenous osteomyelitis, particularly in children, edema may cause increased intramedullary pressure and compromise blood flow. The result is decreased rather than focal increased radiophosphate deposition on delayed images (Fig. 3). Although more difficult to recognize than hyperconcentration, photon deficiency is of equal diagnostic value and has obvious clinical implications (Murray, 1982). Furthermore, growth plate activity in children may obscure minor abnormalities and the importance of meticulous technique cannot be overemphasized. Multiple projections in standard positions with accompanying views of the contralateral side, and exposures at multiple intensity settings to show high and low activity regions and intralesional detail are mandatory (Gilday, 1980). The normal growth plate, although variable in shape, is sharply defined and strict immobilization is needed to avoid motion blurring that may mimic disease.

Animal studies have yielded confusing results. One study paradoxically showed greater sensitivity of radiography (Rinsky et al, 1977) and the applicability of animal models to human disease was questioned. After intramedullary inoculation of heat-killed staphylococci and a sclerosing agent, Tc-99m phosphate blood pool images and gallium images were positive

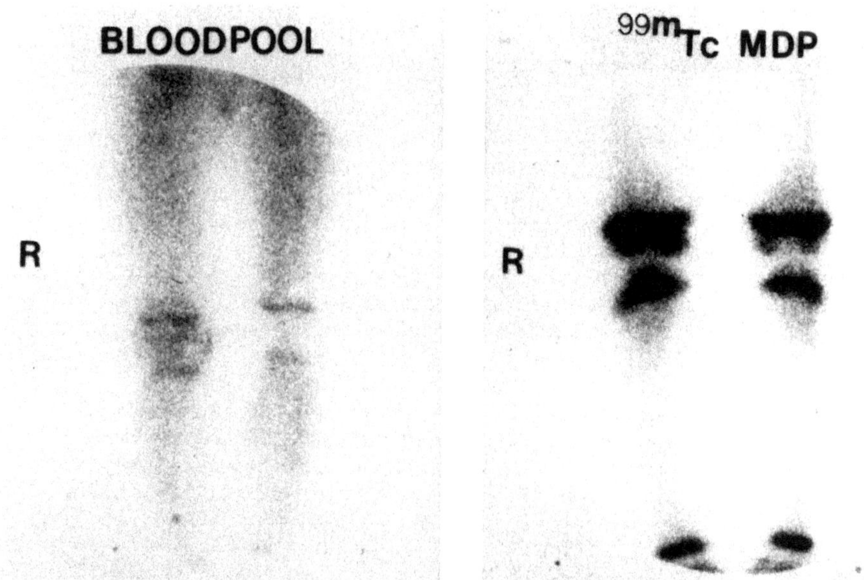

Fig. 2. Septic arthritis: the blood pool image on the left shows diffuse increased activity in the region of the right knee. Delayed technetium phosphate images on the right show diffuse increased activity surrounding the right knee. The activity decreases progressively with distance from the joint but growth plates remain sharply defined. No superimposed focus to indicate associated osteomyelitis

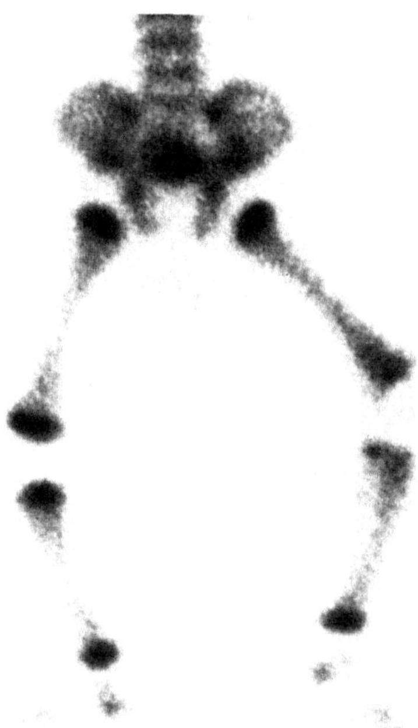

Fig. 3. Septic arthritis of the right knee and osteomyelitis of the distal femur and proximal tibia: The growth plates in the distal femur and proximal tibia cannot be identified in this 10-day old infant, indicating ischemia due to osteomyelitis. Radiographs at the time were normal

early in the course when delayed bone images were either normal or showed photon deficiency (Norris and Watt, 1981). The superior sensitivity of gallium in early infection has also been shown by others (Dye et al, 1979; Norris et al, 1978).

Because of the delay in seeking help and the time of the incubation period, most human studies are positive at the time of presentation. Nevertheless, normal radiophosphate bone scans occur occasionally, particularly in the first 48 hours after onset of clinical symptoms. With negative studies in patients with relatively low-grade symptoms and a short history, repeat examinations after a delay of several days or supplementary imaging with gallium or leukocytes may be indicated (Handmaker, 1980). Neonates in particular present great difficulty and radiophosphate imaging should be applied with caution (Ash and Gilday, 1980).

Although some studies report as low as 52% accuracy of phosphate imaging (Sullivan et al, 1980), with appropriate technique and diagnostic criteria more than 90% accuracy is achievable. This has been demonstrated in several large reviews including both pediatric and adult patients (Gilday et al, 1975; Howie et al, 1983; Rosenthall et al, 1982).

Sequential Technetium Phosphate and Gallium Imaging

Technetium phosphate is the preferred radiopharmaceutical because it shows greater anatomic detail, requires a lower radiation dose, and gives more rapid results. However, when an underlying abnormality is present that would also cause an abnormal radiophosphate study -- eg, fracture, chronic osteomyelitis, surgery or prosthetic devices -- supplementary imaging with gallium is required. The mechanism of gallium localization is complex (Hoffer, 1980). Gallium resembles the ferric ion and, when administered intravenously, binds to transferrin and other iron-binding substances. Localization at sites of inflammation is by transudation of plasma proteins exchange with siderophores in bacteria and lactoferrin in leukocyte granules. Nontransferrin-bound gallium is associated with the mineral phase of bone. Because of this, areas of intense new bone formation will accumulate some gallium even in the absence of inflammation. Interpretation must, therefore, be made in conjunction with the preceding radiophosphate study (Lisbona and Rosenthall, 1977; Rosenthall et al, 1979) and only gallium accumulations that are excessive relative to a reference area of normal bone (disproportionate), or different in distribution from the phosphate study (incongruent) are indicative of a process other than sterile bone reaction (Fig. 4). Inflammation and gallium-avid neoplasms must be differentiated by other means. Using the algorithm in Fig. 5, high accuracy in diagnosis of infection can be maintained even in the presence of associated bone damage. The main difficulties are in the acute postoperative period because of the propensity of gallium to localize in surgical or nonsurgical soft tissue wounds, even in the absence of infection.

Gallium images tend to revert to normal with successful antibiotic therapy (Mendelson et al, 1983). Activity may persist even after sterilization of the process because of uptake in nonspecific inflammation and the reparative process. Although uptake can therefore be expected to lag behind clinical response, a reversion to normal implies successful treatment. Results should not, however, be used to shorten established minimum courses o antibiotic therapy.

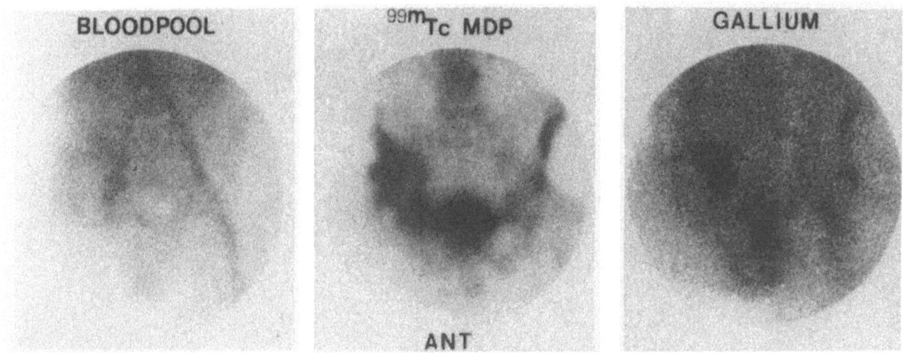

Fig. 4. Osteomyelitis in a patient with previous total hip replacement: The blood pool image (left) shows focal hyperemia in the acetabular region. The delayed technetium phosphate bone image (centre) shows a large area of increased activity with an area of photon deficiency medial to the acetabular component. The gallium image (right) shows intense increased activity in the area of the decreased uptake on the bone images. This is an incongruent pattern indicating active infection

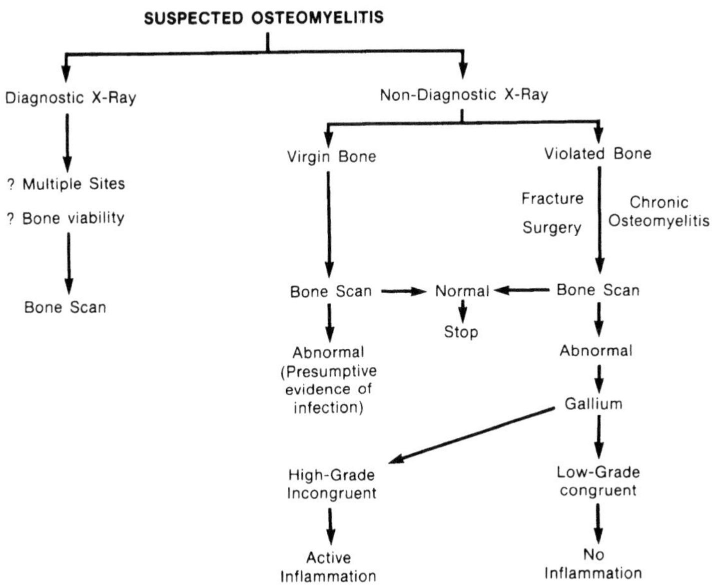

Fig. 5. Algorithm for investigation of suspected osteomyelitis

Indium-111 Labelled Leukocytes

Considerable initial success has been shown in demonstrating sites of acute pyogenic infection with indium-labelled leukocytes (Fig. 6). Sensitivities and specificities in the range of 90% have been reported (Goodwin, 1983; McDougall et al, 1979; Propst-Procter et al, 1982). The technique involves separation of the leukocytes from a 50 mL sample of the patient's blood, incubation with a lipid soluble indium oxine complex and reinfusion of the

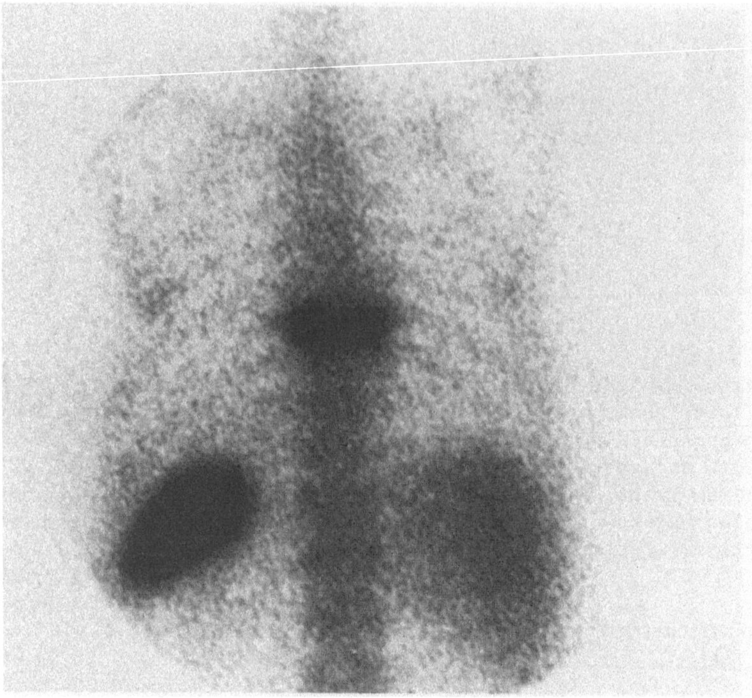

Fig. 6. Osteomyelitis: Intense focal increased uptake of indium-labelled leukocytes indicating active osteomyelitis of the midthoracic spine. The activity in liver and spleen is normal

cells. Most abnormal sites are visible within 24 hours. With acute infection, lesion to background ratios tend to be higher than with gallium and there is normally no activity within the bowel, in recent noninfected surgical wounds, and in sterile bone reaction or neoplasms.

Although leukocyte function is not impaired by the separation and labelling process (Zakhireh et al, 1979), diagnosis and location of sepsis depend on active migration of the cells towards the abnormal focus. With partially treated, chronic or subacute infection, leukocyte migration is reduced and lesion detectability falls significantly (Sfakianakis et al, 1982). Because of different mechanisms of localization, the sensitivity of gallium is less affected and surpasses indium-111 leukocyte scintigraphy in chronic infection and after the first two weeks of acute human and experimental infection (Sfakianakis et al, 1982).

Radiophosphate bone imaging will certainly remain a procedure of choice for uncomplicated osteomyelitis because of its rapidity, anatomic detail, and relatively low radiation dose. Leukocyte studies show promise in acute infection complicating other types of bone injury and in the early postoperative period. Their role as a guide to therapy remains undefined. In violated bone when the clinical condition suggests a low grade chronic infection, sequential phosphate and gallium imaging retains its established role at the present time.

References

1. Ash, J.M. and Gilday, D.L.: The futility of bone scanning in neonatal osteomyelitis: Concise communication. J. Nucl. Med. 21, 417, 1980.
2. Duszynski, D.O., Kuhn, J.P., Afshani, E., and Riddlesberger, M.M., Jr.: Early radionuclide diagnosis of acute osteomyelitis. Radiol. 117, 337, 1975.
3. Dye, S.F., Lull, R.J., McAuley, R.J., Van Dam, B.E., and Young, W.: Time sequence of bone and gallium scan changes in acute osteomyelitis: An animal model. J. Nucl. Med. 20, 647, 1979 (Abstract).
4. Gilday, D.L.: Problems in the scintigraphic detection of osteomyelitis. Radiol. 135, 791, 1980.
5. Gilday, D.L., Paul, D.J., and Paterson, J.: Diagnosis of osteomyelitis in children by combined blood pool and bone imaging. Radiol. 117, 331, 1975.
6. Goodwin, D.A.: Clinical use of In-111 imaging. Clin. Nucl. Med. 8, 36, 1983.
7. Handmaker, H.: Acute hematogeneous osteomyelitis: Has the bone scan betrayed us? Radiol. 135, 787, 1980.
8. Hoffer, P.: Gallium: Mechanisms. J. Nucl. Med. 21, 282, 1980.
9. Howie, D.W., Savage, J.P., Wilson, T.G., and Paterson, D.: The technetium phosphate bone scan in the diagnosis of osteomyelitis in childhood. J. Bone Joint Surg. 65A, 431, 1983.
10. Lisbona, R. and Rosenthall, L.: Observations on the sequential use of ^{99m}Tc-phosphate complex and ^{67}Ga imaging in osteomyelitis, cellulitis and septic arthritis. Radiol. 123, 123, 1977.
11. McDougall, I.R., Baumert, J.E., and Lantieri, R.L.: Evaluation of ^{111}In in whole body scanning. Am. J. Radiol. 133, 849, 1979.
12. Mendelson, D.S., Som, P.M., Mendelson, M.H., and Parisier, S.C.: Malignant external otitis; The role of computed tomography and radionuclides in evaluation. Radiol. 149, 745, 1983.
13. Murray, I.P.C.: Photopenia in skeletal scintigraphy of suspected bone and joint infection. Clin. Nucl. Med. 7, 13, 1982.
14. Norris, S.H., Ehrlich, M.G., McKusick, K., and Provine, H.: The radioisotopic study of an experimental model of disc space infection. J. Bone Joint Surg. 60B, 281, 1978 (Abstract)
15. Norris, S.H. and Watt, I.: Radionuclide uptake during the evolution of experimental acute osteomyelitis. Brit. J. Radiol. 54, 207, 1981.
16. Propst-Proctor, S.L., Dillingham, M.F., McDougall, I.R., and Goodwin, D.: The white blood cell scan in orthopedics. Clin. Orthop. 168, 157, 1982.
17. Rinsky, L., Goris, M.L., Schurman, D.J., and Nagel, D.A.: Technitium bone scanning in experimental osteomyelitis. Clin. Orthop. 128, 361, 1977.
18. Rosenthall, L., Kloiber, R., Damtew, B., and Al-Majid, H.: Sequential use of radiophosphate and radiogallium imaging in the differential diagnosis of bone, joint and soft tissue infection: Quantitative analysis. Diagn. Imaging 51, 249, 1982.

19. Rosenthall, L., Lisbona, R., Hernandez, M., and Hadjipavlou, A.: ^{99m}Tc-PP and ^{67}Ga imaging following insertion of orthopedic devices. Radiol. 133, 717, 1979.

20. Sfakianakis, G.N., Al-Sheikh, W., Heal, A., Rodman, G., Zeppa, R., and Serafini, A.: Comparisons of scintigraphy with In-111s and Ga-67 in the diagnosis of occult sepsis. J. Nucl. Med. 23, 618, 1982.

21. Sullivan, D.C., Rosenfield, N.S., Ogden, J., and Gottschalk, A.: Problems in the scintigraphic detection of osteomyelitis in children. Radiol. 135, 731, 1980.

22. Zakhireh, B., Thakur, M.L., Malech, H.L., Cohen, M.S., Gottschalk, A., and Root, R.K.: Indium-111 labeled human polymorphonuclears: Viability random migration, chemotaxis, bactericidal capacity, and ultrastructure J. Nucl. Med. 20, 741, 1979.

The History of a Patient with an Infected Total Joint Replacement

J. P. McElwain and G. A. Hunter

Introduction

Since the introduction of total hip and total knee replacement as a surgical treatment for irreparably destroyed joints in elderly patients, the infection rate continues to decline. This may be related to better component design, improved technical skills, the use of antibiotics, better patient selection, and improved surgical facilities. As the number of total joint replacements continues to increase and provided the infection rates remain between 1 and 3%, then, undoubtedly, the number of septic prosthetic joints requiring treatment will increase correspondingly.

Deep infection involves the bone and soft tissues adjacent to the implant and cement. It implies the presence of inflammatory tissue (granulation tissue and pus) due to pathogenic organisms. We will discuss the treatment options available to the patient and the surgeon following an established diagnosis of deep infection. Since the symptomatology differs between infected hips and knees, each joint will be discussed individually.

Etiologic Factors

The predisposing factors common to both hip and knee replacement sepsis include:

1. Patient with rheumatoid arthritis (Arden, 1975; Editorial, 1972; Garner et al, 1973; Van Nierkerk and Charnley, 1979).

2. Previous surgery, especially after revision of joint replacement and after sepsis (Cherney and Amstutz, 1983; Fitzgerald et al, 1977; James et al, 1982; Murray, 1982).

3. Patients who have received multiple local steroid injections or are receiving long-term steroid therapy (Garner et al, 1973).

4. Diabetes mellitus and psoriasis (Hood and Insall, 1983; Menon and Wroblewski, 1983).

5. Obesity (Hood and Insall, 1983).

6. Immunodeficient state after renal transplantation (Karas et al, 1984).

7. Urethral instrumentation and dental procedures after joint replacement surgery (Wroblewski and Del Sal, 1980).

Current Concepts of Infections in
Orthopaedic Surgery

8. Local wound problems, such as hematoma and delayed wound healing (Hood and Insall, 1983).

Experimentally, it has been shown that total joint replacement may impair local defence mechanisms and decrease the vitality of the surrounding soft tissues (Blomgren and Lindgren, 1980).

Charnley considered the source of infection to be exogenous, coming from the environment, and this was supported in a recent report by Lidwell et al (1982). Hematogenous spread of infection from a distant source has been shown to occur (Stinchfield et al, 1980).

The effect of ultraclean air in operating rooms on deep sepsis has been studied by Lidwell et al (1982). They have shown that combining an ultra-clean air ventilation system with whole body exhaust ventilation suits and prophylactic antibiotics significantly reduces the incidence of infection in both total hip and total knee replacement.

Hips

If we assume that throughout the world 1,000 total hip replacements are performed daily, with a minimum 1% infection rate, we can expect at least 2,500 infected hips per year (Elson, personal communication, 1978).

Infection may occur early (up to 1 month after operation) or delayed (more than 1 month after operation). Early infection is suspected by one or more of the following symptoms and signs:

a) wound pain and swelling;
b) purulent discharge from the wound;
c) fever;
d) dislocation of the prosthesis.

When infection is suspected, and when the radiograph shows that the prosthesis is not dislocated, the wound should be explored in the operating room and a thorough debridement performed. Gram stain, aerobic, anaerobic, mycobacterial and fungal cultures and sensitivities as well as a direct smear should be obtained from the surrounding fluid and the local soft tissues. Specimens should be inoculated into the appropriate broth and culture media before transport to the laboratory. The prosthesis should be left in place unless it is obviously loose or has been placed in a poor position leading to dislocation. The wound may be closed with suction drainage, or left open and secondary suture carried out a few days later.

If prophylactic antibiotics have not been used, a combination of cephalexin and gentamicin should be prescribed initially until the cultures and sensitivities are available from the laboratory. If antibiotics have been used, the culture may well be sterile and one is forced to treat the patient only on the basis of a strong suspicion of sepsis. If the response is favorable, antibiotics should be prescribed for a minimum of 4-6 weeks. During that period, adverse effects from the antibiotics should be monitored. The patient should not be given a lifetime of antibiotic therapy. The management of infected joint replacement, in both the early and late stages, is predominantly surgical combined with antibiotic therapy. One can never rely on antibiotics alone to control deep sepsis after joint replacement.

If the response is not favorable (ie, pain, profuse wound drainage, or prosthetic dislocation), excision arthroplasty should be offered to the patient, although refusal is likely. At this stage, one has to cope with an angry disappointed patient (and relatives) with possible medicolegal overtones. A second opinion is mandatory to satisfy the patient that excision arthroplasty is the best solution, and the blow can be softened by discussing the value of staged revision hip arthroplasty, once the infection has settled.

Overwhelming septicemia, endangering the life of the patient, is an absolute indication for removal of the prosthesis and cement at this stage.

The recognition of delayed infection rests on a combination of features: wound pain; occurrence of wound sinus; metastatic septicemia, especially in the rheumatoid patient.

It is extremely difficult to distinguish between sterile loosening and deep infection. All infected total joint replacements are not loose, but it should be assumed that every loose joint replacement is infected until proven otherwise.

A high index of suspicion should be aroused if patients have had an infection of the ipsilateral lower extremity, delayed primary wound healing or a postoperative hematoma. Radiographic abnormalities may include periostitis, gross evidence of loosening of the prosthetic-cement or cement-bone interface with extensive bone resorption or dislocation of the prosthesis.

Hip aspiration may be combined with an arthrogram at this stage. Positive needle aspiration varies from 66 to 90% (Dussualt et al, 1977; Patel et al, 1976; Tehranzadeh et al, 1981) and false positive results are frequent. Arthrography is useful in demonstrating abnormalities of the cement-bone interface, abscess cavities, bursae and sinus tracts that communicate with the joint. Negative arthrograms are of little significance.

Three-phase technetium 99m - labelled diphosphonates, gallium 67c citrate, and more recently indium-labelled leukocyte scintography have been reported to be of help in the diagnosis of late infections, but in the authors' opinion they have not been of much value.

If the patient is frail, the wound is dry or draining intermittently, and the pain is controlled by analgesics, the hip prosthesis should be left in situ and the patient reassessed and observed frequently. The risks of disarticulation and death from septicemia are low and can be ignored if the patient is relatively comfortable. If the patient has severe pain and the wound drainage is profuse and offensive, the entire prosthesis should be removed together with as much cement as is possible and practical. We feel that too much emphasis has been placed on bone cement rather than dead bone as a source of persistent wound drainage after excision arthroplasty.

Several alternatives are now available for the patient and the surgeon after excision arthroplasty of the hip.

1. One-stage revision with -

a) Palacos® with gentamicin cement (Buchholz et al, 1981; Elson, 1979).

b) Palacos with gentamicin together with parenteral antibiotics (Carlsson et al, 1978).

c) Conventional cement mixed with antibiotics (James et al, 1982).

2. Two-stage reimplantation -

a) after insertion of Septopal® beads (Hovelius and Joseffson, 1979). At six weeks, the beads may be removed and a second hip replaced using Palacos and gentamicin cement if the bone stock is healthy in the femur and the pelvis.

b) with conventional cement and parenteral antibiotics (Fitzgerald and Bryan, 1981). Two-stage revision does allow observation of the wound, better control of the infecting organisms with appropriate antibiotic therapy, and avoids an extremely long operation. It does, however, mean prolonged hospitalization and two operations for the patient.

3. Permanent excision arthroplasty with traction for six weeks. The wound may be allowed to granulate over or may be closed secondarily in a few days. The surgical technique of this procedure is comprehensively described (Clegg, 1977). The long-term results of excision arthroplasty improve with time (Bourne et al, 1984).

4. Excision arthroplasty combined with trochanteric arthroplasty (Salvati, 1983).

5. Excision arthoplasty followed by hip fusion. This procedure has been described by Kostuik (1983), who reported that 13 out of 14 hips fused. He recommended this procedure for the young patient.

6. Disarticulation (Fenelon et al, 1980). This is a rare alternative chosen only after multiple revisions for sepsis.

Decision making may be extremely difficult and may often be made only at the time of surgery. If the surgeon and the patient are not happy about revision, a trial of excision arthroplasty may be beneficial. If the patient wants a revision and understands the risks involved, the surgeon may remove the Septopal beads at six weeks and implant a new prosthesis. Successful revision depends on the age of the patient, the type of infection, the amount of bone loss, and whether or not there is a discharging sinus. Contraindications to revision surgery would be a persistently elevated erythrocyte sedimentation rate (ESR) in nonrheumatoid patients, a draining sinus, infection with gram-negative, anaerobic or mixed organisms, pelvic or femoral osteomyelitis, loss of bone stock including a recent fracture of the pelvis, and a frail elderly patient who is a poor risk for prolonged elective surgery. We feel happier reoperating on an older patient than a younger patient because of the possibility of further revision if the patient survives more than five years.

The risks involved in revision surgery must be explained to the patient. The number of local complications increases after revision surgery:

1. increased blood loss;
2. fracture of the femoral shaft or acetabulum;
3. dislocation of the prosthesis;
4. trochanteric problems;

5. nerve palsy;
6. increased incidence of deep sepsis.

The long-term results of revision hip arthroplasty for sepsis may be disappointing. To date, the main problems encountered are further loosening, reinfection and loss of bone stock. In the long term, the mechanical bonding can never be as good as the initial arthroplasty. This will lead to increasing radiolucent zones in the femoral shaft and acetabulum with further loosening due to the formation of a fibrous membrane and bone lysis. The risk of reinfection has been reported to be 17% after revision hip surgery for sepsis (James et al, 1982). Following failure, a second excision arthroplasty may be necessary, and with further bone loss, considerable shortening of the lower extremity will occur. Further revision or excision procedures are being increasingly reported after the first revision for sterile loosening or sepsis (Schurman, 1982; Weber, 1981).

Hunter (1982) estimated that if 100 patients with an infected hip replacement were reviewed a few years later, 10-15% of patients would have died, 70% would have the implant excised, and 10% of this group would require further surgery to control infection. The remaining 20% would have the hip implant still in situ but the clinical results would vary. At that time revision arthroplasty was not favored after sepsis, and it is interesting to report that in a multicentre trial reported by Lidwell et al (1982) revision procedures were carried out in less than 40% of the infected hip replacements. We await with interest the long-term results of revision arthroplasty of the hip after sepsis.

Knee

The presentation of early and delayed infection is similar. Infection rates vary from 1-2% (Locht and Hunter, 1983) to 15% (Jones et al, 1979). Perhaps a more realistic figure would be about 5%. Both the early and late infection rates following knee surgery are higher than those of hips (Hood and Insall, 1983).

Delay in wound healing is more likely to lead to infection in knee surgery due to the proximity of the skin incision to the implant (Jones et al, 1979). The type of prosthesis influences the incidence of infection. Reported incidences vary from 1% for surface replacement (Insall et al, 1979) to 12.4% (Arden, 1975) for the Shiers constrained type of prosthesis. When using ultraclean air, the infection rate differs little in patients with hip surgery compared with those after knee surgery (Lidwell et al, 1982). However, Salvati et al (1982) have demonstrated that a horizontal laminar air flow system reduces the infection rate in total hip replacements, but in total knee replacements the infection rate was increased, probably because during the surgery members of the surgical team will stand between the source of the air flow and the open wound.

Early infection

Early infection is usually not difficult to recognize provided its course is not marked by injudicious use of antibiotics. The presenting symptoms and signs are:

a) wound pain and swelling;
b) purulent wound drainage;
c) fever.

Any patient with pain for which no mechanical cause can be found should be suspected of having an infection (Insall, 1982). The white cell count and erythrocyte sedimentation rate (ESR) are usually raised. Aspiration of the knee with strict aseptic precautions should be performed. The aspirate should be sent to the laboratory for direct smear, Gram stain, aerobic, anaerobic, mycobacterial and fungal cultures and sensitivities. Specimens should be inoculated into the appropriate broth and culture media before transport to the laboratory. A high white cell count (25,000 polymorph leukocytes per 1,000,000) high protein and low glucose levels of the aspirated fluid are indicative of an infection. A diagnosis of infection may often not be made without resorting to open biopsy where specimens are taken for the above investigations and for tissue culture. A thorough debridement is recommended at this stage, leaving the prosthesis in situ and closing the wound over wide bore suction drains if the prosthesis is firmly cemented in the correct position.

If the patient is not receiving antibiotics, antibiotic therapy is started and then changed, if necessary, according to the sensitivity of the organisms. If the wound heals and the cultures are negative, antibiotic therapy should be continued for a minimum of four to six weeks. If the clinical course deteriorates, a definite decision on further management must be made, taking into consideration the general condition of the patient and the treatment modalities available. Prolonged antibiotic therapy is not recommended as it may complicate the problem by producing resistant strains, and it may make subsequent culture of the organisms difficult if revision surgery is contemplated.

Late infection

The symptoms and signs of infection may be difficult to distinguish from the symptoms of sterile loosening. There may be evidence of a primary infective focus, the commonest sites being an infected foot lesion, chest infection or urinary tract infection. The investigations are the same as already outlined. A positive culture may not be obtained from needle aspiration or arthrotomy. Infection at the cement-bone interface may only be detected at the time of removal of the prosthesis. It is imperative that if revision surgery is being contemplated, multiple cultures be obtained from around both components as it is not unusual to find more than one infecting organism. Factors to be considered in relation to the further management are the patient's general condition and the other joint involvement, the type of infection, amount of bone loss, type of implant used for the initial arthroplasty, the integrity of the surrounding skin and soft tissue sleeve, and the availability of multiple components of varying constraints including custom-made prostheses.

Attempts at retaining the prosthesis by debridement and suction irrigation have been reported. Petty et al (1975) reported on ten patients with early and late infection, with an average follow-up of 15 months following debridement, suction irrigation and systemic antibiotics. However, three of the ten knees had to be revised at an early stage due to loosening, fracture, or instability. Initially, eight patients were considered to have a good result at preliminary follow-up, but Broderson et al (1979) reported from the same institute that a formal arthrodesis had to be performed on all ten knees.

Woods et al (1983) reviewed 27 knees treated in a similar manner. Only three had retained the prosthesis and all had unsatisfactory results because of pain and continuous drainage. Sixteen knees had satisfactory formal arthrodesis. Two of the remaining eight fused spontaneously. The remaining six patients had unsatisfactory results.

Clearly, from the results of this treatment method, the chances of retaining a functional pain-free knee prosthesis after sepsis in the long term are negligible. With or without wound drainage, satisfactory retention of an implant is rare (Locht and Hunter, 1983), and the patient will usually require removal of the implant with as much cement as possible and practical. Following removal of the knee implant, the patient and the surgeon are faced with the following possibilities:

1. excision and early reimplantation (Rand and Bryan, 1983);
2. excision and delayed reimplantation (Insall et al, 1983);
3. excision and fusion with or without electrical stimulation (Bigliani et al, 1983);
4. excision without attempted fusion (Kaufer and Matthews, 1981);
5. amputation (Hunter and Arciszewski, 1984).

The results of revision will be presented later. The remainder of this review will concentrate on the results of alternative treatment methods.

Arthrodesis

Successful arthrodesis of an infected knee can be difficult to achieve and a stiff knee in full extension is a significant problem for a marginally ambulatory patient or a patient with polyarthropathy.

Hagemann (1974) reviewed 14 patients with failed total knee replacement. Solid fusion was obtained in only 64% compared with 95% of patients undergoing primary arthrodesis.

The type of prosthesis used for the initial arthroplasty is directly related to the success of the arthrodesis. Broderson et al (1979) have reported an 81% fusion rate following failure of a minimally or partially constrained prosthesis, compared with a 56% fusion rate in the failed hinged arthroplasty group. Similar observations were made by Stulberg (1982). Locht and Hunter (1983) reported on seven attempted fusions. Only four of these were successful, and all followed the use of minimally or partially constrained implants. In the series reported by Woods et al (1983), all but one infected knee fused on the first attempt. He recommends early bone grafting, preferably at three months, provided free of infection.

The indications for arthrodesis are a chronically infected total knee replacement with gram-negative or resistant organisms and a failed total knee replacement with inadequate soft tissue coverage (Thornhill et al, 1982).

Resection arthroplasty

Kaufer and Matthews (1981) reported on 17 knees in which the prosthesis-cement composite was removed and no attempt was made to obtain an arthrodesis. Twenty-three percent were nonambulatory. Eighteen percent required a brace or splint, and 25% could walk without external support. They suggest that resection arthroplasty is preferable to arthrodesis as an initial procedure to control sepsis. By today's standards, it would be more appropriate to use this procedure with a view to performing a delayed secondary reimplantation.

Amputation

Amputation following infected total knee replacement has not been given much attention. In 160 deep infections reported in the literature following total knee arthroplasty, amputation was carried out in 28 knees, an incidence of 17.5% (Hunter and Ardiszewski, 1984). Most of the implants were fully constrained arthroplasties of the spherocentric or hinged type. Although the chances of amputation being necessary after an uncomplicated total knee arthroplasty are less than 1%, the risk increases considerably when an infection develops and a revision procedure is performed using a hinged type prosthesis.

Summary

In infections complicating total joint replacement, antibiotics may suppress the symptoms of infection and may be used as a temporizing measure if surgery is contraindicated due to associated medical problems or if the patient refuses to consider further surgery. However, antibiotics alone are unlikely to cure the infectious process.

If an infection involving an implant is diagnosed, the ideal treatment is early, adequate, and prolonged antibiotic therapy combined with incision, drainage, debridement, and removal of the prosthesis. If revision hip and knee surgery is being contemplated, consideration should be given to the age of the patient, the state of the bone to be operated on, the type of organisms present and whether or not mechanical stability including firm fixation of components is possible to achieve.

Successfully revised joints do not perform as well as a good primary arthroplasty. Pain relief following revision is not comparable to initial arthroplasty. The range of movement and overall function is reduced and the incidence of local complications increases including infection. The need for early subsequent revisions is increasing.

Late infection is more common in knee replacements. Because the knee is a more superficial joint, skin healing may be difficult to obtain, particularly in cases of numerous previous incisions. The close proximity of the implant to the skin renders it more susceptible to pressure necrosis. Because the knee depends on its surrounding ligaments for constraint, revision with a nonconstrained prosthesis in the presence of gross instability may be impossible.

References

1. Arden, G.P.: Total replacement of the knee. J. Bone Joint Surg. 57B, 119, 1975.
2. Bigliani, L.U., Rosenwasser, M.P., Schink, C.W., and Bassett, C.A.L.: The use of pulsating electromagnetic fields to achieve arthrodesis of the knee following failed total knee arthroplasty. A preliminary report. J. Bone Joint Surg. 65A, 480, 1983.

3. Blomgren, G., and Lindgren, U.: The susceptibility of total joint replacement to hematogenous infection in the early post-operative period. An experimental study in the rabbit. Clin. Ortho. Rel. Res. 151, 308, 1980.

4. Bourne, R.B., Rorabeck, C.H., Hunter, G.A., and Macnab, J.: A 6 year follow-up of infected total hip replacement by resection arthroplasty. (In press)

5. Broderson, M.P., Fitzgerald, R.H. Jr., Peterson, L.F.A., Coventry, M.B. and Bryan, R.S.: Arthrodesis of the knee following failed total knee arthroplasty. J. Bone Joint Surg. 61A, 181, 1979.

6. Buchholz, H.W., Elson, R.A., Engelbrecht, E., Lodenkämper, H., Rotger, J., and Siegel, A.: Management of deep infection of total hip replacement. J. bone Joint Surg. 63B, 342, 1981.

7. Carlsson, A.S., Josefsson, G., and Lindberg, L.: Revision with gentamycin impregnated cement for deep infections in total hip arthroplasties. J. Bone Joint Surg. 60A, 1959, 1978.

8. Cherney, D.L. and Amstutz, H.C.: Total hip replacement in the previously septic hip. J. Bone Joint Surg. 65A, 1256, 1983.

9. Clegg, J.: The results of pseudarthrosis after removal of ain infected total hip prosthesis. J. Bone Joint Surg. 59B, 298, 1977.

10. Dussualt, R.G., Goldman, A.B., and Ghelman, B.: Radiological diagnosis of loosening and infection in hip prosthesis. J. Canad. Assoc. Radiol. 28, 119, 1977.

11. Editorial: Infections in rheumatoid disease. Brit.med.J. 2, 549, 1972.

12. Elson, R.A.: Personal communication, 1978.

13. Elson, R.A.: The management of deep infection involving joint implants. J. Bone Joint Surg. 61B, 118, 1979.

14. Fenelon, G.C.C., Von Foerster, G., and Engelbrecht, E.: Disarticulation of the hip as a result of failed arthroplasty. A series of 11 cases. J. Bone Joint Surg. 62B, 441, 1980.

15. Fitzgerald, R.H.Jr., Nolan, D.R., Ilstrup, D.M., Van Scoy, R.E., Washington, J.A., and Coventry, M.B.: Deep wound sepsis following total hip arthroplasty. J. Bone Joint Surg. 59A, 847, 1977.

16. Fitzgerald, R.H.Jr., and Bryan, R.S.: Indirect exchange of the infected hip implant. Course in Traumatic and Reconstructive Surgery of the Adult Hip at Harvard Medical School, Boston, September 1981.

17. Garner, R.W., Mowat, A.G., and Hazlemann, B.L.: Wound healing after operations on patients with rheumatoid arthritis. J. Bone Joint Surg. 55B, 134, 1973.

18. Hagemann, W.F., Woods, G.W., and Tullos, H.S.: Arthrodesis in failed total knee replacement. J. Bone Joint Surg. 60A, 790, 1978.

19. Hood, R.W., and Insall, J.N.: Infected total knee joint replacement arthroplasties. In, Evarts, C.W. (Ed.): Surgery of the Musculo-Skeletal System, Vol. 4. Churchill Livingstone, 1983, pp 173-188.

20. Hovelius, L. and Josefsson, G.: An alternative method for exchange operation of infected arthroplasty. Acta Orthop. Scand. 50, 93, 1979.

21. Hunter, G.A.: The natural history of the patient with an infected total hip replacement. In, Frankel, V.H. (Ed.): Instructional Course Lecture. American Academy of Orthopaedic Surgeons, Vol. XXXI. C.V. Mosby Co., 1982, pp. 38-41.

22. Hunter, G.A. and Arciszewski, C.: Amputation - A rare complication following infected total knee arthroplasty (in press).

23. Insall, J.N.: Infection in total knee arthroplasty. In, Frankel, V.H. (Ed.): Instructional Course Lecture. American Academy of Orthopaedic Surgeons, Vol. XXXI. C.V. Mosby Co., 1982, pp 42-48.

24. Insall, J.N., Scott, W.N., and Ranawat, C.S.: The total condylar knee prosthesis. A report on 220 cases. J. Bone Joint Surg. 61A, 173, 1979.

25. Insall, J.N., Thompson, F.M., and Brause, B.D.: Two-stage re-implantation for the salvage of infected total knee arthroplasty. J. Bone Joint Surg. 65A, 1087, 1983.

26. James, E.T.R., Hunter, G.A., and Cameron, H.U.: Total hip revision arthroplasty. Does sepsis influence the results? Clin. Orthop. Rel. Res. 170, 88, 1982.

27. Jones, E.C., Insall, J.N., Inglis, A.E., and Ranawat, C.S.: Guepar knee arthroplasty results and late complications. Clin. Orthop. Rel. Res. 140, 145, 1979.

28. Karas, S.E., Gebhardt, E.M., Kenzora, J.E., and Thornhill, T.S.: Total hip arthroplasty for osteonecrosis following renal transplantation. Presented at the American Academy of Orthopaedic Surgeons, Atlanta 1984.

29. Kaufer, H., and Matthews, L.S.: Resection Arthroplasty: An alternative to arthrodesis for salvage of infected total knee arthroplasty. Orthop. Transactions 5, 413, 1981.

30. Kostuik, J.P.: Hip arthrodesis for failed hip arthoplasty. Orthop. Transactions 7, 388, 1983.

31. Lidwell, O.M., Lowbury, E.J.L., Whyte, W., Blowers, R., Stanley, S.T., and Lowe, D.: Effect of ultraclean air in operating rooms on deep sepsis in the joint after total hip or knee replacement. A randomized study. Brit.med.J. 285, 10, 1982.

32. Locht, R.C. and Hunter, G.A.: Deep sepsis after cemented total knee replacement. Infections in Surgery. 1983, pp 219-224.

33. Menon, T.J. and Wroblewski, B.M.: Charnley low-friction arthroplasty in patients with psoriasis. Clin. Orthop. Rel. Res. 176, 127, 1983.

34. Murray, W.R.: Treatment of the established deep wound infection after total hip arthroplasty: A report on 65 cases. In, Leach, Hoaglund, Riseborough (Eds.): Controversies in Orthopaedic Surgery. W.B. Saunders, 1982. pp 382-398.

35. Patel, D., Karchmer, A., and Harris, W.H.: Role of pre-operative aspiration of the hip prior to total hip replacement. In, Proc., 4th Open Scientific Meeting of the Hip Society, St. Louis. C.V. Mosby Co. 1976, pp 219-223.

36. Petty, W., Bryan, R.S., Coventry, M.B., and Peterson, L.F.A.: Infection after total knee arthroplasty. Orthop. Clin. North Am. 6, 1005, 1975.

37. Rand, J.A. and Bryan, R.S.: Re-Implantation for the salvage of an infected total knee arthroplasty. J. Bone Joint Surg. 65A, 1081, 1983.

38. Salvati, E.A.: Infected total hip replacement. In, Evarts, C.W. (Ed.) Surgery of the Musculo-Skeletal System. Vol. 4. Churchill Livingstone 1983, pp. 153-172.

39. Salvati, E.A., Robinson, R.P., and Zeno, S.M.: Infection rates after 3175 total hip and knee replacements performed with and without a horizontal unidirectional filtered air-flow system. J. Bone Joint Surg. 64A, 525, 1982.

40. Schurman, D.J.: Personal communication, 1982.

41. Stinchfield, F.E., Bigliani, L.W., Neu, H.C., Goss, T.P., and Foster, C.R.: Late hematogenous infection of total joint replacement. J. Bone Joint Surg. 62A, 1345, 1980.

42. Stulberg, S.D.: Arthrodesis in failed total knee replacement. Orthop. Clin. North Am. 13, 213, 1982.

43. Tehranzadeh, J., Schnider, R., and Freiberger, R.H.: Radiological evaluation of painful total hip replacement. Radiol. 141, 355, 1981.

44. Thornhill, T.S., Dalziel, R.E., and Sledge, C.B.: Alternatives to arthrodesis for the failed total knee arthroplasty. Clin. Orthop. Rel. Res. 170, 131, 1982.

45. Van Niekerk, A., and Charnley, J.: Post-operative infection of the Charnley low-friction arthroplasty of the hip. J. Bone Joint Surg. 61B, 252, 1979.

46. Weber, B.G.: Total hip replacement revision surgery: Surgical technique and experience. In, The Hip. Proc. 9th Open Scientific Meeting of The Hip Society. C.V. Mosby, 1981, pp 3-14.

47. Woods, G.W., Lionberger, D.R., and Tullos, H.S.: Failed total knee arthroplasty: Revision and arthrodesis for infection and noninfectious complications. Clin. Orthop. Rel. Res. 173, 184, 1983.

48. Wroblewski, B.M. and Del Sal, H.J.: Urethral instrumentation and deep sepsis in total hip replacement. Clin. Orthop. Rel. Res. 146, 209, 1980.

Joint Replacement Infections: Prophylaxis, Diagnosis and Treatment

E. A. SALVATI

Introduction

The widespread use of total joint replacements has brought the problem of ensuing sepsis to the fore. In contrast to the highly successful outcome of such surgery without complications, the development of deep infection almost always leads to pain and septic loosening, generally requiring extensive surgery. Removal causes large skeletal defects, extremity shortening, and marked disability (Fig. 1a, 1b).

The cost of hospital care for such patients is extremely high. Based on our own experience, the cost of hospitalization averages about $30,000, ie, four times the cost of the primary prosthetic joint replacement. A reasonably conservative estimate of the current incidence of deep infection is between 1% and 2%. Approximately 100,000 total hip and 40,000 total knee replacements are performed annually in the United States. Thus, roughly 1400 to 2800 infections occur per year in hip and knee replacement surgery at an approximate cost of 42 to 84 million dollars for hospitalization alone.

Prophylaxis

Clean air

The incidence of infection can be reduced by prophylactic measures. Sir John Charnley reduced exogenous surgical wound contamination by means of an enclosure, unidirectional airflow, ultrafiltered air, rapid air changes, ultrafine fabrics for clothing and draping, and air exhaust systems for the surgical team (Charnley, 1979).

We have studied the effect of clean air at The Hospital for Special Surgery. The air flowing over the wounds of patients undergoing surgery in the enclosure with horizontal unidirectional filtered airflow was shown to be five-fold cleaner bacteriologically than without airflow. Moreover, within the enclosure, wound culturing before closure showed significantly less contamination when horizontal unidirectional filtered airflow was used. Coagulase-negative staphylococci were most frequently isolated from incisions, surgical field, and air flowing over the wound (Aglietti et al, 1974).

In 1982, a comprehensive study was published on the efficacy of ultraclean air (Lidwell et al, 1982). In a multicenter, randomized, prospective study of sepsis over a seven-year period after more than 8,000 total hip or knee replacements, Lidwell et al demonstrated that the infection rate

Current Concepts of Infections in
Orthopaedic Surgery

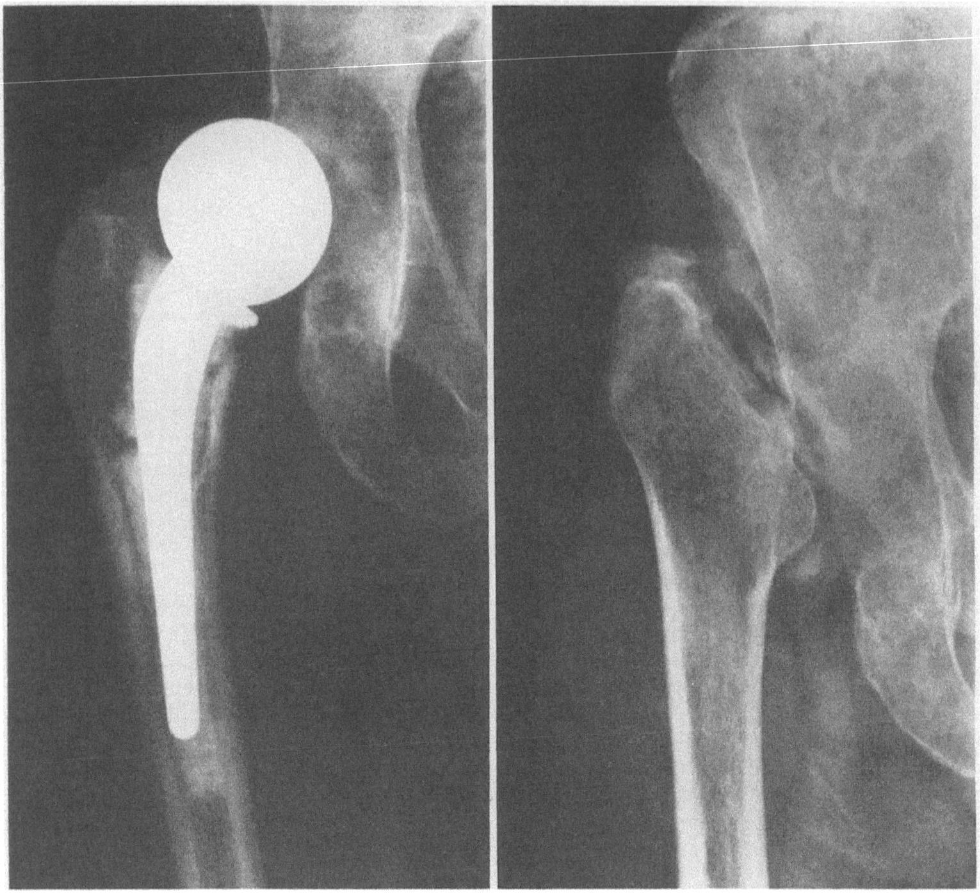

a b

Fig. 1. a) Radiograph of an infected cemented bipolar implant with subluxation. b) Radiograph after removal of prosthetic components and acrylic cement

in ultraclean air systems was about one-half of that encountered in conventional operating rooms. Furthermore, when whole body exhaust-ventilated suits had been worn in the theater ventilated by an ultraclean air system, the incidence of spesis was about one-quarter of that found in conventional operating rooms. A significant reduction of infections was also observed in patients who received antibiotics prophylactically (Lidwell et al, 1982).

However, a study performed by us in 1982 at The Hospital for Special Surgery demonstrated that horizontal laminar airflow may produce either beneficial or adverse effects, depending on whether the surgical procedure can be performed in accordance with the theory of operation of the airflow system. We demonstrated a significant reduction of infections in total hip replacements, whereas in total knee replacements the infection rate was increased. This was probably due to the fact that the surgical team must stand between the source of the horizontal laminar airflow and the open wound. As surgeons did not use whole body-exhaust ventilated suits, they were probably shedding their own microbes onto the open wound during total knee replacement (Salvati et al, 1982).

Antibiotics

Our own experience and that of others has definitely shown that antibiotics administered prophylactically are highly efficacious. At The Hospital for Special Surgery, a prophylactic program of antibiotic treatment was instituted in December 1969 because our early experience with total hip replacement had been associated with a high incidence of infection, particularly of the latent deep type (Wilson et al, 1972). As most of these infections were due to gram-positive organisms, particularly coagulase-negative *Staphylococcus epidermidis*, a semisynthetic penicillin, oxacillin, was selected to control beta-lactamase-producing organisms. In patients allergic to penicillin (delayed reactions), intravenous cefazolin was administered. So far, we have not encountered any significant difficulty due to cross-sensitivity. Cefazolin is also preferred in patients with a history of urinary tract infection or requiring catheterization. Of all the first generation cephalosporins, cefazolin reaches a higher serum peak and has the longest half-life (1.8 hours); since its renal clearance is slower and it is more highly bound to serum proteins, it can be administered at a lower dosage of q 8 h (Schurman et al, 1978).

A prospective, double-blind, randomized, placebo-controlled study performed on 2137 total hip arthroplasties demonstrated that cefazolin significantly reduced the infection rate from 3.3% to 0.9% (Hill et al, 1981). The reduction of infection, however, was not statistically significant in patients whose operations were performed in ultraclean operating rooms.

Extensive experimental and clinical investigations have shown that the prophylactic short-term use of bactericidal antibiotics in clean surgery lowers the infection rate. In a literature survey, Sandusky has reported a reduced infection rate in over 30 studies using prophylactic antibiotics; he recommends their routine use before implant procedures (Sandusky, 1980).

By means of a dermal model, Burke (1961) was able to show the most effective time to administer antibiotics prophylactically. His work showed that antibiotics, to be effective, must reach adequate tissue concentrations before microbial invasion, thereby preventing exponential microbial growth and allowing the host to eradicate the infection.

The pharmacokinetics of these antibiotics require their administration one hour preoperatively. They should be discontinued after 24 to 48 hours when the drainage tubes and intravenous lines are removed (Wiggins et al 1978).

Bone penetration by antibiotics

High serum levels of bactericidal antimicrobial agents also penetrate bone by readily traversing capillary membranes. Bone levels of most antibiotics approximate 10-30% of serum levels.

Antimicrobial dosage regimens for bone infections are usually calculated to produce bactericidal serum concentrations several multiples higher than the minimal inhibitory concentrations. It has been a comforting clinical axiom that a bactericidal serum titer of 1:8 constitutes effective antimicrobial therapy for osteomyelitis although no data have yet been published substantiating this assertion (Coleman et al, 1982).

Antibiotic penetration of joints, synovia and hematoma.

Most antimicrobial agents easily diffuse into infected joint spaces. Bactericidal levels in synovial fluid have a linear relationship to bactericidal serum activity. In synovial fluid, antibiotic levels are substantially higher in infected joints than in noninfected joints (Parker and Schmid, 1971). Antibiotics administered intravenously penetrate hematomas up to four days after their formation, depending on their size. Larger hematomas may not have demonstrable antibiotic concentrations (Wilson et al, 1971).

Local antibiotics

As antimicrobial agents diffuse readily into infected joints, it is not necessary to administer intra-articular antibiotic therapy for the standard treatment of septic arthritis.

Intra-articular antibiotics can be irritants to the synovium, inducing a severe chemical synovitis. In addition, intra-articularly administered antibiotics are readily absorbed systemically which can result in high toxic serum levels. Moreover, intra-articular administration may predispose to contamination and superinfection in the involved joint. These problems may also arise postoperatively when antibiotics are used in irrigation tubes.

The rapid microbial penetration into deep wound foci appears to defeat the purpose of surface therapy. Recent studies have shown that antibiotic solutions failed to eradicate microbes from wounds even when irrigation was begun one minute after contamination (Petty, 1979).

Surgical technique

The importance of meticulous, gentle surgical technique cannot be overemphasized. Good aseptic technique is absolutely essential and requires strict discipline by the surgical team. The following precautionary measures are crucial in the reduction of infection risks:

1) Surgical time should be kept to a minimum without jeopardizing the quality of surgery.
2) Gentle tissue handling: a) maintenance of moist tissue surfaces by repeated irrigation and antibiotic-soaked sponges; b) avoidance of tissue-crushing clamps, rough or excessive retraction, unnecessary use of electrocautery; c) frequent lavage to remove clots and tissue particles (we find the water pik most helpful).
3) Careful hemostasis and suction drainage to avoid hematoma.
4) Meticulous closure to obliterate dead space (but without excessive tension).

Diagnosis

During the last two decades, great improvements have been made in prosthetic design, materials, cementation, and surgical techniques of total joint replacement. These factors have been reflected in good to excellent results reported in over 90% of patients (Charnley, 1979).

Persistent symptoms after total joint replacement in the absence of a clear mechanical explanation should alert the surgeon to the possibility of infection. While diagnosing severe infections based on local and constitutional symptoms poses no particular problem, latent infections can manifest themselves mainly by joint pain with mild or no systemic symptoms. The wound may look benign, and the usual laboratory tests and radiologic findings may not be decisive, including white blood cell count, differential left shift, and erythrocyte sedimentation rate.

Metastatic or hematogenous infections can produce acute and severe symptoms resembling early deep infections despite their late onset. Some patients may suffer from preceding infections at sites remote from the prosthetic joint such as skin ulcers, lungs, gastrointestinal and genitourinary tract, or teeth. In these cases, a transient bacteremia most likely seeds the prosthetic joint (Blomgren and Lindgren, 1983). Thus, before performing a joint replacement, the patients should be carefully searched for foci of infection and, if present, these should be treated. After joint replacement, patients must be instructed to seek immediate medical advice if infections develop.

Plain radiographs, studied serially, are a most informative method of evaluation, particularly when obtained with standardized position and technique. The original postoperative radiographs provide the baseline for future comparison with radiographs obtained at yearly intervals (O'Neil and Harris, 1984).

Joint aspiration

The recommended procedure to establish the presence of infection is a joint aspiration performed under strict antiseptic precautions, preferably under fluoroscopic control. The patient should not have had antibiotic treatment within the last few weeks. The fluid aspirated has to be sent immediately to the bacteriology laboratory for direct smear, Gram stain, aerobic, anaerobic, mycobacterial and fungal cultures and sensitivities. To increase bacterial growth, the aspirate should be inoculated as soon as possible into the appropriate broth and culture medium. We favor the use of a culture medium that supports the organisms during the time of transport. We believe that so-called "sterile infections" (a contradictory term) are due to difficulty in culturing fastidious and anaerobic types of organsims. Occasionally, organisms cannot be isolated despite all precautions and repeated aspirations.

If enough fluid is aspirated, a complete cell count and differential WBC may also give valuable information. If the complete count shows more than 25,000 leukocytes/mL and the differential count reveals that more than 25% are polymorphonuclear cells, infection should be suspected. Obviously, the higher the number of polymorphonuclear leukocytes the greater the possibility of infection. Fluid should also be analyzed for glucose and protein levels. In the normal synovial fluid, protein levels are about one-third those of serum levels, while in infection they approach serum levels. Glucose values in synovial fluid are similar to those of plasma. In the presence of infection, synovial glucose levels are lower due to the presence of organisms and cells which utilize sugar for their metabolism. Thus, a low glucose and a high protein level are suggestive of infection.

Elevated lactic acid assays in synovial fluid are useful in the diagnosis of septic arthritis, and of particular diagnostic value in patients in whom antibiotic therapy was started before joint aspiration. Sequential measurements can be helpful in assessing the response of septic arthritis to treatment (Riordan et al, 1982). We are currently studying lactic acid levels in the diagnosis of infected prosthetic replacements.

Arthrography

Having confirmed intra-articular position of the needle, arthrography can demonstrate loosening of prosthetic components, abscessess, bursae, etc (Salvati et al, 1971; 1974). The communication of sinus tracts with the intra-articular space may be better demonstrated by arthrography than by sinogram.* However, false negative arthrograms can be observed despite radiographic evidence of loosening. This is due to the presence of granulation tissue at the bone cement interface preventing penetration of the contrast agent. When abscesses are present, the contrast agent tends to collect at these sites and does not penetrate at the bone cement interface (Fig. 2). Injection of a larger quantity of contrast agent could outline the loosening, but in infection the increased pressure is contraindicated as it can cause septicemia.

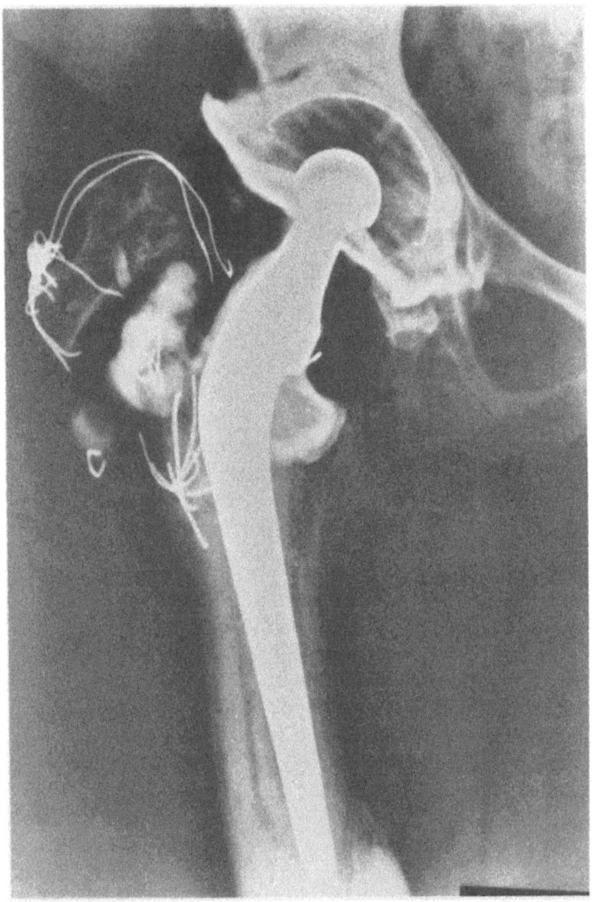

Fig. 2. Arthrogram of an infected total hip replacement. Despite evidence of acetabular loosening, the contrast agent does not outline it, as it collects in the trochanteric nonunion. The intra-articular hip aspirate of this joint was negative. Once the arthrogram depicted the abscess at the trochanteric nonunion, a needle was introduced into this site, obtaining a positive aspirate from which organisms were cultured

---

* Cultures obtained from draining sinuses are unreliable as they frequently grow mixed flora and not necessarily the main pathogen causing the deep periprosthetic infection.

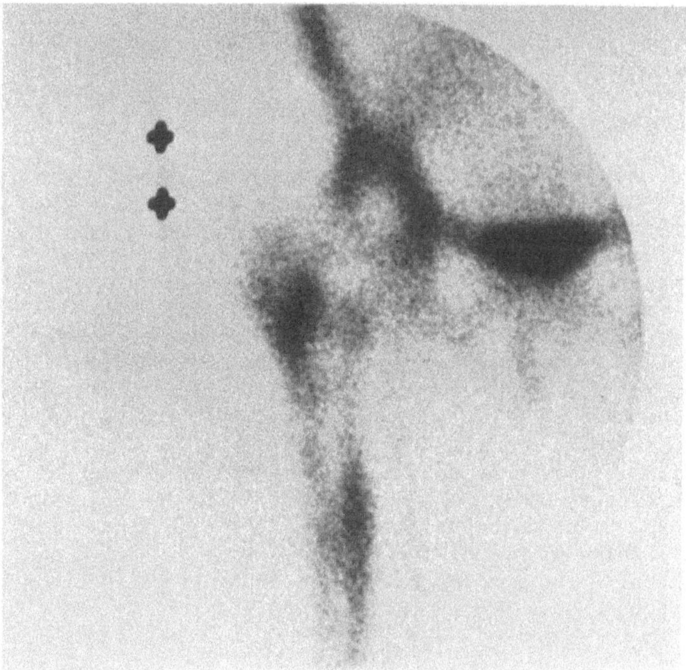

a

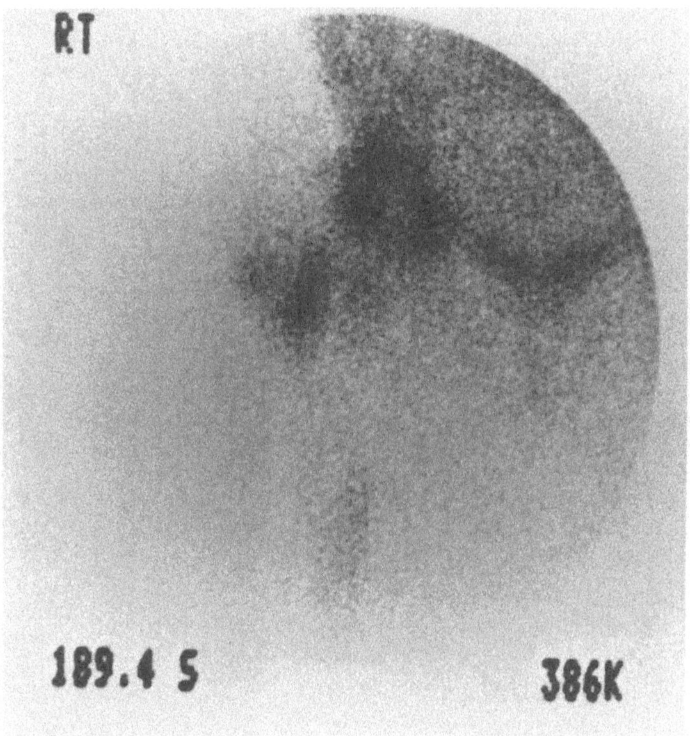

b

Fig. 3. Gallium scan of an infected total hip replacement. a) Increased uptake is observed at 24 hours, and b) persists even after 72 hours

A negative culture following aspiration in which fluid was obtained should exclude the possibility of infection, provided adequate bacteriologic techniques were used without delay.

Radioactive isotope scanning

The use of bone scanning has been advocated to aid in the diagnosis of the painful endoprosthesis. Combined technetium and gallium scanning has been reported as an accurate and reliable method of demonstrating infection (Rushton et al, 1983). Technetium^{99} diphosphonate is believed to be absorbed into the hydroxyapatite crystal of bone and its uptake is proportional to the degree of vascularity and rate of bone remodeling. Its uptake is usually increased in the presence of mechanical loosening or infection, while gallium^{67} uptake is increased in the presence of infection due to its affinity to polymorphonuclear leukocytes (Fig. 3a, 3b). It has been also helpful in evaluating osteomyelitis (Deysine et al, 1975).

"Three-phase" bone scan in infection demonstrates increased uptake on the early vascular phase and diffuse uptake around the components in the static phase (Maurer et al, 1981). The leukocyte scan in which the patient's polymorphonuclear cells are labeled with indium^{111} appears to be sensitive and specific in the diagnosis of infection (Merkel et al, 1984; Propst-Proctor et al, 1982). A negative bone scan should rule out the possibility of infection.

Biopsy and reoperation

If the diagnosis is still unclear once all this information is gathered, and if the clinical suspicion of infection is strong, a biopsy might be indicated, either open or closed with needle, trocar or with arthroscopic techniques. However, in most instances we have established the final diagnosis at the time or reoperation. Antibiotics should not be given before surgery to maximize the chances of isolating and identifying the infecting organism. Antibiotics are given intravenously as soon as several cultures have been obtained from joint fluid and suspicious tissue specimens. At the time of surgery, frozen tissue sections will give a good idea of the severity of the inflammation. More than five polymorphonucleocytes per high power field in the tissues, excluding those found in fibrin, is generally considered a reliable indication of infection. Repeated Gram staining cultures of joint fluid, and several tissue specimens, the macroscopic appearance of the wound, and histopathologic findings (demonstrating inflammatory granulation tissue) should provide diagnostic and definitive bacteriologic information.

Treatment

The management of the infected endoprosthesis at The Hospital for Special Surgery is based on the time and mode of presentation, virulence, infecting organism, antibiotic sensitivity, the patient's clinical status, and the condition of the hip.

Early infections are treated by immediate incision, debridement, and primary closure over closed suction irrigation (for 2-3 days only). In these early infections, the bone cement interface is most likely still intact, not yet invaded by sepsis. If recognized early, with adequate surgery there is a chance of salvaging the prosthetic arthroplasty, particularly if the microbe is highly sensitive to antibiotic therapy.

Late, open, and acute purulent infections are being treated by thorough debridement, including removal of all foreign material and primary closure over closed tube suction irrigation. In severely inflamed cases, we use open packing, followed a few days later by delayed primary closure over closed suction irrigation. In these patients, reconstruction considerations are secondary to controlling the infection. Although, occasionally, primary torchanteric reconstructions are being performed, simple resection followed by skeletal traction for three to four weeks have predominated (Bourne et al, 1984) (Fig. 1a, 1b).

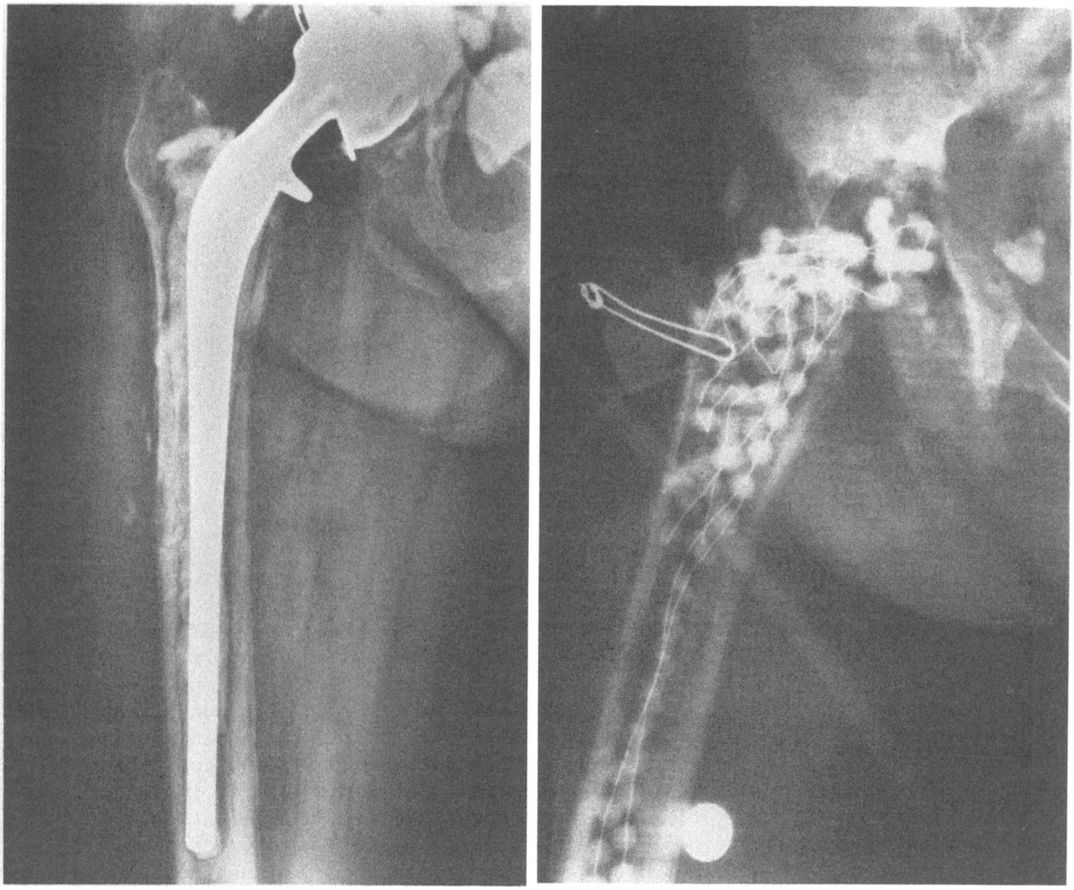

a b

Fig. 4. a) Radiograph of a septic loosening following a long-stem total hip replacement, with a deficient medial acetabular wall and a mass of intrapelvic cement. b) Radiograph after removal of prosthetic components and acrylic cement, and implantation of gentamicin impreganted beads. c) Reimplantation performed six weeks after removal of prosthetic components and acrylic cement. An autogenous bone graft was used to cover the medial acetabular defect, supplemented by an acetabular ring fixed with screws to the ilium. Gentamicin-impregnated acrylic cement was used to cement both components

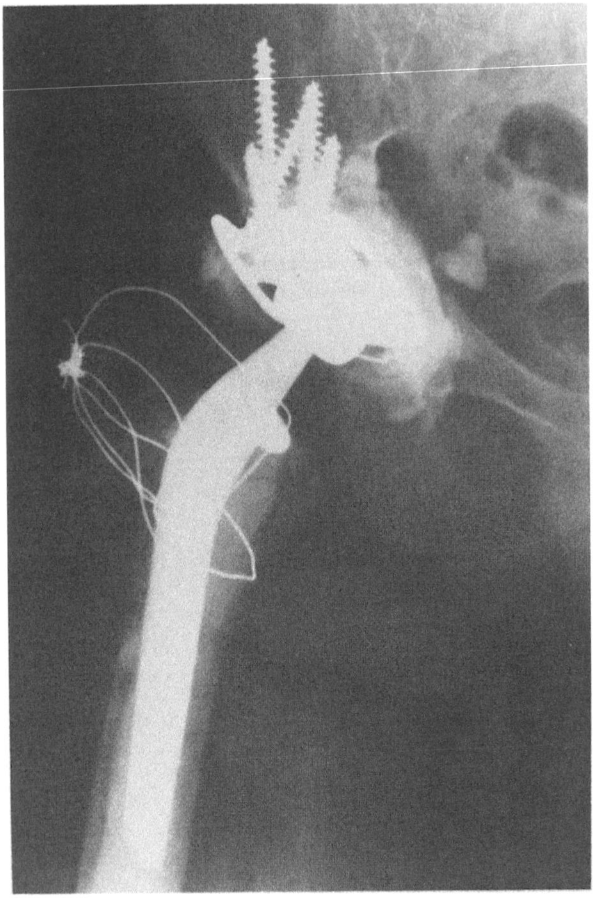

Fig. 4c

Late, closed subacute infections are also treated by extensive debridement, removal of all foreign material, followed by a second total hip replacement at the same stage or, preferably, at a second stage after a minimum interval of six weeks. During this period, under the supervision of a consultant from Infectious Diseases, intravenous antibiotic therapy is administered for six weeks, aiming for at least 1:8 peak bactericidal serum concentrations. Inability to obtain 1:8 peak bactericidal serum levels, immunodeficiency, frailty of the patient, limited potential for rehabilitation, poor soft tissues, and severe bone loss precluding an adequate biomechanical reconstruction, are considered contraindications for reimplantation. Careful preoperative planning before reimplantation to obtain a stable and adequate reconstruction is essential. Special prosthetic components and sophisticated techniques of revision surgery are frequently necessary (Fig. 4a, 4b, 4c).

Bactericidal oral antibiotic (suppressive) therapy may enable prosthesis retention when surgery is contraindicated in the old patient, provided the infection is at an early stage, with no systemic manifestations nor prosthetic loosening, and the causative microbe is avirulent and sensitive to oral antibiotic therapy. These prerequisites are rarely all present and, thus, suppressive antibiotic therapy is infrequently used by us.

The appearance of resistant micröorganisms is posing an increasing challenge; *S. epidermidis* resistant to the semisynthetic penicillins is being identified occasionally (fortunately they are still sensitive to vancomycin). Recently, some strains of both *Staphylococcus aureus* and *S. epidermidis* have been tolerant, a new form of resistance, generally occurring when the difference is large between the minimal inhibitory concentration (MIC) and the minimal bactericidal concentration (MBC).

References

1. Aglietti, P., Salvati, E.A., Wilson, P.D. Jr., and Kutner, L.J.: Effect of surgical unidirectional filtered air-flow unit on wound bacterial contamination and wound healing. Clin. Orthop. 101, 99,1974.
2. Blomgren, G.,and Lindgren, V.: In, Elson, R.A. (Ed.): Revision Arthroplasty 2. Proc. Symposium held in Harrogate, England, March 2-4, 1983. Franklin Scientific Publications, 1983, pp 46-49.
3. Bourne, R.B., Hunter, G.A., Rorabeck, C.H., and Macnab, J.J.: A six year follow-up of infected total hip replacements managed by Girdlestone's arthroplasty. J. Bone Joint Surg. 66B, 340, 1984.
4. Burke, J.: The effective period of preventative antibiotic action in experimental incisions and dermal lesions. Surgery 161, July 1961.
5. Charnley, J.: Low-friction Arthroplasty of the Hip: Theory and Practice. Springer-Verlag, 1979.
6. Coleman, D.L., Horwitz, R.I., and Andriole, V.T.: Association between serum inhibitory and bactericidal concentration and therapeutic outcome in bacterial endocarditis. Am. J. Med. 73, 260, 1982.
7. Deysine, M., Rafkin, H., Russell, R., Teicher, I., and Aufses, A.H. Jr.: The detection of acute experimental osteomyelitis with 67 ga. citrate scannings. Surg. Gynec. Obstet. 141A, 40, 1975.
8. Hill, C., Mazas, F., Flamant, R., and Evrard, J.: Prophylactic cefazolin versus placebo in total hip replacement. Lancet i, 795, 1981.
9. Lidwell, O.M., Lowbury, E.J.L., Whyte, W., Blowers, R., Stanley, S.J. and Lowe, D.: Effect of ultraclean air in operating rooms on deep sepsis in the joint after total hip or total knee replacement: A randomized study. Brit. Med. J. 285, 10, 1982.
10. Maurer, A.H., Chen, D.C.P., Camargo, E.E., Wong, D.F., Wagner, H.N., Jr., and Alderson, P.O.: Utility of three-phase skeletal scintigraphy in suspected osteomyelitis: Concise communication. J. Nucl. Med. 22, 941, 1981.
11. Merkel, K.D., Fitzgerald, R.H., Jr., and Brown, M.L.: Scintiographic examination of total hip arthroplasty: Comparison of indium with gallium-technetium in the loose and infected canine arthroplasty. The Frank Stinchfield Award Paper. The Hip Society, Twelfth Open Scientific Meeting, Feb. 8, 1984, Atlanta, Georgia.
12. O'Neil, D.A., and Harris, W.H.: Failed total hip replacement: Assessment by plain radiographs, arthrogram, and aspiration of the hip joint. J. Bone Joint Surg. 66A, 540, 1984.
13. Parker, R.H., and Schmid, F.R.: Antibacterial activity of synovial fluid during therapy for septic arthrits. Arthrit. Rheum. 14, 96, 1971.

14. Petty, W.: Quantitative determination of the effect of antimicrobial irrigating solutions on bacterial contamination of experimental wound. Trans. Twenty-Fifth Annual Meeting, Orthopaedic Research Society 4, 9, 1979.

15. Propst-Proctor, S.L., Dillingham, M.F., McDougall, I.R., and Goodwin, D.: The white blood cell scan in orthopaedics. Clin. Orthop. 168, 157 1982.

16. Riordan, T., Doyle, D., and Tabaqchali, S.: Synovial fluid lactic acid measurement in the diagnosis and management of septic arthritis. J. Clin. Pathol. 35, 390, 1982.

17. Rushton, N., Coakley, A.J., Tudor, J. and Wraight, E.P.: The value of technetium and gallium scanning in assessing pain after total hip replacement. J. Bone Joint Surg. 64B, 313, 1983.

18. Salvati, E.A., Freiberger, R.H., and Wilson, P.D., Jr.: Arthrography for complication of total hip replacement. J. Bone Joint Surg. 53A, 701, 1971.

19. Salvati, E.A., Ghelman, B., McLaren, T., and Wilson, P.D., Jr.: Subtraction technique in arthrography for loosening of total hip replacement fixed with radiopaque cement. Clin. Orthop. 101, 105, 1974.

20. Salvati, E.A., Robinson, R.P., Zeno, S.M., Koslin, B.L., Brause, B.D., and Wilson, P.D., Jr.: Infection rates after 3175 total hip and total knee replacements performed with and without a horizontal unidirection filtered air-flow system. J. Bone Joint Surg. 64A, 525, 1982.

21. Sandusky, W.R.: Use of prophylactic antibiotics in surgical patients. Surg. Clin. North Am. 60, 83, 1980.

22. Schurman, D.J., Hirshman, H.P., Kajiyama, G., Moser, K., and Burton, D.S.: Cefazolin concentrations in bone and synovial fluid. J. Bone Joint Surg. 60A, 359, 1978.

23. Wiggins, C.E., Nelson, C.L., Clarke, R., and Thompson, C.H.: Concentration of antibiotics in normal bone after intravenous injection. J. Bone Joint Surg. 60A, 93, 1978.

24. Wilson, F.C., Worchester, N.N., Coleman, P.D., and Byrd, W.E.: Antibiotic penetration of experimental bone hematomas. J. Bone Joint Surg. 53A, 1622, 1971.

25. Wilson, P.D., Jr., Amstutz, H.C., Czerniecki, A., Salvati, E.A., and Mendes, D.G.: Total hip replacement with fixation by acrylic cement: A preliminary study of 100 consecutive McKee-Farrar prosthetic replace ments. J. Bone Joint Surg. 54A, 207, 1972.

Prevention of Infection in Total Hip Replacement

H. W. BUCHHOLZ

In 1970, I published the early results of our total hip replacements with a minimum two year follow-up. The infection rate recorded in this paper was highly underestimated at an overall 1% in 1,352 patients (Buchholz, 1970). Subsequently, the deep infection rate rose to about 7%. During this time we were administering perioperatively systemic antibiotics. I was aware that Charnley (1969) had experienced the same problem with his hip replacements and as a result had developed the clean-air enclosure. Because of the heavy work load of general and traumatic surgery with which we had to cope, this method was not possible at our hospital and it was partly for this reason that the concept was developed of adding an antibiotic to the cement. It was recognized that any special measure to combat deep infections would be worthless unless other more general aspects of the aseptic ritual were rigidly observed. This we attempted in an average conventional operating theatre. It was our impression that hematoma formation, aggravated by the necessity to use prophylactic anticoagulation, contributed to our rising infection rate.

Charnley pursued the clean-air technique and did not use systemic antibiotics. Likewise, as we became more confident in the antibiotic-loaded cement and were anxious to assess its value apart from other methods, we did not use systemic antibiotics. It is perfectly clear from other reports that prophylactic systemic antibiotics are beneficial for both deep and superficial infections. It should also be borne in mind that in the past some investigators had even suggested that the prophylactic use of antibiotics could actually increase the incidence of infections. Thus, I cannot speak authoritatively about the effects of systemic antibiotics and only present the results of the prophylactic use of gentamicin-Palacos® cement used in a conventional operating room of average good quality.

During our early work in 1970, we happened to be using Palacos cement and it was for this reason, almost by chance, that our first experiments were performed with this particular cement. Subsequent comparisons with other cements (Wahlig and Dingeldein, 1980) have shown that most antibiotics elute at higher concentrations for longer periods from Palacos than from other brands. This is due to differences in chemical properties. All the cements are of roughly equal mechanical quality.

At first, penicillin and erythromycin were chosen. These antibiotics led to a definite improvement of deep infection rates and no deleterious effects were observed. Nevertheless, with respect to allergy, I had confidence in the safety of gentamicin whereas I was not so sure about penicillin.

Current Concepts of Infections in
Orthopaedic Surgery

The ideal antibiotic for prophylactic purposes should possess the following qualities:

1) adequate elution quantitatively and timewise;
2) broad-spectrum activity against gram-positive and gram-negative organisms common in bone diseases;
3) the minimal bactericidal and minimal inhibitory concentrations should be similar;
4) a low rate of resistance development;
5) low protein binding;
6) low sensitizing potential;
7) high water solubility;
8) overall chemical stability (especially against heat)
9) a low allergenic potential.

Many antibiotics have been tested against several kinds of cement. There is no doubt that the aminoglycosides are most appropriate, and of these gentamicin was chosen. In the beginning, we were conscious of the dangers of its toxic properties but numerous tests thereafter have shown that blood levels are never dangerously high and in many thousands of joint replacement operations, no toxicity or adverse effects have been observed. To my knowledge, no report of such complication has ever been published.

We hoped that the long-lasting elution of gentamicin could protect the field from late hematogenous contamination. There is no doubt that tissue concentrations of gentamicin can be detected years after the operation (Wahlig et al, 1984). These concentrations are variable and in some instances cannot be measured. They vary from place to place in the same surgical field, and presumably some areas of cement can become exhausted before others depending on the extent of exposed surface. Undoubtedly, hematogenous infections do occur and late infections may arise from the hematogenous route or originate at the perioperative period. Animal studies, while confirming the efficacy of gentamicin-Palacos in controlling infections from an artificial contaminated wound, have not substantiated protection against late hematogenous contamination (Blomgren, 1981).

Results of Prophylaxis

Between 1968 and 1975, a total of 4,697 hip replacements were performed. The results of these hip arthroplasties with respect to the onset of subsequent deep infection are shown in Table I. Obviously, a number of these patients died, but if they were examined not less than three years from the time of operation and found to have no evidence of deep infection, they were included in the series. Otherwise the histories and examinations of the patients are up-to-date, the follow-up having been completed in 1983. It should be emphasized that this is a relatively long-term assessment in a significant series of patients. The incidence of superficial infections has not been included. During the whole period under study, the same technique was used under conventional operating room conditions, the same surgical team performing the operations.

Table I shows that Group A comprises joint replacements performed during 1968 and 1969 when no antibiotic was added to the cement but prophylactic systemic antibiotics were used. In 1970 and 1971, in Group B patients, erythromycin or penicillin mixed with cement was used. From 1972 to 1975, in Group C operations, gentamicin, 1/2 g, was added to the Palacos cement (40 g of powdered polymer). Table II is a breakdown of each year according to the diagnosis for which operations were performed. A study of these figures reveals that the incidence of infections was higher in secondary osteoarthritis (trauma, old infection, or previous surgery) and rheumatoid disease than in primary osteoarthritis.

Table I. Deep infection in 4,697 total hip arthroplasties (THR) (1968-1975)

		A	B	C
Primary osteoarthritis THR		627	1,096	845
Secondary osteoarthritis THR		363	524	704
Rheumatoid arthritis THR		164	268	106
Total number of	operations:	1,154	1,888	1,655
	infections:	71	68	27
	%:	6.1	3.4	1.6

Group A: (1968-1969) - Plain Palacos cement
Group B: (1970-1971) - 1 mega penicillin or
0.5 g erythromycin-loaded Palacos cement
Group C: (1972-1975) - 0.5 g gentamicin-loaded Palacos cement

Table II. Deep infection in total hip arthroplasty (THR) performed 1968 to 1975 at the St. Georg Hospital, Hamburg. Follow-up completed December 1983

Type of THR	1968	1969	1970	1971	1972	1973	1974	1975
Primary osteoarthritis								
Number of operations	295	332	564	532	304	188	177	173
Deep infections (%)	7.5	6.6	4.4	3.2	1.3	1.0	1.7	0.6
Secondary osteoarthritis								
Number of operations	127	236	281	303	179	212	171	142
Deep infections (%)	2.4	3.8	5.7	1.6	2.2	0.5	0.6	4.9
Rheumatic disease								
Number of operations	67	97	113	95	26	31	31	18
Deep infections (%)	6.0	11.3	2.6	2.1	7.7	3.2	3.2	0.0
Total:								
Number of operations	489	665	958	930	512	431	379	333
Number of deep infections	29	42	44	24	10	4	5	8
%	5.9	6.3	4.6	2.6	1.9	0.9	1.3	2.4

1968/69 plain cement
1970/71 erythromycin or penicillin in cement
Since 1972 0.5 g gentamicin-loaded Palacos cement

Throughout, there is a reduction in infection rate following the use of gentamicin-loaded Palacos cement. This decrease is particularly satisfactory for primary osteoarthritis in which an infection rate of approximately 1% has been achieved. The late infection rates for secondary osteoarthritis and rheumatic disease vary somewhat and are particularly poor for the former in 1975. These variabilities are difficult to explain.

In an appraisal of this declining infection rate, which we attribute to gentamicin-Palacos cement, the same problems arise as were faced by Charnley in the assessment of the clean-air enclosure. These relate to progressive improvements in technique and general surgical expertise. I suspect, for example, that our tissue care and wound closure improved. Nevertheless, there were no gross changes that we could identify, and I believe that the figures are valid. The generally long follow-up period is important. Most deep infections are diagnosed during the first two years postoperatively but thereafter the hazard of hematogenous contamination persists, and while it appears to be relatively infrequent considering the number of occasions when bacteremia can occur, specific cases certainly exist. Even a long time after an operation, a proportion of late deep infections are associated with perioperative contamination.

Of the deep infections that have occurred after the use of gentamicin-Palacos cement, about one-half were due to organisms sensitive to some degree to gentamicin. Of those following hematogenous spread, most were gentamicin-resistant organisms.

In conclusion, I submit that the use of an appropriate antibiotic-loaded acrylic cement bears no risks in any way and that it contributes significantly to a reduced incidence of deep infections. Clean air operating environment and systemic antibiotics are also effective. There is no question of competition between these measures and each has its part to play in the prevention of infection, the most serious complication of joint replacement surgery. I emphasize again the importance of a long-term assessment of deep infection rates which will probably show in most instances an average of about 2%.

References

1. Blomgren, G.: Haematogenous infection of total joint replacement. Acta Orthop. Scand. 52, 187, 1981.
2. Buchholz, H.W.: Modification of the Charnley artificial hip joint. Clin. Orthop. 72, 69, 1970.
3. Charnley, J.: Total prosthetic replacement of the hip. Reconstr. Surg. Traumat. 11, 9, 1969.
4. Wahlig, H., and Dingeldein, E.: Antibiotics and bone cements. Acta Orthop. Scand. 51, 49, 1980.
5. Wahlig, H., Dingeldein, E., Buchholz, H.W., Buchholz, M., and Bachman, F.: Pharmacokinetic study of gentamicin-loaded cement in total hip replacements. Comparative effects of varying dosage. J. Bone Joint Surg. 66B, 175, 1984.

Prophylactic Effect of Gentamicin Cement

L. LINDBERG

We have known for some time from the work of Professor H.W. Buchholz in Hamburg, Germany and his coworkers that gentamicin-containing bone cement has a prophylactic effect against postoperative infections in total joint replacement surgery (Buchholz and Engelbrecht, 1970; Röttger et al, 1979). It is not possible, however, to draw definite conclusions about the prophylactic effect of gentamicin-containing cement based on the above mentioned investigations since they were not controlled. Therefore, to investigate the prophylactic effects of the gentamicin-containing cement in greater detail, a large-scale study was started in Sweden in 1976 (Josefsson et al, 1981). This study was undertaken by the Departments of Orthopaedic Surgery at nine Swedish hospitals to enlarge the patient population sufficiently for an evaluable assessment. It was a prospective, controlled study, completed in 1979. The purpose of this investigation was to compare the generally accepted prophylactic effect of systemic antibiotics with gentamicin cement whose prophylactic effects were, at that time, somewhat questionable.

All operations were performed in conventional operation theatres. The operations were randomly assigned to two groups of patients -- one operated with plain cement and administered systemic antibiotics for prophylaxis, and a second group was operated with gentamicin-containing cement without any additional antibiotic therapy. Systemic antibiotic prophylaxis was already a routine procedure in all nine hospitals before the investigation. For practical purposes, each hospital continued its own routine and systemic prophylaxis was therefore not a completely uniform measure in all of the nine centres. It is, however, important to point out that antibiotic prophylaxis in all centres was started before the operation, and administered for 7 to 14 days, the times differing among hospitals.

The series consisted of 1,685 consecutively operated total hip replacements in 1,596 patients. After a dropout of 52 patients, the final number was 812 total hips in the antibiotic group and 821 in the gentamicin cement group. The patients were examined 3, 6 and 12 months after the operation, consisting of a clinical examination, radiograms, and erythrocyte sedimentation rate determinations. Each problem patient in whom an infection was suspected was seen by one particular surgeon to render the assessment more uniform. All patients have been regularly followed since the start of this investigation.

Results

Table I shows the results of the infection rate after a follow-up of from 1 - 3½ years.

Current Concepts of Infections in
Orthopaedic Surgery

Table I. Infection rates following use of gentamicin cement

	Antibiotic group		Gentamicin cement group
Total number of total hip replacements	812		821
Superficial infections	49 (6.0%)	$p < 0.05$	71 (8.7%)
Deep infections	13 (1.6%)	$p < 0.01$	3 (0.4%)

In the group of 812 total hip replacements that had received systemic antibiotics 49 superficial infections (6.0%) were encountered. In the gentamicin cement group, 71 (8.7%) occurred. The superficial infections thus seem to be more common in the gentamicin cement group than in the antibiotic group. The explanation might be that the cement obtains an insufficient antibiotic concentration in the superficial part of the wound. It is impor tant to point out, however, that all these superficial infections have healed without any further problems. Of the deep infections, however, 13 (1.6%) were found in the antibiotic group in contrast to only three (0.4%) in the gentamicin cement group. This difference is statistically significant (p =<0.01). A second review of the patients with a minimum observation time of five years is now going on and the preliminary results point in the same direction.

No side effects of the gentamicin cement have yet been observed. In Sweden we have data on several thousand patients and in Germany over ten thousand reports exist. The serum and urine concentrations of gentamicin achieved with the cement are so low and of such short duration that no toxic effects are expected (Lindberg, 1982; Nelson and Bergman, 1984). Allergic reactions have not yet been reported. They may occur if other antibiotics except gentamicin are mixed with the cement. Development of bacteriologi resistance has not yet been observed in Sweden. This risk appears to be minimal but must naturally not be overlooked.

Our conclusion is that the prophylactic effect of the gentamicin cement against deep infection in total hip arthroplasties is at least as good as that of systemic antibiotics and has fewer side effects. This conclusion is certainly universally applicable and based not only on the results of Swedish investigations but also supported by the results of many other investigators (Elson, 1979; Röttger et al., 1979 ; Thierse, 1979; Wannske and Tscherne, 1979).

References

1. Buchholz, H.W., and Engelbrecht, E.: Über die Depotwirkung einiger Antibiotika bei Vermischung mit dem Kunstharz Palacos. Chirurg 41, 511, 1970.

2. Elson, R.A.: Prophylaktische Verwendung von Gentamicin-Palacos in Northern General Hospital, Sheffield, England. In, Burri, C., and

Rüter, A. (editors): Aktuelle Probleme in Chirurgie und Orthopädie. Lokalbehandlung Chirurgischer Infektionen, Verlag Hans Huber, Bern. 12, 206, 1979.

3. Josefsson, G., Lindberg, L., and Wiklander, B.: Systemic antibiotics and gentamicin-containing bone cement in the prophylaxis of postoperative infection in total hip replacement. Clin. Orthop. 159, 194, 1981.

4. Lindberg, L.: Infection and antibiotics in relation to bone cement. In, Williams, D.F. (editor): Biocompatibility of Orthopaedic Implants. Vol. II, pp 25-47. CRC Press, Boca Raton, FLA, 1982.

5. Nelson, C.L., and Bergman, B.R.: Antibiotic-impregnated acrylic composites. In, Eftekhar, N. (editor): Infection in total joint replacement. pp 267-280. C.V. Mosby Company, St. Louis-Toronto-London, 1984.

6. Röttger, J., Buchholz, H.W., Engelbrecht, E., and Siegel, A.: Ergebnisse beim Prothesenwechsel unter Verwendung von Refobacin-Palacos in Hamburg. In, Burri, C., and Rüter, A. (editors): Aktuelle Probleme in Chirurgie und Orthopädie, Lokalbehandlung Chirurgischer Infektionen, Verlag Hans Huber, Bern. 12, 211, 1979.

7. Thierse, L.: Erfahrungen mit Refobacin-Palacos im Hinblick auf die tiefen Spätinfektionen nach Hüftendoprothesenoperationen. Z. Orthop. 116, 847, 1979.

8. Wannske, M., and Tscherne, H.: Ergebnisse prophylaktischer Anwendung von Refobacin-Palacos bei der Implantation von Endoprothesen des Hüftgelenkes in Hannover, Aktuel Probl. Chir. Orthop. 12, 210, 1979.

Open Fractures - Is Primary Stabilization Desirable?

M. TILE, C. B. BEAUCHAMP, and J. F. KELLAM

Introduction

Treatment of the open fracture has undergone a considerable change in the past decade, related in no small measure to improved techniques of internal and external fixation. More skill is required by the orthopedic surgeon in the management of an open fracture than in most of his other endeavors, especially skill in decision making. Mindless dogma has no place in the management of such a fracture, only careful logical thinking.

Union of the fracture is not the primary aim of fracture care, but function of the extremity. Significant loss of function of the extremity is unacceptable despite fracture union. Once function has been restored to the extremity union may be obtained secondarily, maintaining the functional status of the limb. Therefore, the complications of delayed or nonunion can be easily managed provided the limb has maintained satisfactory function. The reverse, however, is not true; that is, once function is lost in a joint, it is extremely difficult to regain by secondary reconstructive procedures and physiotherapy.

Most fractures may be managed by closed means, but there are specific indications for open reduction and internal fixation to improve the final functional result. These indications are listed below:

Indications for open reduction and internal fixation:

1. Displaced intra-articular fractures.
2. Metaphyseal compression fractures with axial malalignment (lower extremity).
3. Select diaphyseal fractures.

   a) *The forearm* - Displaced fractures of the forearm require anatomic reduction, stable internal fixation, and early motion for optimal results. It is generally agreed that almost all fractures of the forearm in adults are best treated by open reduction (Anderson et al, 1975; Tile and Petri, 1970).

   b) *The femur* - Although femoral fractures can be managed in skeletal traction, most of the recent literature supports the use of intramedullary nailing as optimal treatment to restore early full function to the extremity (Hansen and Winquist, 1979). As has been clearly demonstrated, internal fixation of a femoral fracture in a polytraumatized patient is beneficial to both the fracture and the patient.

Current Concepts of Infections in
Orthopaedic Surgery

c) *The tibia* - Although most tibial fractures may be managed nonsurgically, specific indications for tibial stabilization include:

i) fractures into either the ankle or knee joint,
ii) fractures with neurovascular injuries,
iii) inability to maintain length or reduction of the fracture,
iv) fractures associated with compartment syndromes,
v) unstable segmental fractures.

d) *The humerus* - The humerus is rarely an indication for surgical stabilization. However, in our Trauma Unit, humeral fractures associated with severe chest trauma are stabilized internally to facilitate chest care of the patient. The results have been uniformly excellent (Bell and McMurtry, 1984).

4. Miscellaneous indications
   a) the polytraumatized patient
   b) the polytraumatized limb
   c) vascular injury
   d) medical indications -- eg, hip fractures.

What about the open fracture -- should it also be stabilized? Orthopedic opinion has been undecided on this issue. Therefore, the issue is yet another example of cyclic orthopedics. Stabilization of open fractures has had periods when it was recommended; during other periods this technique was considered heretical -- for example, during the Vietnam War. At the present time, this method is again in favor. To answer the above question, it is important to look at the natural history of the open fracture.

Natural History of Open Fracture

The natural history of an open fracture depends on many factors:

1) the patient and his injury -- the age and medical state of the patient, and the degree of violence that caused the fracture;
2) the limb -- its vascular and neurologic state;
3) the fracture itself -- its anatomic location, whether it involves a joint, its degree of instability, displacement, and comminution

are all important in the natural history.

Therefore, it is important to carefully define the personality of the specific injury before treatment. Nicol, in 1964, described 705 tibial fractures of which 144 were open. He classified these tibial fractures into different personality types depending on the nature of the jury. The open fractures caused by high energy had 34% delayed union, 14% infection, and 60% significant functional disability, compared with the good personality types which were closed injuries, low energy, spiral, with an insignificant functional disability rate treated by closed means.

This paper, describing the various personality types of tibial fractures, contains an accurate account of the natural history of these injuries. Most reports on the care of open fracture without surgical stabilization do not comment on function. They comment only on union and sepsis, with infection rates usually between 6 and 10%. Treatment is often prolonged; therefore, function of adjacent joints and the limb may be compromised, as noted in Figure 1. To improve function, surgical stabilization of some open fractures is therefore indicated.

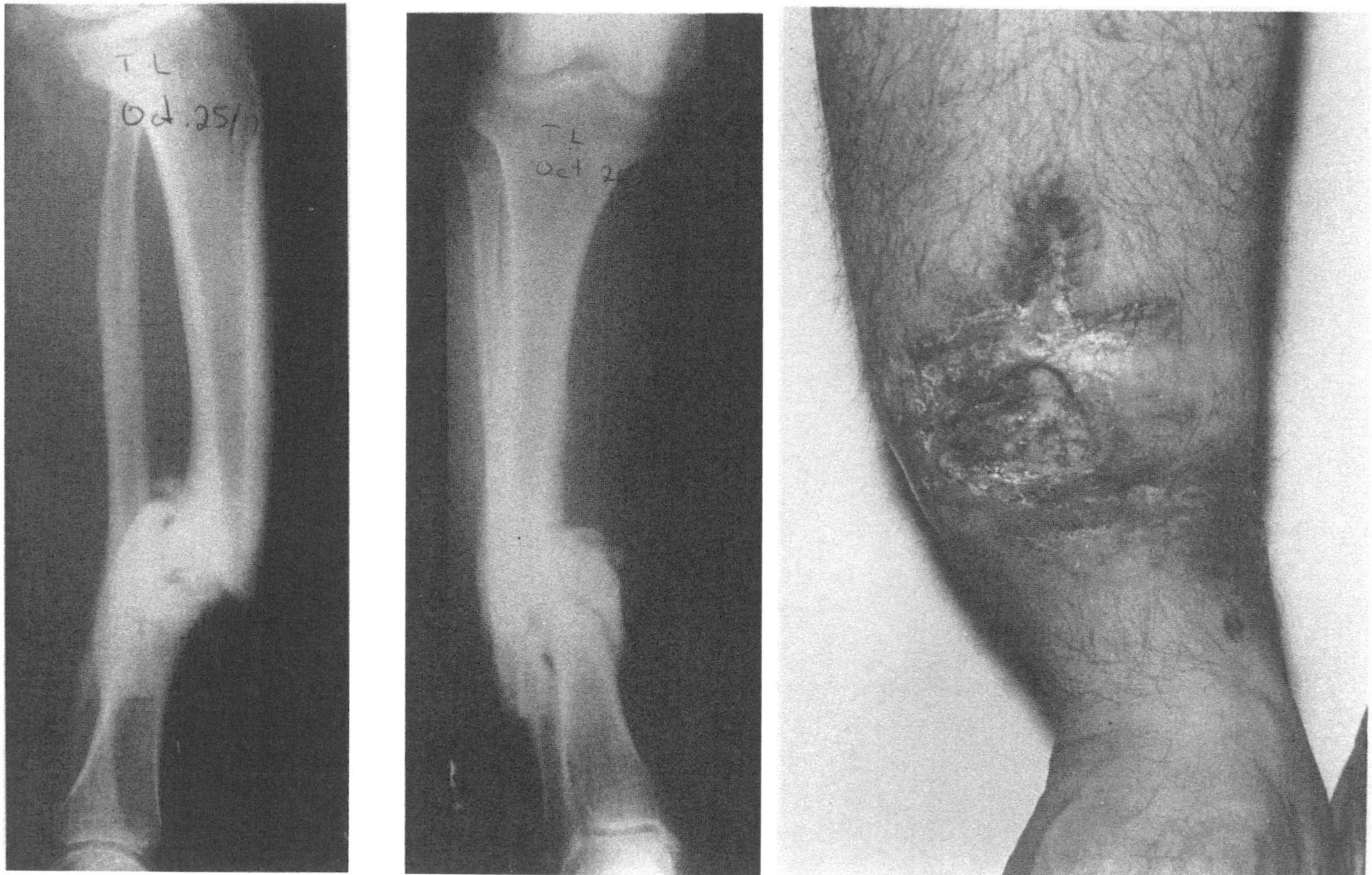

a b c

Fig. 1. a,b Lateral and anteroposterior radiographs of a 21 year old man 2 years following an open fracture of the tibia and fibula in a motorcycle accident. Original treatment consisted of debridement, plaster cast fixation and early weight bearing. The fracture failed to heal, became septic, and required several bone grafting procedures, all of which failed. c Indicates the condition of the skin and the extremity at this time

Management of The Open Fracture

Decision making

In practice, when confronted with an open fracture, two situations may be encountered: 1) an open reduction and internal fixation of the fracture may definitely be indicated; or 2) the indication may not be firm.

Displaced intra-articular fractures, fractures of the forearm, reimplantation (the ultimate open fracture) are all firm indications for open reduction and internal fixation. Therefore, in this group of patients, primary surgical stabilization is indicated, whether the fracture is open or closed. There would be little argument that the ankle fracture in Figure 2 requires open reduction and internal fixation for an optimum functional result.

The patients without a definite indication for surgical stabilization may be managed by closed means. However, experience gained with open reduction and surgical stabilization in other types of injury allows us to look beyond this statement to improve the function of some of these patients.

General principles of management

The general principles in the management of open fractures are widely accepted. These include:

a) *Cleansing the wound* - a careful cleansing of the wound is performed with copious amounts of solution.

b) *Debridement* - a careful debridement of all devitalized tissue and foreign bodies is essential.

c) *Antitetanus prophylaxis and antibiotics* - while the use of antibiotics is still a controversial issue in many centres, most surgeons favor the use of a broad-spectrum antibiotic (cephalosporin) in contaminated areas.

The controversial aspects in the management of open fractures concern the most effective methods of managing the skeletal injury and the soft tissue.

Management of the bony injury

We believe that surgical stabilization of the bone in open fractures is desirable to rest the soft tissues, to reduce the patient's pain, and to allow early restoration of limb function. The form of fixation, that is internal versus external, depends on a careful assessment of the injury. The surgeon must choose the most effective form of stabilization for the situation at hand.

Open reduction and internal fixation are indicated for injuries involving the articular cartilage, for fractures of the metaphysis with bone loss and axial malalignment, for some diaphyseal fractures and reimplantations (Fig. 3). In general, we do not favor internal fixation with plates in open tibia fractures with massive soft tissue involvement. In that situation, external fixation is a better choice. External fixation is indicated in severely comminuted fractures of the midshaft of the tibia, with or without bone loss and with major soft tissue involvement. External fixation of the femur may be used under similar circumstances but usually only as a temporary fixation.

Combined external fixation with minimal internal fixation is effective in some patients. Interfragmental compression with screws may be used to fix a short oblique fracture, whereas the fracture may be neutralized with an external fixation device.

Also, when internal fixation is being carried out, careful preoperative planning is essential. Where possible, major implants, such as plates, should be buried under muscle layers, so that if the wound is left open, the metal is covered by adequate soft tissue.

Management of the soft tissues

Wound management will depend on whether there is only a skin laceration with no skin loss, whether there is skin loss, skin and muscle loss, or skin, muscle and bone loss, and whether a vascular injury is superimposed.

Postoperatively, open care of the wound is favored since this is generally the safest course; therefore, wound closure should be dealt with as a secondary procedure. The wound is left open with a wetting solution to protect the soft tissues.

Some recent reports (Patzakis et al, 1983) indicate that in the absence of skin or soft tissue loss, and when the wound is not grossly contaminated, primary skin closure will not increase the incidence of infection. However, the safest route is to leave the wound open.

Secondary management of the wound depends on the condition of the soft tissues. When no skin loss has occurred, direct closure by steri-strips or sutures is indicated provided the wound is clean and granulating, usually on the fifth postoperative day.

If there has been some skin loss but no underlying soft tissue loss, a split thickness skin graft is indicated when the wound is granulating, again usually on the fifth to tenth day.

In patients with major soft tissue loss, the use of various flaps is indicated. These include local or regional flaps and, especially in the tibia, the gastrocnemius flap. The latter allows excellent coverage of the bone surface, brings local blood supply to the bone, and should be performed early when the wound is clean and granulating.

Finally, free flaps of a composite nature may be indicated for major bone loss in rare situations. Most often, bone loss may be managed with an autogenous bone graft.

Ongoing care

It is important to stress to the patient that the first operation of an open fracture is only the beginning, not the final treatment. Aggressive early care is essential, which includes further debridement of the wound, early bone grafting, and early skin coverage. Therefore, the patient may require multiple anesthetics and procedures in the early period.

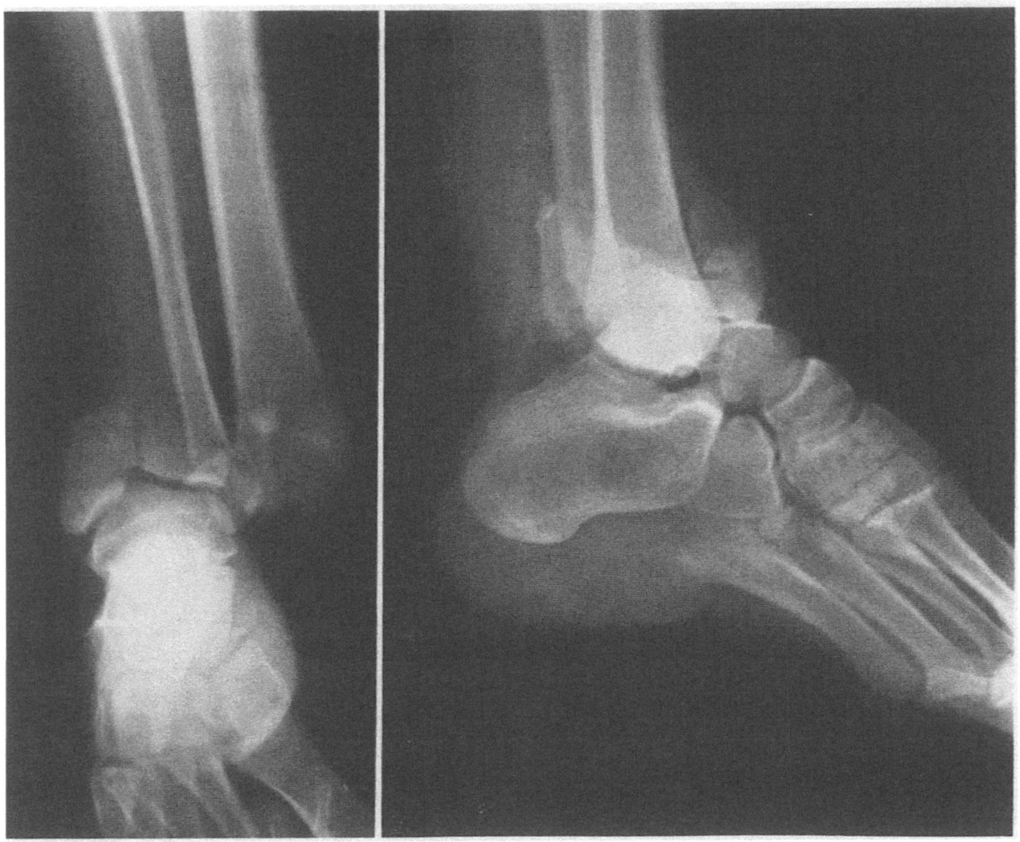

Fig. 2. a) Anteroposterior radiographs and b) lateral radiographs of an 18 year old boy injured in a motor vehicle accident. c) The bone is protruding through the medial skin incision, the missing medial malleolus hidden posteriorly in the wound. The neuromuscular structures and the tibialis posterior tendon were impacted between the tibia and fibula. The joint was thoroughly cleansed, debrided, the neurovascular structures reduced, and the ankle internally fixed as seen in d) the anteroposterior and e) lateral radiographs. The reduction was anatomic. The wound was left open and closed secondarily at 5 days with a good result

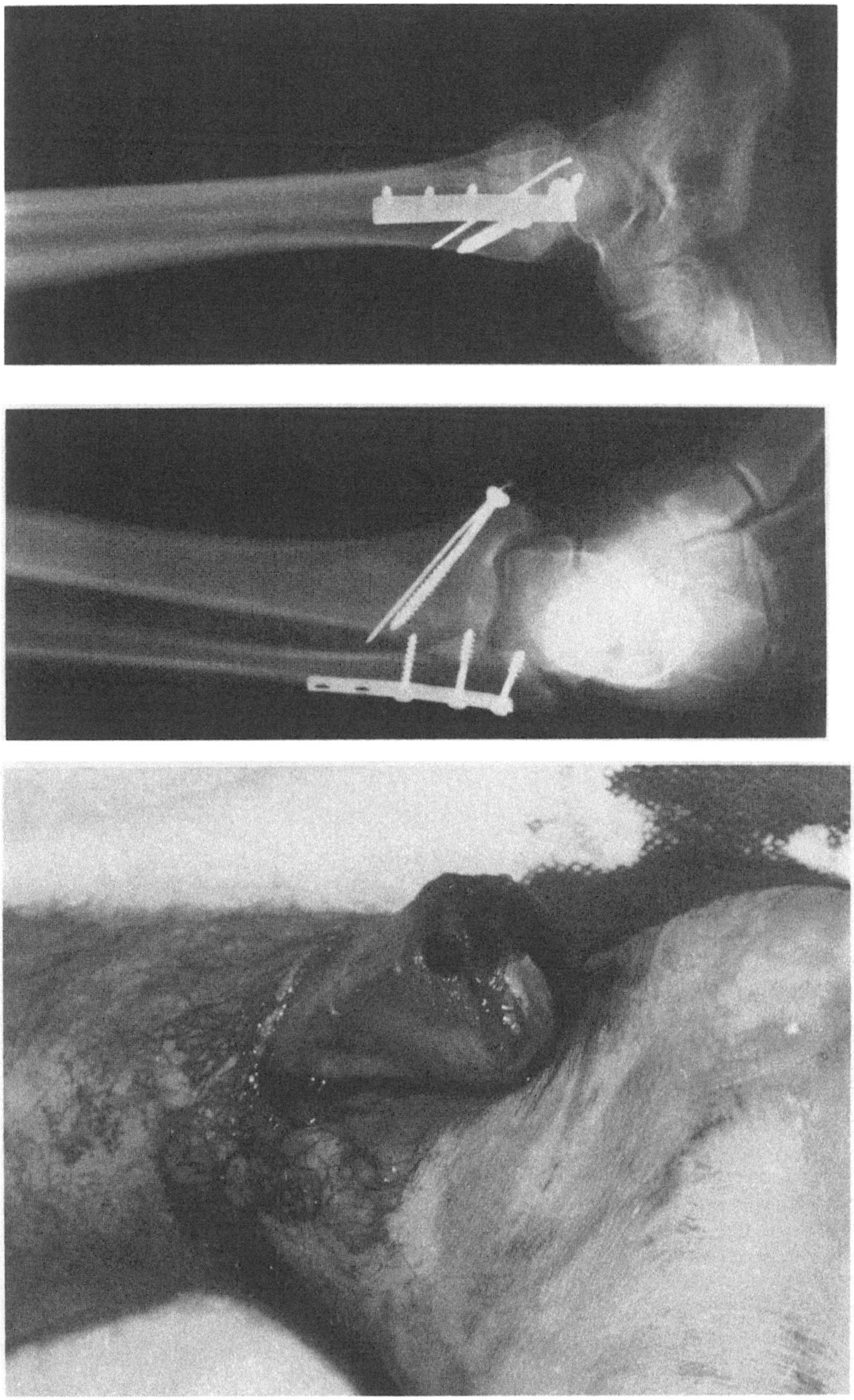

c d e

Fig. 2c-e

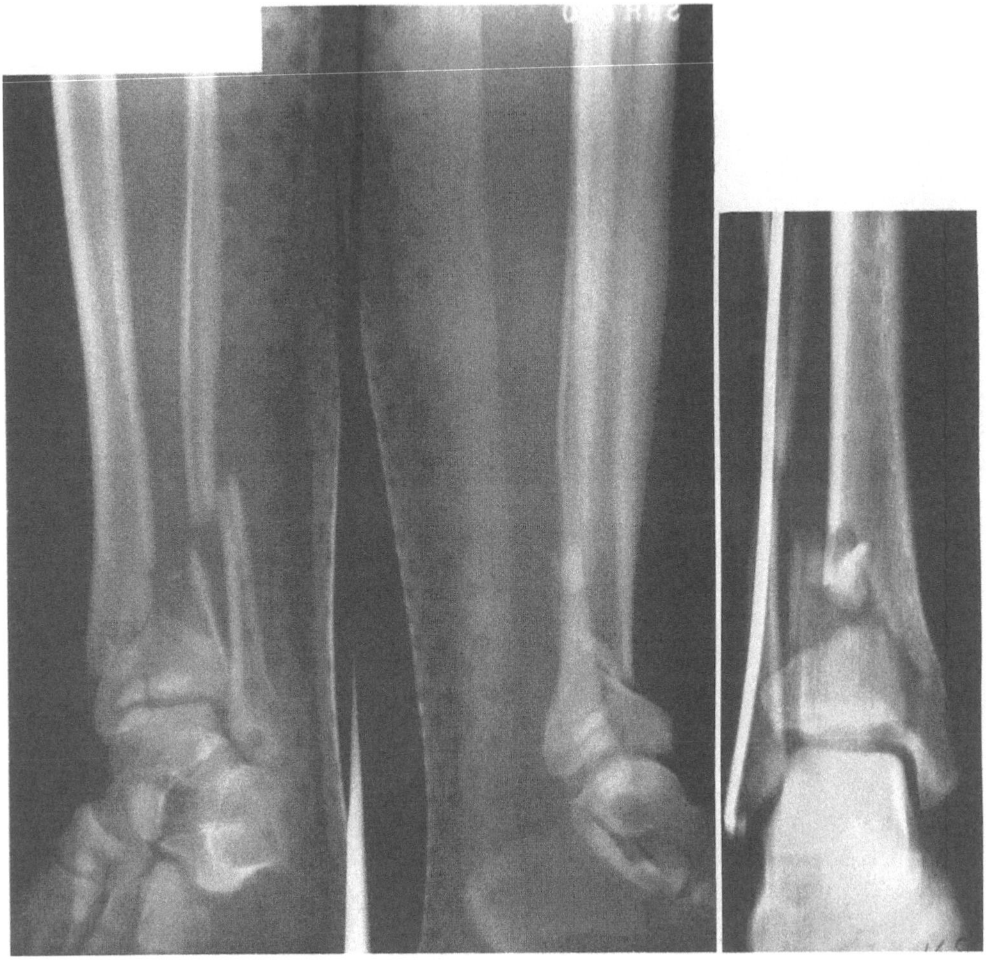

a b

Fig. 3. a) Anteroposterior radiograph of a 43 year old man with a severe open fracture of the distal tibia into the ankle joint (pilon fracture). The major wound was on the medial aspect of the joint. On the night of injury it was debrided and left open. The fibular fracture was fixed with a Rush pin to maintain length as noted on b) the anteroposterior radiograph. On the 5th postoperative day, with a granulating clean wound, internal fixation of the tibial fracture and the joint component was carried out. The distal wound was closed, the original wound left open and c) subsequently closed with steristrips on the 10th postoperative day. d) The final appearance of the ankle joint with wound healing and a good ankle. Note the bony syndesmosis between the tibia and fibula. e) No infection developed, the wound healed per primam, and the range of ankle motion was from 5° of dorsiflexion to 25° of plantar flexion

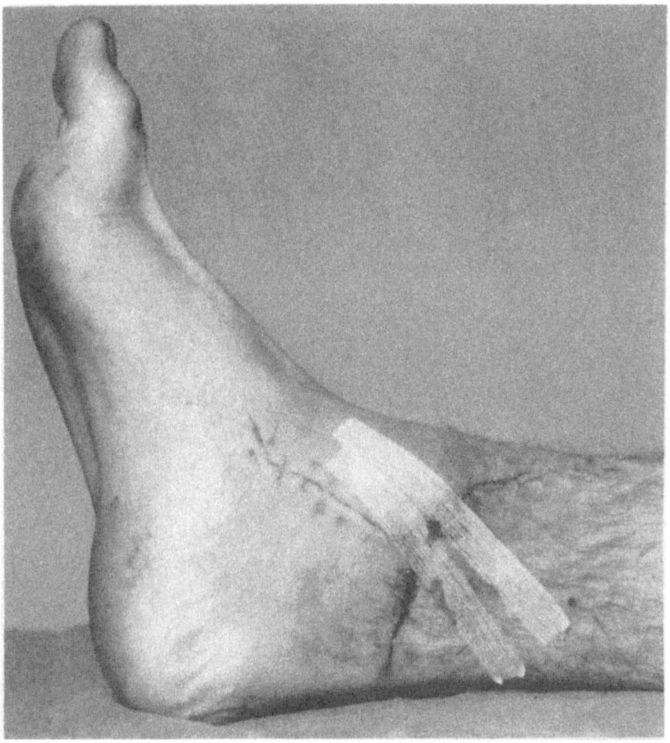

Fig. 3c

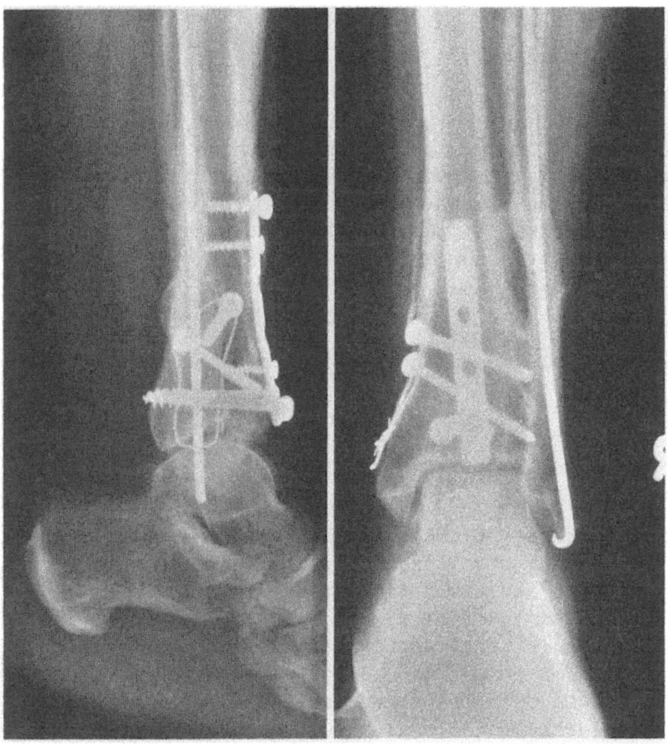

Fig. 3d

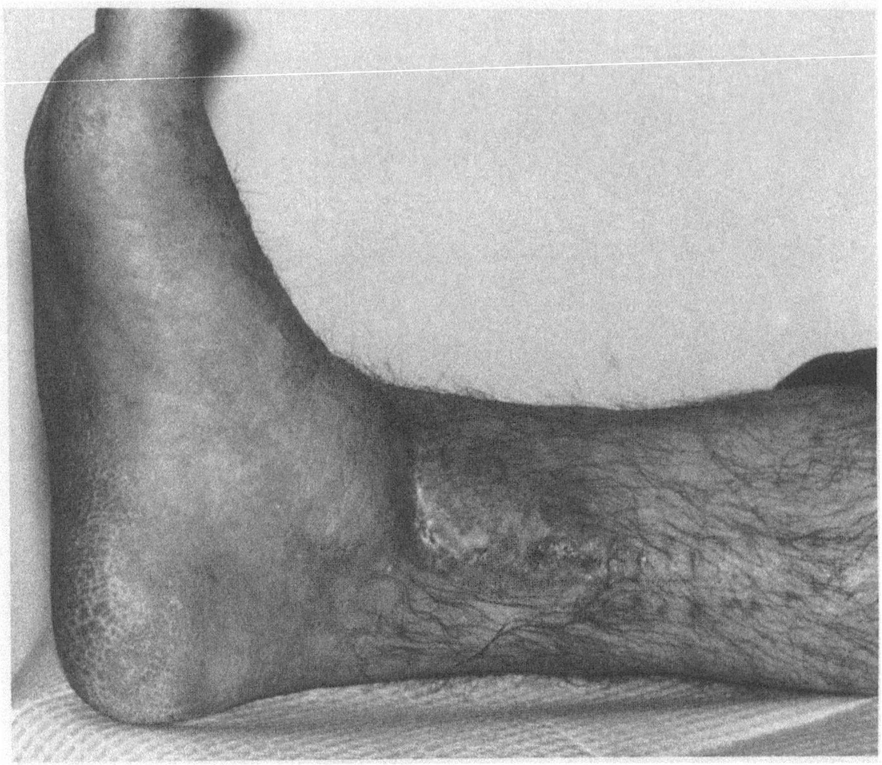

Fig. 3

Early bone grafting

In comminuted fractures, fixed either with open reduction and internal fixation or especially with external frames, early bone grafting is advisable to ensure union and to avoid losing the race between implant failure and bone union. Autogenous bone may be placed through the open wound, but in the tibia we favor the posterolateral approach. The procedure is done electively, usually three weeks after the original trauma.

Early soft tissue coverage

This aspect has already been discussed in the section on management of the soft tissues.

Discussion

Is there a price to pay for surgical stabilization in open fractures? If our hypothesis is correct, surgical stabilization will result in better function of the extremity without increased risk of sepsis. In reviewing the literature, open reduction and internal fixation (ORIF) for open fractures have resulted in a 15% sepsis rate, approximately, but most settled down after implant removal. Function was generally good. A review of publications on external fixation in open fractures indicated an 8% sepsis rate but few articles mentioned the functional result. However, most literature reviews unfortunately compare different types of injuries, and are therefore difficult to assess.

At Sunnybrook Medical Centre, we have reviewed our open fractures and classified them according to their Grade -- I, II or III -- and whether vascular injury was present.

a) *Forearm* - 34 open fractures were treated by primary open reduction and internal fixation with interfragmental compression and plates. At review (Tile and Petrie, 1970), 90% had full function. There was one delayed union and no infections.

b) *Humerus* - 14 open fractures of the humerus in polytraumatized patients were treated by primary ORIF (Bell and McMurtry, 1984). Thirteen of 14 patients regained full function. All fractures united primarily with one superficial infection which cleared subsequently.

c) *Tibia* - 38 open fractures of the tibia were treated by open reduction and internal fixation (Beauchamp et al, 1984). Thirty-six of 38 have united with a 10% infection rate. Full function, meaning normal ankle and foot motion, was recorded in 23 of 38 patients, more than 80% function in nine of 38, and less than 80% in three patients. Since the Grade III wounds associated with a tibia fracture had an unacceptably high sepsis rate, we do not recommend this treatment and prefer external frames for that injury.

d) *Femur* - at the time of this publication, we have not completed our review of femoral fractures. In the 12 fractures reviewed, all have united, one has a chronic infection, and only three have less than 90% knee function.

We therefore conclude that the results of surgical stabilization for upper extremity open fractures are excellent. The results in the tibia depended on the soft tissue wound and the type of bone injury. In general, precise attention to detail produced excellent functional results with a 10% sepsis rate equal to patients with nonsurgical care; however, as mentioned above, in the presence of a Grade III wound, external fixation is a safer choice.

The femur obviously presents problems. Most of our cases occurred in polytraumatized patients. For the isolated femur, we feel that the wound should be dealt with primarily, the patient placed in skeletal traction and a delayed primary nailing carried out when the wound has adequately healed. For the polytraumatized patient, where stabilization is important, we use either an external fixator or plate depending on the size of the soft tissue wound.

Treatment Protocol

We therefore recommend the following treatment protocol:

Carefully assess the personality of the injury, and begin immediate general care of the traumatized patient. As soon as possible, the wound should be thoroughly cleansed and debrided in an operating theatre. Small fragments of devitalized bone should be removed and discarded, whereas large fragments of bone necessary for stabilization should be retained if possible. The bone should be surgically stabilized by the appropriate method, open reduction and internal fixation being indicated for joint fractures, fractures around the metaphysis and the forearm; whereas external fixation is preferred for massively comminuted fractures of the tibia with bone loss and major tissue loss. We recommend open wound care followed by aggressive postoperative management, which includes further debridement, early cancellous bone grafting, and early attention to soft tissue closure, either by delayed primary closure, split thickness skin grafting or a flap. This management protocol will yield excellent functional results with no apparen increase in sepsis or delayed union. However, a careful assessment to define "personality" of the fracture is essential. The surgeon must have all forms of fixation devices available to him and he must exercise sound judgment for the particular situation at hand.

The actual techniques used are beyond the scope of this article (see suggested reading, 1980, 1981). Generally, interfragmental compression with lag screws should be used when possible, and the major fragments neutralized with dynamic compression plates or an external fixator. Intramedullary nails are rarely used primarily except in Grade I type fractures of the femur. After fracture management, follow-up care of the soft tissues must be exemplary.

Finally, care of the injured must be individualized according to well accepted principles. We must not forget our primary aim in the management of all fractures, that is, the return of the limb to full function at the earliest possible moment and with the fewest complications.

References

1. Anderson, L.D., Sish, T.D., Tooms, R.E., and Park, W.I.: Compression plate fixation in acute diaphyseal fractures of the radius and ulna. J. Bone Joint Surg. 57A, 287, 1975.
2. Beauchamp, C.G., Clifford, R.P., Webb, J.K., Kellam, J.F., and Tile, M.: Functional results after immediate internal fixation of open tibia fractures. Presented at Canadian Orthopaedic Association, Winnipeg, Canada, June 1984.
3. Bell, M., and McMurtry, R.H.: Excellent results with plating of humeral shaft fractures in multiply injured patients. Presented at Canadian Orthopaedic Association, Winnipeg, Canada, June 1984.
4. Hansen, S.T., and Winquist, R.A.: Closed intramedullary nailing of the femur. Clin. Orthop. Rel. Res. 138, 56, 1979.
5. Nicol, E.A.: Fractures of the tibial shaft. A survey of 705 cases. J. Bone Joint Surg. 46B, 373, 1964.
6. Patzakis, M.J., Harvey, J.P., and Tillman, M.M.: Comparing the incidence of infection in primary and delayed primary closure of open fracture wounds. American Academy of Orthopaedic Surgeons, March 1983.
7. Tile, M., and Petrie, D.: Fractures of the radius and ulna - using AO technique. Canadian Orthopaedic Association Annual Meeting 1970.

Suggested Reading

Schatzker, J., and Tile, M.: The AO (ASIF) method of fracture care. American Academy of Orthopaedic Surgeons Instructional Course Lectures. C.V. Mosby, 1980.

AO/ASIF Instrumentation Manual of Use and Care. Springer-Verlag, Berlin, Heidelberg, New York, 1981.

Compound Fractures: The European Approach

I. KEMPF

Introduction

The open fracture requires immediate therapeutic management since infection can lead to post-traumatic osteitis. Our approach has undergone a radical change over the last 30 years. Traditionally, open fractures were treated by repair of soft tissues and, if possible, by wound closure.

Immediate internal fixation was considered contraindicated and condemned. Internal fixation was carried out after complete skin healing. Nowadays, the situation is seen in a totally different light. Absolute stability of the bone fragments is considered a prerequisite for uneventful healing of the soft tissue. Consequently, we routinely proceed with an internal fixation of the fracture and try to obtain skin closure but do not consider it an absolute necessity.

Current European Approach

Treatment of soft tissue damage

We will limit our discussion to skin, fascia, and muscles, and exclude neurovascular lesions since they necessitate special surgical measures. Immediate amputations as well as reimplantations will also not be considered because these procedures merit a special chapter.

The classical principles of wound debridement followed, if possible, by wound closure remain the basis of soft tissue treatment. Their proper execution requires a thorough appreciation of the extent and gravity of the damage. A classification into three grades based on anatomopathologic criteria has been adopted by the majority of trauma surgeons and is universally accepted. A recent study in Germny (Oestern and Tscherne, 1982) outlined some additional considerations. These authors add a Grade IV to the classification that corresponds to a quasi-amputation or to an amputation which may require reimplantation. Furthermore, they classify closed fractures into three grades. Grade II indicates a localized contusion of soft tissue and skin abrasions, whereas Grade III denotes an extensive contusion, detachment, hematoma, and avulsion of muscles and fascia overlying a severe comminution. Both conditions may cause complications, especially skin breakdown.

When there are compound fractures with major damage of soft tissue, the simplest management is always the best treatment: debridement, excision of necrotic tissue, and, if suture is impossible, immediate free thin skin

Current Concepts of Infections in
Orthopaedic Surgery

grafting. In such conditions, extensive cutaneoplasties are contraindicated as long as the extent of the damage is still undetermined. Close observation of the healing process is required during the next several days before planning future complementary measures, ie, additional debridement, grafting, covering of soft tissue loss by the latest grafting technique: myocutaneous pedicled flaps, fascia-cutaneous flaps, or free flaps with microvascular anastomosis.

Treatment of skeletal injuries

Treatment consists predominantly of stable internal fixation, although traditional conservative methods still have a place as adjunctive therapy but rarely as the main treatment. Reduction of the fracture followed by immobilization in a plaster of Paris remains a simple and efficient method. It not only permits putting the extremity to rest but it also allows optimal skin healing and contributes to the prevention of infection. Plaster casts can still be used in:

1) Grade I and II fractures which are not too extensive and which have minimal displacement;
2) children;
3) certain compound intra-articular fractures.

The plaster cast still remains an excellent method, particularly in the presence of unstable osteosynthesis.

In Europe, skeletal traction is considered an insufficient means of treating open fractures. It is certainly capable of aligning the fragments, but it cannot immobilize sufficiently to ensure uneventful healing of the soft tissues. In compound leg fractures, traction can increase the chances of skin breakdown. Traction, however, is an excellent auxiliary method either in its original setup or as balanced traction in cases of unstable internal fixation. It also permits easy access to wounds. As such it is used when alignment nailing has been done.

Internal fixation

The advantages of this procedure are well known; its modalities are numerous. We consider screws, encircling wires, or isolated Kirschner wires methods of minimal internal fixation or as adjuncts, for example, to fixing separated fragments. They never result in a stable fixation and require additional methods such as plaster casts and skeletal traction. However, they may be indicated in children (Fig. 1a, 1b).

Encircling and Kirschner wires are excellent when using the tension wiring principle at specific sites: olecranon, greater trochanter, patella, malleoli, etc.

Essentially, there are three basic modes of fixation: plate fixation, intramedullar rodding in its various forms, and external fixation. Their exact place in fracture treatment has not reached a consensus in Europe. The use of the various compression plates and blade plates has been advocated by the Swiss AO group in the treatment of compound fractures. We firmly oppose their use in diaphyseal fractures of femur and tibia since they can cause serious problems in skin closure and healing and since intramedullar rods are biomechanically superior at these two sites (Fig. 2a, 2b).

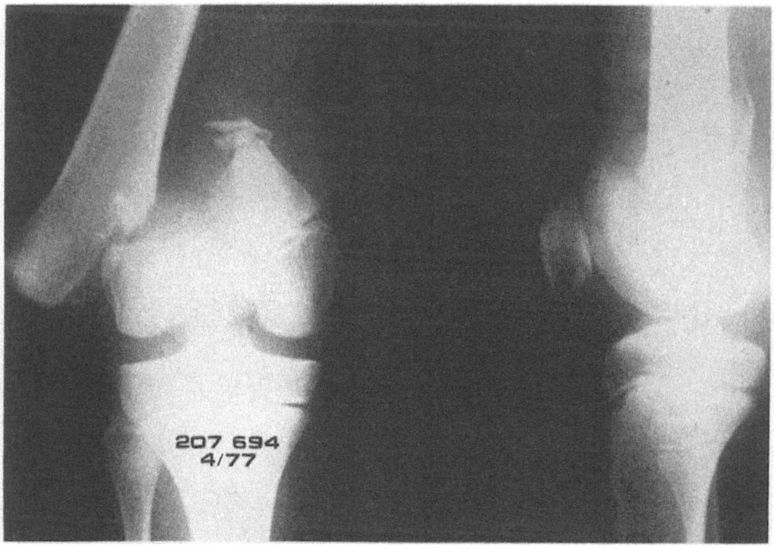

a

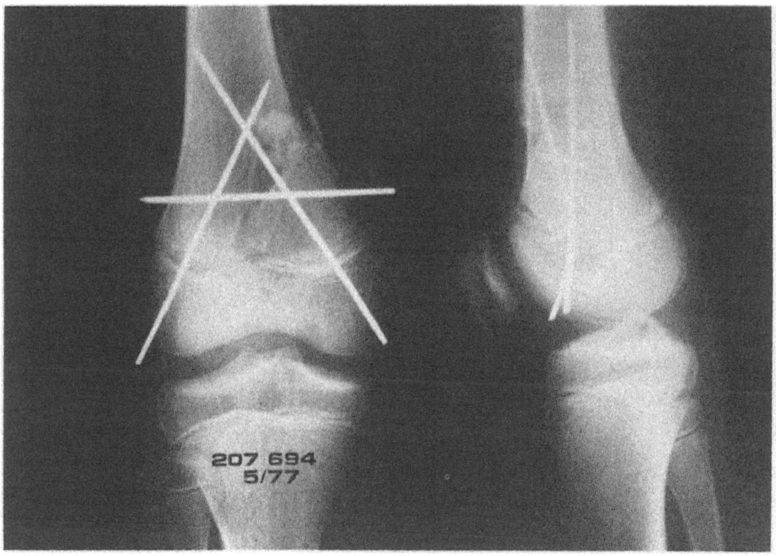

b

Fig. 1. a) Open fracture going through the distal femoral growth plate in 13-year old child. b) minimal fixation with wires supplemented by a plaster cast

We use these methods for humeral and forearm fractures (Fig. 3). Here, intramedullar rodding has been disappointing. Another accepted use is for various epiphyseal fractures.

Methods of closed intramedullar nailing

It sounds paradoxical when we state that we treat an open fracture by a closed method, but, as a matter of fact, we are debriding and closing the wound and proceed thereafter on a fracture table with closed intramedullar nailing. The Küntscher nail is our method of choice. Its use in the

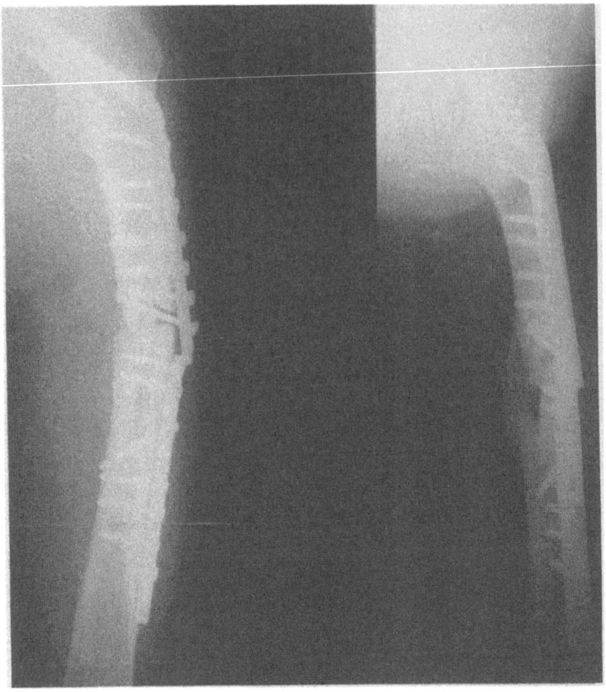

a

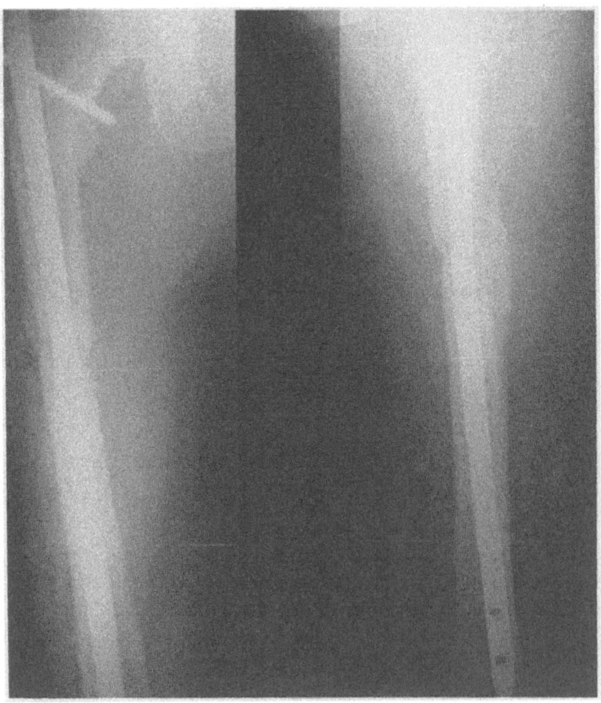

b

Fig. 2. a) Breakage of plate used for a comminuted femur fracture. b) Reoperation and fixation with dynamic locking nail

treatment of compound fractures, however, is still debated. Some surgeons rigidly follow Küntscher's teaching and nail only secondarily after healing of the soft tissues. We believe that such an approach does not prevent later complications due to delayed skin healing. Moreover, delayed inter-

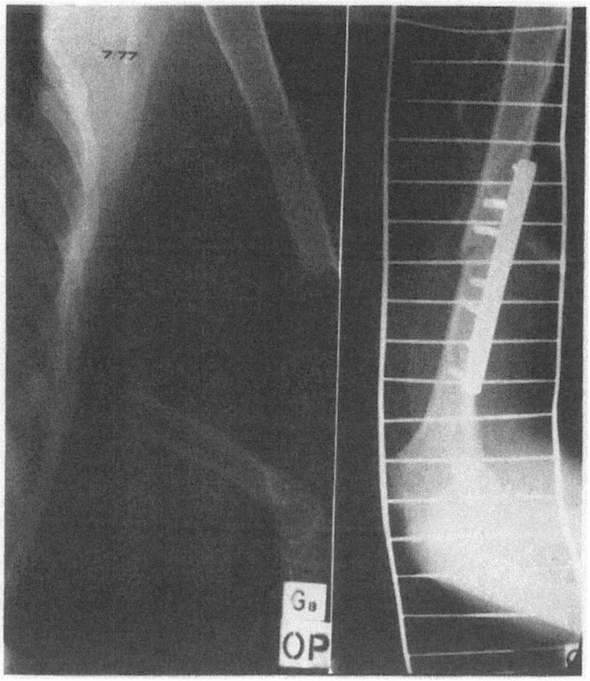

Fig. 3. Grade III open fracture of humeral shaft. Internal fixation with compression plate

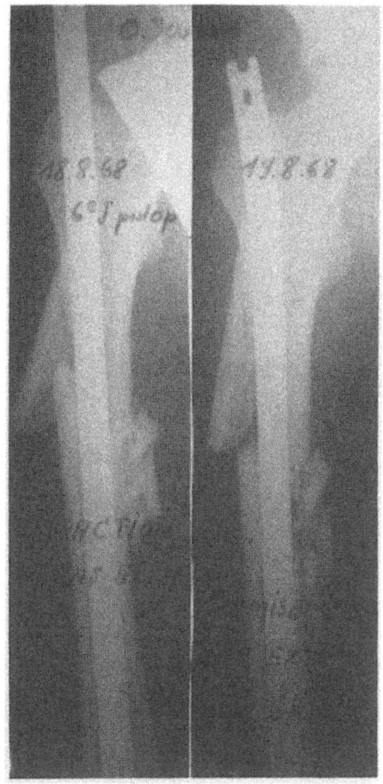

Fig. 4. Alignment nailing of comminuted proximal femur fracture: telescoping of fragments necessitating additional skeletal traction

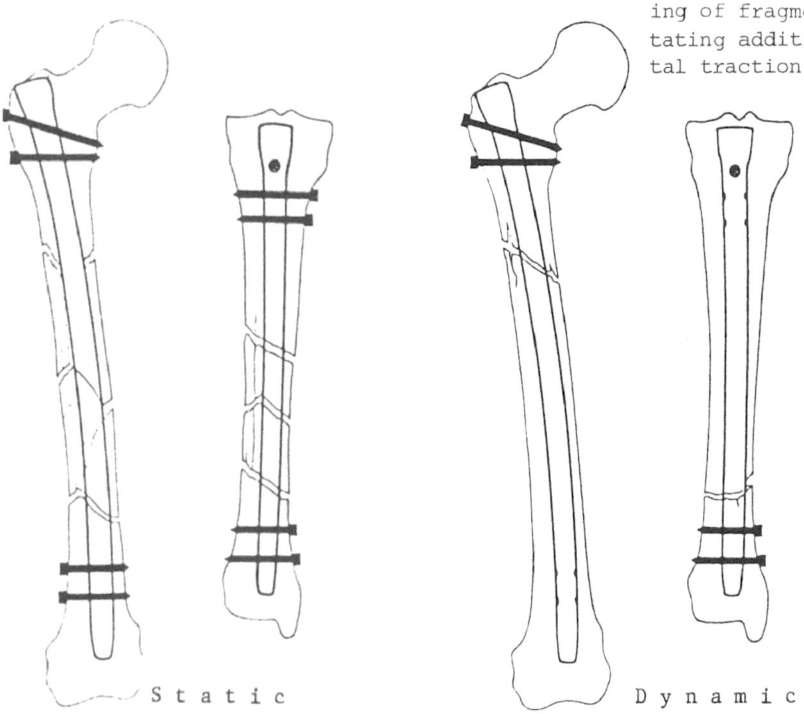

Fig. 5. Intramedullar locked nailing. Principles

Fig. 6. a) Grade III compound fracture of femoral shaft with loss of bone. b) Static locked nailing

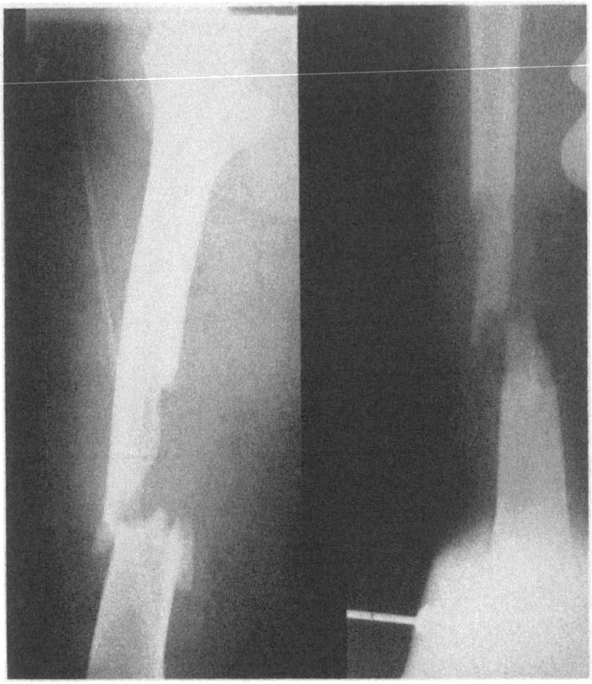

a

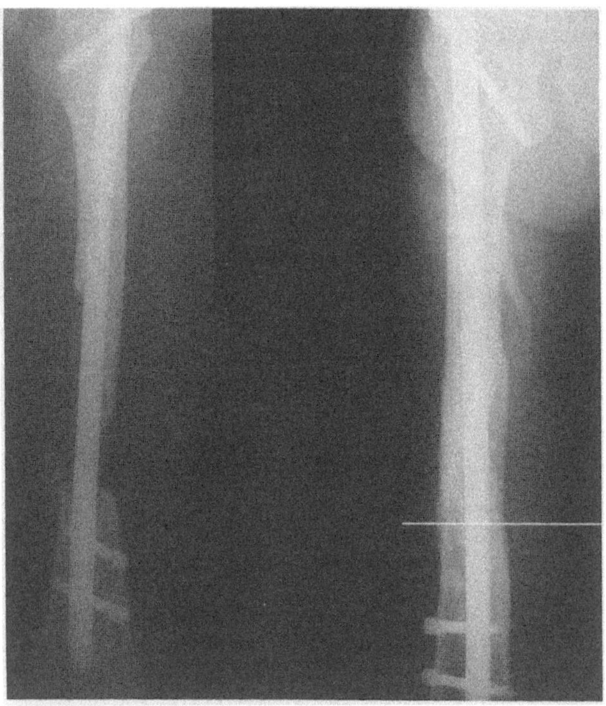

b

nal fixation causes serious inconveniences, particularly in polytraumatized patients. We therefore advocate immediate nailing of compound fractures of all grades of the femur and of Grades I and II of the tibia. Nailing can be done in three different ways.

1) Classic nailing for simple fractures - for example, transverse midshaft fractures.
2) Alignment nailing (Fig. 4) for complex comminuted fractures. This method combines a conventional rod of medium calibre with prolonged postoperative skeletal traction. This is an excellent method of a limited, immediate internal fixation. Unfortunately, it necessitates prolonged bedrest. We used it for quite a time, but have abandoned it in favor of:
3) Locked nailing, which not only controls rotation by dynamic locking but also prevents shortening by static locking (Fig. 5). This is the method of choice for severely comminuted fractures and bone loss. It also permits a broader scope for nailing, including distal and proximal diaphyseal fractures (Fig. 6a, 6b).

While contemplating this method it must be remembered to include in the armamentarium the bundle nailing of Hackethal, a simple and effective method for tibial fractures and sometimes humeral fractures, which is often overlooked. Furthermore, the possible use of Ender's nails, for example in children, should be considered.

External fixation

This method has a definite precise place in the treatment of compound fractures, where it does not compete with the locked nail. It is the only method for the treatment of extensive, dirty, and contaminated Grade III fractures. Here, the use of nails or plates would carry too great a risk of osteitis. We have adopted the Hoffmann system, one of the oldest in Europe, extensively used and constantly being improved. The ease of application and its versatility make it the method of choice in the treatment of serious compound fractures. Moreover, we should not forget its possible use in extensive comminuted intra-articular fractures by bridging the joint.

Antibiotic therapy

Antibiotics are an indispensable adjunct to carefully planned and executed surgical treatment. They can be administered systemically or locally. Only in extensively contaminated wounds do we use antibiotics locally in the form of chains of polymethylmethacrylate (PMMA) gentamicin beads. They are applied before wound closure and the end of the chain is brought out through a separate stab wound. We mobilize the chain at the fourth postoperative day, and remove it progressively after 15 to 20 days. We never use antibiotics locally in powder or liquid form.

Broad-spectrum antibiotics in high dosage are used systemically, beginning on the first day. The antibiotic may be changed once we have received the results of the culture and sensitivity studies of swabs taken during surgery. Specific universally accepted measures are taken for the prevention of tetanus and gas gangrene.

Indications

Our indications for the use of various methods depend on the extent of soft tissue damage and on the anatomic site.

Grade I and limited Grade II damage

Treatment of choice: internal fixation by plate and screws, intramedullar rodding, or tension band wiring.

Conservative treatment, or limited internal fixation in specific instances only: children or medical contraindications for extensive surgery, etc.

Extensive Grade II and Grade III damage:

When good skin closure is possible: intramedullar rodding or plates.

When conditions do not allow skin closure: external fixation.

Indications depending on site

Diaphysis:

- upper extremity - humerus and both bones of forearm: plate and screws.
- lower extremity - femur: intramedullar rodding, even in Grade III fractures, since conditions usually permit soft tissue coverage. Moreover, external fixators (used only in extreme cases) do not stabilize the femur sufficiently and cause important muscle trauma at sites of transfixation.

  Tibia: Usually intramedullar rodding, except in Grade III fractures when the external fixator is used, mostly due to problems relating to skin coverage.

Epiphyseal sites:

- Grade I, II and III, well covered: screws, plates, blade plates, on the condition that the bone can be reconstituted.

  In special cases - olecranon, greater trochanter, patella, malleoli: tension band wiring.
- Serious Grade III with extensive comminution: external fixator spanning the joint.

  Resection arthrodesis is rarely indicated.

Reference

1. Oestern and Tscherne: Unfallheilkunde 85, 111, 1982.

Subacute Osteomyelitis in Children

R. M. LETTS

In 1832, Sir Benjamin Brodie described his first experience with subacute osteomyelitis (Brodie, 1832). He amputated the leg of a man who had suffered from intractable pain for a number of years. On examination of the specimen he found "a cavity the size of a walnut filled with dark colored pus." "The bone immediately surrounding the cavity was whiter and harder than the surrounding bone. The inner surface of the cavity presented an appearance of high vascularity." Since then, low grade pyogenic abscess of the bone has frequently been called a Brodie's abscess.

Childhood hematogenous osteomyelitis occurs in the metaphysis of long bones. Hobo in 1921 demonstrated that branches of nutrient arteries "reach the growth plate, make hairpin turns on themselves and terminate in wide calibre sinusoids, which in turn drain into the marrow." (Hobo, 1921-22) Hobo and Trueta suggested that this results in stasis of blood (Hobo, 1921-22; Trueta, 1959). When bacterial emboli are present, they settle in the periphery of the flow and result in thrombosis of the veins. In the sinusoids the phagocytic cells are either absent or inactive (Rang, 1969). Any obstruction of these blood vessels results in avascular necrosis and abscess formation.

It has been postulated that repeated minor trauma of the lower limbs in children occurs most frequently in the knee region. This results in microfractures in the trabeculae, mild hemorrhage and necrosis without clinical symptoms.

Lennert observed a schematic arrangement of cells in concentric zones in osteomyelitis (Lennert, 1965). The predominance of one zone over the other determines the histologic picture of the disease:

1) *Central zone* consisting of necrotic tissue, fibrin deposits and massive polymorphonuclear infiltration.

2) *Surrounding area* showing little sign of acute inflammation but consisting of granulation tissue, lymphocytes and plasma cells.

In acute osteomyelitis, the picture is that of localized suppuration and abscess formation but little or no scar tissue nor sclerotic bone.

In Brodie's abscess, little necrosis is present and a few pus cells are seen in the center of the lesion. The bony cavity is invaded by granulation tissue and surrounded by dense fibrous tissue, and sometimes by a narrow ring of sclerotic bone.

Current Concepts of Infections in
Orthopaedic Surgery

In rare cases of Garré's sclerotic nonpurulent osteomyelitis, there is little granulation tissue, no necrosis and no purulent exudate. However, there is intense proliferation of periosteum resulting in new bone formation.

Literature Review

A review of the literature since the inception of antibiotics does not reveal any large series of subacute osteomyelitis of the long bones in children. However, in 1938 Brailsford reported on 62 patients with chronic bone abscess in all age groups (Brailsford, 1938). Since then, Harris and Kirkaldy-Willis (1965) have written a paper based on their experience of 75 patients in East Africa, in whom subacute osteomyelitis was the main form of osteomyelitis. King and Mayo (1969), Kendal and Mankin (1973) and Gledhill (1973) have produced reviews of small series of 25, 8, and 9 patients respectively (Table I).

Table I. Review of Brodie's abscess

	Source	No. of patients (age group)
1938	Brailsford	62 (all ages)
1965	Harris and Kirkaldy-Wallis	75 (all ages)
1969	King and Mayo	25 (all ages)
1973	Kendal and Mankin	8 (children)
1973	Gledhill	9 (children)

The purpose of this review is to question whether the nature of osteomyelitis has changed in recent years and whether, perhaps, subacute and chronic clinical presentations are becoming more common.

A review of the case records at the Childrens Hospital, Winnipeg, between 1970 and 1980 revealed 20 patients who met the criterion for the diagnosis of subacute osteomyelitis (Table II).

Diagnosis Criteria for Subacute Osteomyelitis

Only patients who had histologic as well as radiologic findings consistent with the diagnosis of subacute osteomyelitis were included in this series. Patients who had a history of treated osteomyelitis, surgery, open fracture or foreign body were excluded.

Age and Sex

The ages ranged from eight months to 15 years, the average age being nine years. There was predominance of 12 boys to eight girls.

Table II. Subacute osteomyelitis diagnosed at Childrens Hospital, Winnipeg, 1970-1980

Patient	Age	Sex	Complaints	Duration (weeks)	Site	ESR	WBC	Polymorphs/ lymphocytes	Culture	Treatment
1 J.G.	12	M	Pain and swelling	103	Distal tibial metaphysis	75	8,400	69/24	*S.aureus*	* † § ¶
2 C.W.	8 mo	F	Pain and swelling; limp	2	Distal femoral metaphysis	75	12,000	36/51	negative	* † § ¶
3 S.S.	1	M	Pain; limp	28	Distal femoral metaphysis	27	7,300	35/51	negative	* † § ¶
4 S.K.	6	F	Pain	1	Tibial diaphysis	50	7,300	61/25	*S.albus*	* † § ¶
5 A.T.	11	F	Pain	2	Radial metaphysis	23	7,900	45/37	*S.aureus*	* † §
6 L.S.	15	M	Pain and swelling	24	Distal femoral metaphysis	21	10,300	52/30	*S.aureus*	* † § ¶
7 T.C.	10	M	Pain	12	Distal tibial metaphysis	92	10,000	53/21	*S.aureus*	* † § ¶
8 G.A.	8	M	Pain; limp	12	Femoral neck	15	4,400	36/49	negative	* † § ¶ Thomas splint
9 S.S.	11	M	Pain and swelling	24	Distal tibial metaphysis	12	5,500	44/47	*S.aureus*	* † § ¶
10 A.S.	10	M	Pain and swelling	52	Distal femoral metaphysis	44	4,800	56/38	*S.aureus*	* † § ¶

Table II continued

Patient	Age	Sex	Complaints	Duration (weeks)	Site	ESR	WBC	Polymorphs/ lymphocytes	Culture	Treatment
11 A.S.	13	M	Pain	4	Distal femoral metaphysis	59	5,600	37/43	*S. aureus*	* † § ¶
12 H.W.	13	M	Pain	1	Femoral diaphysis	65	3,900	37/55	negative	* † § ¶
13 D.H.	11	F	Pain and swelling	2	Distal femoral metaphysis	110	12,100	82/25	negative	* † § ¶
14 A.D.	5	F	Pain	104	Distal femoral metaphysis	33	6,600	48/40	*S. aureus*	* † § ¶
15 P.O.	10	M	Pain and swelling	4	Distal tibial metaphysis	60	6,900	56/26	*S. aureus*	* † § ¶
16 C.K.	2	M	Pain	6	Distal femoral metaphysis	25	7,400	24/46	negative	* † § ¶
17 L.H.	11	F	Pain	3	Proximal tibial metaphysis	15	8,600	56/35	negative	* † § ¶
18 M.G.	12	F	Pain and swelling	12	Humeral diaphysis	20	6,900	74/11	*S. aureus*	* † §
19 E.L.	4	M	Pain and swelling	24	Proximal tibial diaphysis	-	8,500	57/20	negative	* † § ¶
20 J.W.	10	F	Pain	20	Proximal tibial diaphysis	-	-	-	negative	* † § ¶

* biopsy; † antibiotics; § curretage; ¶ plaster cast

History

Subacute osteomyelitis is characterized by an insidious onset and a long delay between the onset of pain and diagnosis. Systemic reaction is characteristically absent and the disease is localized. Pain was the commonest complaint, being present in all patients. Pain was often more severe at night. The history revealed limping in eight patients, local swelling in eight, and local tenderness in 18. Three patients gave a history of trauma to the affected limb 3-24 months before diagnosis of the abscess.

Nine patients gave a history of associated infection and had been treated with antibiotics during the 12 months before diagnosis of Brodie's abscess. Four of these had an upper respiratory tract infection or urinary tract infection. One had an umbilical stump infection. The remaining four had musculoskeletal infections, two after injuries, and two were thought to have had septic joints which were inadequately treated (one hip joint, one knee joint).

Duration of Symptoms

The abscess may be present for years before it is discovered. In this series, many patients were symptomatic for prolonged periods before the diagnosis was finally made (Table III)

Table III. Duration of symptoms

	No. of patients
5 - 24 months	8
1 - 3 months	6
1 - 3 weeks	6
Total patients	20

Site of Lesion

The most common site of Brodie's abscess as reported in the literature is the distal tibia. However, in our series, the commonest site was the distal femoral metaphysis, followed by distal metaphysis of the tibia, and then proximal metaphysis of the tibia (Table IV).

Roentgenographic Findings

The usual radiologic picture shows a clearly defined radiolucent lesion in the metaphysis or diaphysis of a long bone with varying amounts of reactive bone formation (Fig. 1).

Two patients had marked cortical thickening with new bone formation. These appearances could have readily been confused with osteoid osteoma. They were diagnosed as Garré's sclerosing osteitis (Table V).

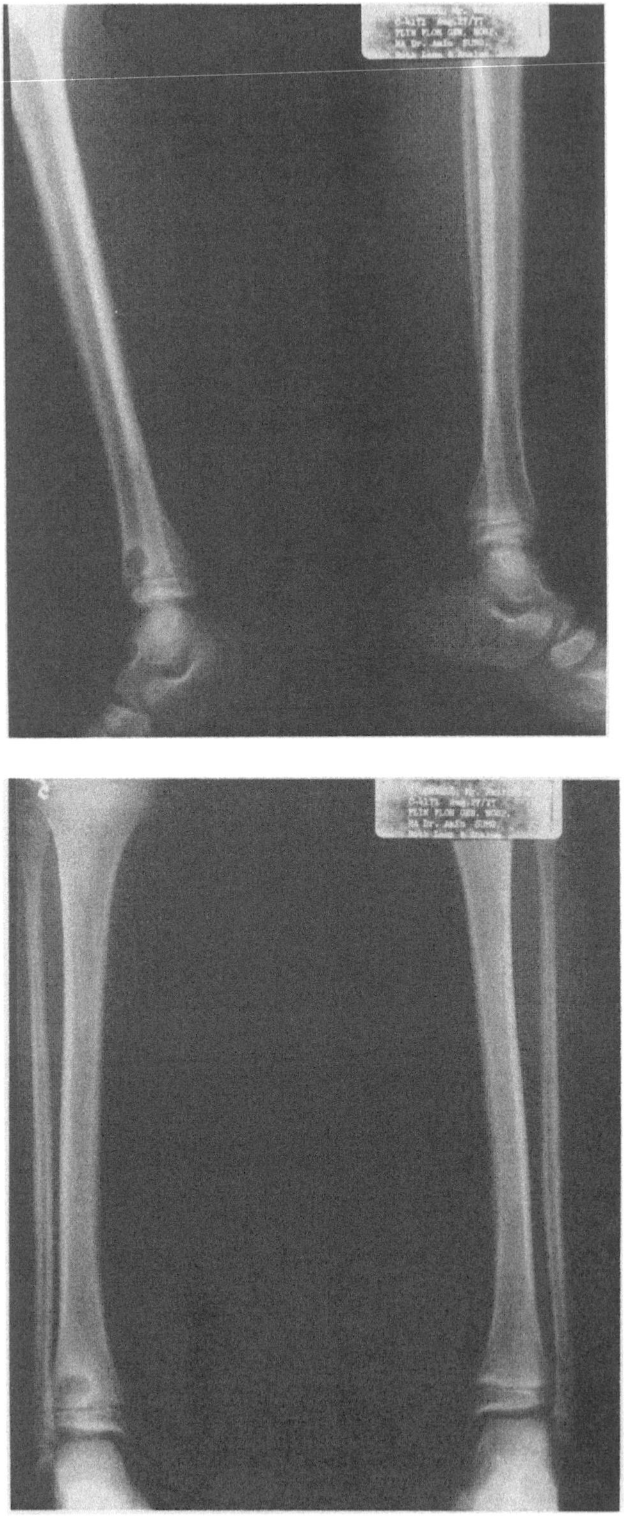

Fig. 1. Typical appearar of subacute osteomyelitis in distal tibia

Table IV. Site of lesion

Site	No. of patients
Femoral	
Metaphysis	8
Diaphysis	1
Neck	1
Tibial	
Metaphysis	5
Diaphysis	3
Humeral	
Diaphysis	1
Radial	
Metaphysis	1
Total	20

Table V. Radiographic findings

	No. of patients
Lucent defect with sclerotic margins	16
Defect with marked sclerosis	2
Excessive cortical thickening of sclerosing osteomyelitis of Garré	2
Total	20

In two patients, destruction of the distal tibial epiphysis was evident. Follow-up has not demonstrated any limb length discrepancy.

Laboratory Studies

White blood cell count in most patients was below 10,000 and was not diagnostically significant. However, the erythrocyte sedimentation rate (ESR) was elevated in 75% of the patients. This was a higher rate than reported elsewhere (Table VI).

Histologic Findings

The fluid content of the cavity may be purulent, oily, or even mucoid or slimy. Histologically, most specimens showed similar features of chronic inflammatory exudate with presence of neutrophils, lymphocytes, and plasma cells. Moderate fibroblastic response and remnants of necrotic tissue were found.

Table VI. Sedimentation rate

	No. of patients
Over 30 mm	10
20 - 30 mm	5
Below 20 mm	3
Not done	2
Total	20

Bacteriologic Findings

In ten patients, *Staphylococcus aureus* was cultured from the specimen taken at operation; one grew *Staphylococcus albus*, and the remaining nine showed no growth.

Treatment

All patients had a surgical drainage procedure, followed by appropriate antibiotic therapy.

Discussion

A review of the literature suggests that the nature of osteomyelitis has changed during recent years and that the subacute and chronic presentations are becoming more common. During a 10-year period at the Childrens Hospita in Winnipeg, 20 patients with subacute osteomyelitis were diagnosed as compared with 237 with acute osteomyelitis, an incidence of 8.8%. A statistical comparison with the years 1950-60 has revealed 253 patients admitted with osteomyelitis as opposed to 16 with subacute osteomyelitis, an incidence of 6.3%. Kendal and Mankin (1973) in their review found 400 patients with acute osteomyelitis compared with eight with subacute osteomyelitis. Few other centers have published figures comparing the acute with subacute osteomyelitis rates. Our yearly averages show that during the last ten years, subacute osteomyelitis at the Childrens Hospital has remained constant. In our experience, therefore, no evidence supports the belief that subacute bone infections are on the increase.

The organism mainly responsible for acute and subacute bone infections is *Staphylococcus*. It remains an enigma why the same organisms can produce a localized infection on the one hand and a fulminating osteomyelitis on the other.

Kirkaldy-Willis (1965) found that in East Africa subacute osteomyelitis was the chief form of osteomyelitis. Africans would seem to have an increased incidence of foot infections because many of them walk barefoot, giving them increased resistance to staphylococcal infections. Kirkaldy-Willis also suggested that the lesions found in East Africa were caused by less virulent organisms. A large portion of the African population has not been exposed to antibiotics.

In our review, of considerable interest was the finding that 75% of patients with Brodie's abscess became symptomatic during the winter months. Another finding was that 45% of the patients had taken antibiotics before the diagnosis of Brodie's abscess was made. As with infections in general, infection in bone depends on the interplay between the microorganisms and the immune mechanism of the host.

Genetic variations in staphylococci are known to occur in the presence of penicillin. Variants known as Minute G and Minute L forms have been isolated and they are relatively avirulant. Upper respiratory tract infections are more common in winter, and antibiotics are more frequently prescribed both to the very young and the elderly. The lifestyle during long winter months predisposes to certain types of infections. It is possible that when the resistance is low, the body becomes vulnerable to infection by relatively avirulent commensal or deviant forms of staphylococci. A virile form of the staphylococcus would perhaps cause full blown osteomyelitis.

In conclusion, our review of a relatively stable population group in Manitoba revealed only a slight increase in incidence of subacute osteomyelitis over the past 30 years.

References

1. Brailsford, J.F.: Brodie's abscess and its differential diagnosis. Brit. Med. J. 2, 119, 1938.
2. Brodie, B.: An account of some cases of chronic abscess of the tibia. Trans. Med. Clin. Society 17, 238, 1832.
3. Gledhill, R.: Subacute osteomyelitis in children. Clin. Orthop. Rel. Res. October, 1973
4. Harris, H.N. and Kirkaldy-Willis, W.H.: Primary subacute pyogenic osteomyelitis. J. Bone Joint Surg. 47B, 526, 1965.
5. Hobo, T.: Zur Pathogenese der akuten hematogenen Osteomyelitis mit Berücksichtigung der Vitalfärbungslehre. Acta Sch. Med. Univ. Kioto 4, 1, 1921-22.
6. Kendal, S. and Mankin, A.: Pyogenic abscess of long bones in children. Clin. Orthop. Rel. Res. October, 1973
7. King, D.M. and Mayo, K.M.: Subacute hematogenous osteomyelitis. J. Bone Joint Surg. 51B, 458, 1969.
8. Lennert, K.: Grundprobleme der Osteomyelitis. Verh. Dtsch. Orthop. Ges. 51, 27, 1965.
9. Rang, M.: The Growth Plate and Its Disorders. E.S. Livingston, Ltd., 1969, p. 78.
10. Trueta, J.: The three types of acute hematogenous osteomyelitis. J. Bone Joint Surg. 41B, 671, 1959.

Modern Trends in the Investigation and Treatment of Chronic Osteomyelitis

L.-J. Papineau

Introduction

In the past, wars have always contributed to the advancement of surgery. After the First World War, patients suffering from chronic osteomyelitis were treated by the Orr method (saucerization and open drainage (Orr, 1939) or by the Baer method using maggots for adequate debridement of the bony lesion and of the soft tissues (Baer, 1931).

After the Second World War, Kelly and Shannon popularized the technique of extensive saucerization followed by a split thickness skin graft (Armstrong and Jarman, 1936; Kelly, 1946; Shannon and Woolhouse, 1954).

However, despite these improvements, less than 25 years ago, the treatment of chronic osteomyelitis requiring saucerizations or segmentary resections was always despairingly slow for the patient as well as for the surgeon. Amputation was often used for a rapid and inexpensive but most unsatisfactory result.

Investigations

Many technologic developments in radiology and nuclear medicine have contributed to the early diagnosis of osteomyelitis. Moreover, new radiologic tools have helped to adapt the planning of operations (incision site, magnitude of saucerization) to the condition of each patient.

Radiology

1. Simple roentgenograms sometimes suffice to obtain a proper diagnosis and to plan treatment, the cavities and sequestrae being clearly demonstrated. However, it is often better to carry out investigations with more thorough techniques.

2. Tomography will give us information on the size, number and layout of the sequestrae and their place in connection with the cortex. Bone cavities and sequestrae not evident otherwise may show up more clearly.

3. In fistulography, the opacification of the sinus tracts, sometimes quite distant from the site of infection, might help to delineate the exact site of infection, the size of the bone cavities and the presence of the sequestrae. An incision site more appropriate for the initial surgery and for subsequent operations can then be chosen (Fig. 1).

Current Concepts of Infections in
Orthopaedic Surgery

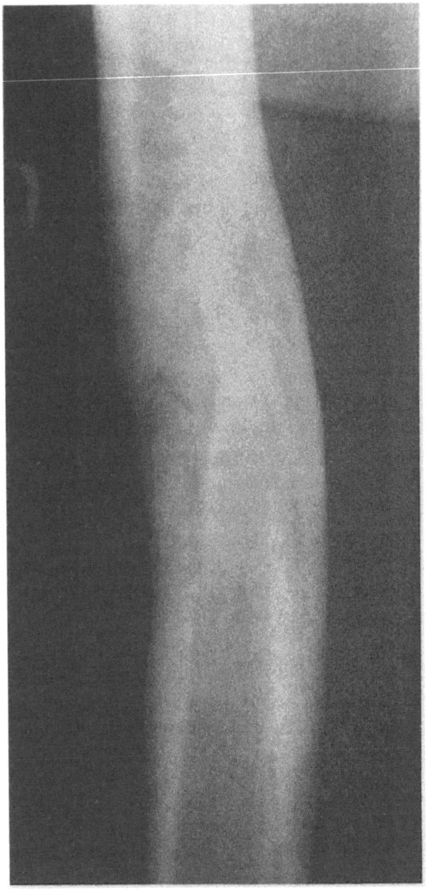

Fig. 1. Simple roentgenogram and fistulography

4. Mammographic techniques applied to the investigation of the osteomyelitic lesions of the small bones has given more precise pictures and permitted the localization and treatment of residual lesions.

5. Computerized tomography shows clearly the narrowing of the medullary cavity by granulation tissue and dead bone, subperiosteal bone reaction, sometimes the presence of gas as well as cortical apertures. Soft tissue abscesses will also be detected (Wilson et al, 1978).

Nuclear medicine

In nuclear medicine, the radiopharmaceutical agents most often used have been technetium diphosphonate, gallium citrate and, more recently, indium.

The investigation with gallium is positive in the presence of active osteomyelitis and negative in the presence of inactive osteomyelitis, while the investigation with technetium is positive in both cases.

We use bone scans not only to obtain a more precise diagnosis but also in cases of recurrences hidden by dense bone to determine their exact site (Goldstein, 1983; Vallières et al, 1977).

Treatment

Based on the exact knowledge of the infectious agent or agents, the treat- must begin with:

Bacteriologic investigations (Papineau, 1979)

During the course of our study the search for pathogens was conducted systematically and repeatedly on superficial preoperative samples and more thoroughly with deep cultures taken at the time of surgery.

The following table shows the most commonly encountered microbes, predominantly staphylococci.

Table I.

Microbes	Incidence
*Staphylococcus aureus**	75%
*Pseudomonas aeruginosa**	40%
Escherichia coli	15%
Klebsiellae species	12%
Streptococcus faecalis	13%
Mycobacterium tuberculosis	2%

* The combination of *S. aureus* and *P. aeruginosa* was found in 40% of our patients

Antibiotic therapy (Papineau et al, 1979)

In the early phase of the open sky excision graft technique, we used prolonged and continuous antibiotic therapy (4 - 6 mos).

With experience, the quality of our saucerizations improved. Consequently, we could shorten antibiotic administration, limiting it to the surgical periods during the different stages. Only the patients with a heavy purulent discharge after adequate saucerization still received prolonged antibiotic therapy.

The antibiotics most commonly used are cloxacillin and dicloxacillin (Table II).

Surgical treatment

1. Open sky excision and grafting (Papineau, 1973; Papineau et al, 1979)

As early as 1957, we discussed the possibility of shortening the traditionally long treatment of chronic osteomyelitis, necessitating an extensive bone resection (Table III).

Confronted with recurrent bone infections with an uncertain prognosis and requiring several months if not years of treatment, we devised two techniques. They were intended to supply healthy cancellous bone at an earlier

Table II

Antibiotic	Use
Cloxacillin or Dicloxacillin	87%
Chloromycetin	40%
Penicillin	35%
Tetracycline	35%
Ampicillin	30%
Lincomycin	22%
Erythromycin	21%
Gentamicin	1%

All patients received at least two of these antibiotics during the course of treatment

Table III. Stages of classical treatment before weight bearing

Saucerization	1/2	mo
Temporary cutaneous covering	1/2	mo
Waiting period	3 - 6	mos
Permanent cutaneous covering	2	mos
Waiting period	2 - 3	mos
Bone construction	3 - 6	mos
Total treatment time - Minimum	13	mos
Maximum	18	mos

phase in functionally insufficient saucerization defects. The skin covering was intentionally delayed.

The first of these techniques deals with the filling of the cavities structurally weakened by saucerization. The stages are diagrammatically outlined in Table IV.

The second technique consists of a segmental bone reconstruction necessitated by the saucerization-resection, used especially in the treatment of infected pseudarthroses. An osteosynthesis is then necessary to prevent shortening and to assure stability (Table V).

Thus, there are three different surgical stages:

1) extensive excision or debridement - wound left open;

2) autogenous open sky cancellous bone grafting after osteosynthesis if necessary;

3) delayed skin covering (Fig. 2).

Table IV. Stages of the technique on weakened bone in continuity

Chronic osteomyelitis
↓
Saucerization without closure
↓
Waiting 7 to 14 days
↓
Autogenous cancellous bone grafting
(wound left open)
↙ ↘
secondary healing | delayed skin graft on granulation tissue

Intermittent antibiotic therapy

Table V. Stages of the technique for treatment of segmental resections

Infected pseudarthrosis
↓
Saucerization without closure (segmental resection)
↓
Waiting 7 to 14 days
↓
Osteosynthesis and autogenous cancellous bone grafting
(wound left open)
↙ ↘
healing of the pseudarthrosis and of the cutaneous wound | healing of the pseudarthrosis skin graft to hasten healing of the skin

Intermittent antibiotic therapy

These new treatments applied to an infected site appeared, at first, paradoxical. However, they were based on known scientific facts:

1) radical excision of the infected site;

2) the known resistance to infection of an autogenous cancellous bone graft;

3) the bacteriostatic action of granulation tissue and its capacity for metaplasia;

and based on established surgical principles:

1) adequate drainage (delayed skin closure);

2) adequate stabilization (osteosynthesis);

3) appropriate antibiotic therapy preventing septicemia in the course of treatment and recurrences of osteomyelitis.

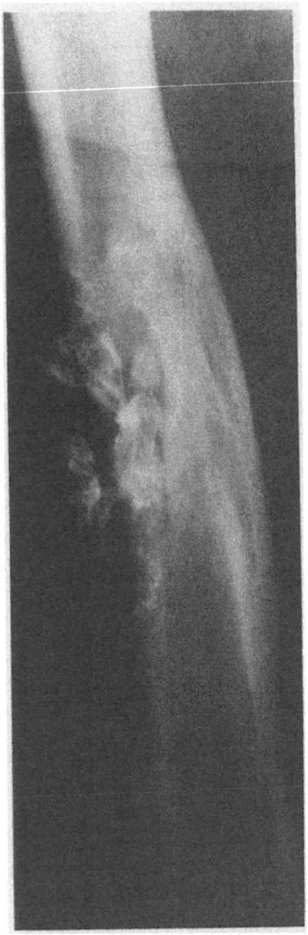

Fig. 2. Infected pseudarthosis. Resection, osteosynthesis and bone grafting

Having used these techniques from 1960 to 1970, we have obtained good results in 93% of our patients. These results were later confirmed in other orthopedic centers. In the lower limb, the duration of treatment up to weight bearing averaged eight months.

Indications for Surgery

Over the years, the scope for the use of these two surgical techniques has greatly increased. Actually, we use them in the following conditions:

Chronic osteomyelitis

1) bone reconstruction for insufficient saucerization;

2) reconstruction after segmental bony resection for infected pseudarthrosis.

Miscellanous indications

1) Musculocutaneous bony losses of long bones: motor bike accidents, bullet wounds. Although not really infected, those losses can be immediately

treated by this method of open sky osteosynthesis and grafting (Papineau et al, 1979; Vidal et al, 1978).

2) Musculocutaneous bony loses of short bones (tarsus, carpus, secondary to gun shots) can also be treated by this technique. The debridement is followed by a filling with cancellous bone and by a delayed skin graft (Hazlett, 1954; Papineau et al, 1979).

3) The method can also be used for open-sky arthrodesis in complications of septic arthritis (Papineau et al, 1979; Roy-Camille et al, 1978)

From 1970 to 1984, we particularly endeavored to find answers for the remaining unfortunate 7% of patients who had not been cured by the previously described technique. With these patients, the unsuccessful results could be attributed to either the failure of soft tissue healing or insufficient bone strength. To solve the nonhealing of the soft tissues we used the following techniques:

a) The muscle pedicle graft (Papineau et al, 1979)

This method has been used to cover the cancellous bone chips used for the treatment of cavities or for nonunions of deep bones (femur, humerus) that are surrounded by muscles.

The continuous use of antibiotic-impregnated gauze prevents the invasion of the bone graft by granulation tissue. It is easy to dissect a muscle pedicle from the adjacent muscle mass and rotate it over the bone graft. The pedicle is fixed in place with a few chromic catgut sutures. The skin and subcutaneous tissue are left open, permitting proper drainage. A split thickness skin graft can be used later.

b) Restarting the granulation phase (Papineau et al, 1979)

In subcutaneous bone, like the tibia, the new skin tends to cover the granulation tissue before the latter has time to cover all of the bone graft. It is then necessary to restart the granulation process by undermining the skin edges and packing the wound with antibiotic-impregnated gauze. The granulation tissue will grow again covering the bone. Spontaneous epithelialization will follow or a split thickness skin graft will be applied.

c) The myocutaneous graft at the leg level (soleus, gastrocnemius) combines both previously described techniques, assuring the revascularization of the bone graft and the skin coverage.

d) Microanastomosed skin graft; taken from the inguinal region, it can be used in certain cases of major skin deficit or for delayed replacement of an unsatisfactory split thickness skin graft (Taylor and Watson, 1978).

To enhance the bone healing we have used the following techniques:

a) A second open sky cancellous bone grafting (Hazlett, 1954)

b) The osseous scarification of Colchero (Cholchero, 1981).

This technique can be used in cases where one wants to limit the extent of the bone resection. It consists of a daily or every other day petalization of the exposed bone near the edge of the granulation tissue. The bone is gradually revascularized. This technique can be done on the ward without anesthesia.

c) The microanastomosed bone or skin-bone graft (Brice and Mialhe, 1982; Taylor and Watson, 1978)

As a first attempt in cases with more than 8 cm defect, or after a failure of the open sky excision-graft technique, the Taylor technique can be employed, using the anterior iliac crest and a branch of the iliac artery.

Brice (1982) also described an interesting technique using the posterior iliac crest vascularized by a branch of the gluteal artery.

d) Electrical treatment of osteomyelitis

The treatment is based on the antibacterial action of silver (Becker, 1983). A low voltage electrical current passed through a silver electrode releases ions of silver into the bone and surrounding soft tissues. Patients are treated first with an extensive debridement and with antibiotics. This treatment is still considered experimental and should be reserved for patients with major problems.

Conclusions

1. During the past 30 years, the investigative technology and treatment of chronic osteomyelitis has advanced impressively.

2. Tomography, fistulography, computerized tomography and bone scanning have all been of help for planning systematic and individualized treatment of the osteomyelitic bone lesions (Arger et al, 1983).

3. Open sky excision/resection and bone/skin grafting are being used for a faster solution to the problems of bone and soft tissue healing.

4. Further advancements have been made in the treatment of skin and bone failures by using myocutaneous grafts, or microanastomosed skin or skin and bone grafts (Brice and Mialhe, 1982; Taylor and Watson, 1978).

5. In selected cases, the electrical treatment of osteomyelitis has been useful.

References

1. Arger, P.H., Coleman, B.G., and Dalinka, M.K.: Computed tomography in orthopedics. Orthop. Clin. North Am. 14, 217, 1983.
2. Armstrong, B. and Jarman, T.F.: A method of dealing with chronic osteomyelitis by saucerization followed by skin grafting. J. Bone Joint Surg. 18:387, 1936.
3. Baer, W.S.: The treatment of chronic osteomyelitis with the maggot. J. Bone Joint Surg. 13, 438, 1931.
4. Becker, R.O.: Electrical treatment of osteomyelitis. In, Evarts (Ed.) Surgery of the Musculo-Skeletal System. Churchill Livingston, 1983. pp. 197-208.

5. Brice, M. and Mialhe, C.: Les transferts osseux libres vascularisés (T.O.L.V.) en milieu infecté. Rev. Chir. Orthop. Rep. 68 (Suppl.II): 24, 1982.

6. Colchero, R.F.: Infecciones oseas. Tratamiento abierto con escarificaciones. In, Trans. VII International Trauma Symposium: Infecciones del apparato locomotor. d. Mapfre, Madrid, 1981, pp 341-360.

7. Hazlett, J.W.: The use of cancellous bone grafts in the treatment of subacute and chronic osteomyelitis. J. Bone Joint Surg. 36B, 584, 1954.

8. Goldstein, H.A.: Bone scintigraphy. Orthop. Clin. North Am. 14, 243, 1983.

9. Goldstein, H.I.: Maggots in the treatment of wound and bone infections. J. Bone Joint Surg. 13, 476, 1931.

10. Kelly, R.P.: Skin grafting in the treatment of osteomyelitic war-wounds J. Bone Joint Surg. 28, 681, 1946.

11. Orr, H.W.: Compound fractures. Am. J. Surg. 46, 733, 1939.

12. Papineau, L.J.: L'excision-greffe avec fermeture retardée délibérée dans l'ostéomyélite chronique. Nouv. Presse Méd. 2, 2753, 1973.

13. Papineau, L.J., Alfageme, A., Dalcourt, J.P., and Pilon, L.: Ostéomyélite chronique: excision et greffe de spongieux à l'air libre après mises à plat extensives. Int. Orthop. 3, 165, 1979.

14. Roy-Camille, R., Reignier, B., Berteaux, D., and Saillant, G.: Papineau-arthrodèse. Ann. orthop. l'Ouest 10, 120, 1978.

15. Shannon, J.G., and Woolhouse, F.M.: Treatment of chronic bone infection. J. Bone Joint Surg. 36A, 841, 1954.

16. Taylor, G.I. and Watson, N.: One stage repair of compound leg defects with free revascularized flap of skin and iliac bone. Plast. Reconst. Surg. 61, 494, 1978.

17. Vallières, B.J., Johnston, G.S., Jones, A.E. and Line, B.R.: Scintigraphie and citrate de gallium-67. Union Méd. Canada 106, 1382, 1977.

18. Vidal, J. et al.: Utilisation de la technique de Papineau dans le traitement des fractures ouvertes récentes avec perte de substance osseuse. Ann. Orthop. l'Ouest 10, 122, 1978.

19. Wilson, J.S., Korobkin, M., Genant, H.K., et al: Computed tomography of musculo-skeletal disorders. Am. J. Roentgenol. 131, 55, 1978.

Acute Suppurative Joint Infections in Children

J. J. WILEY and W. M. MCINTYRE

The capability of microbes to ravage a synovial joint is widely recognized. The patterns of infection, the character of the microbes, host reactions, and treatment modalities, however, have changed somewhat in recent decades.

This paper comprises a study of 110 consecutive cases of pediatric joint sepsis managed at the Children's Hospital of Eastern Ontario from 1974-1984.

Because of the variations of sepsis patterns in different age categories, the children in this series were divided into three age groups (Wiley and Fraser, 1979).

Group I (9 patients) birth to 6 months of age - As well as showing a low incidence of sepsis in infants, this group presented the most puzzling diagnostic problems, the most difficulties with management, and had the worst prognosis.

Group II (46 patients) 6 months to 4 years of age - Sixty percent of infections involved *Haemophilus influenzae* infections (Jackson and Nelson, 1982; Nelson, 1966; Wall and Hunt, 1968).

Group III (55 patients) 4 years to 16 years of age - This older group was more commonly infected by staphylococcal species. Perhaps because of injudicious antibiotic use before diagnosis, many of the patients present with atypical clinical profiles and few abnormal laboratory findings.

Joint Involvement (Table I)

Of the 117 joints affected, 89 (76%) involved the major weight-bearing joints. Hip joint involvement was surprisingly common in Group III, knee infections more common in Group II patients.

Pathogenesis

Sixty-two patients (56%) had a predisposing infection, most commonly a urinary tract or ear infection. Nine patients had a communicable disease (eg, meningitis) with accompanying septic arthritis. Five patients had infected skin lesions.

Twenty-three (30%) described contusions to the region of the affected joint, some sport-related, including skiing, skating, hockey, judo, baseball, tobogganing and sprinting.

Current Concepts of Infections in
Orthopaedic Surgery

Table I. Joint involvement - 117 joints in 110 patients

Joint (no.)	Age groups I 0 - 6 mo	II 6 mo - 4 yr	III 4 yr - 16 yr
Hip (43)	3	12	28
Knee (40)	4	22	14
Elbow (10)	2	5	3
Ankle (6)	1	4	1
Shoulder (5)	2	2	1
Sacroiliac (4)		1	3
Metatarsophalangeal (4)			4
Wrist (2)	1	1	
Proximal interphalangeal (1)			1
Interphalangeal (1)			1
Talonavicular (1)			1

In ten patients, joint sepsis followed a puncture wound, usually inflicted by a nail or glass fragment. One case of hip sepsis followed cardiac catheterization, a known complication of femoral artery or vein puncture (Chacha, 1971; Lunseth and Heiple, 1979). Two patients had postoperative wound infections involving joints, one following knee ligament reconstruction, the other complicating a hip pinning.

Clinical Presentations

The clinical presentation is dictated by many circumstances, most relevant being the anatomic location of the joint involved, eg, a concealed (hip) joint or an unconcealed (knee) joint. Infection in a concealed joint frequently presented in unusual fashion, hardly conforming to the textbook description of joint sepsis. In only a few patients could specific systemic signs or symptoms provide a reliable indication as to the seriousness of the problem. For example, 54% of the patients had temperature readings of 38.5°C (101.3°F) or over. However, 30% (33 patients) had temperature readings of 38°C or less (<100.4°F), hardly reflecting evidence of the serious infectious process.

Compounding the diagnostic problems was the misuse of antibiotics before diagnosis. Thirty-one patients received empirical antibiotic therapy, commonly an oral preparation, before the actual manifestation of joint sepsis. In spite of this therapy, a pathogen was cultured in 26 of these 31 patients either from the joint, blood or other sites. The cultured pathogen was sensitive to the administered drug in only 16 patients, and resistant in seven patients. Sensitivity testing was not performed in three instances. Appropriate therapy in these cases was dictated by positive Gram stain of the aspirate.

Five of these patients were hospitalized for treatment of an infectious disease (eg, meningitis) when the septic arthritic joint became manifest. In only one patient (ankle joint - Group B *Salmonella typhimurium*) was the pathogen cultured from the joint aspirate.

Thirty-eight patients presented with a septicemia (positive blood culture). In retrospect, the septicemia had little effect on the initial clinical presentation and minimal impact on initial laboratory investigation values. It can, however, yield valuable evidence as to the offending pathogen in many cases.

Other than the erythrocyte sedimentation rate (ESR), the usual hematologic screening determinations proved to be of confirmatory value only. The average leukocyte count was $12.7 \times 10^9/l$ (range $4.6\text{-}35.7 \times 10^9/l$). The average percentage of polymorphonuclear leukocytes in the differential count in all patient groups was 63.8%. The most relevant of all screening laboratory tests was the ESR, averaging 41.8 mm/h (range 10-68 mm/h). Although 94% of patients had an elevated ESR (above 20 mm/h), a normal sedimentation rate does not entirely rule out a septic process.

Diagnosis

A definitive diagnosis is confirmed by positive culture of the joint aspirate (Table II). In this series, the positive yield was 63% (72 positive joint cultures), this percentage comparing favorably with other studies (Fink et al, 1977; Nelson, 1972).

Table II. Joint culture - 63% positive yield (72 joints positive)

Microbiology (No. joints)	Group I 0 - 6 mo	Group II 6 mo - 4 yr	Group III 4 yr - 16 yr
Staphylococci (31)	5	3	23
Haemophilus influenzae (17)	2	15	
β-*hemolytic streptococcus* (7)	3	2	2
Streptococcus pneumoniae (5)	2	1	2
Pseudomonas species (3)			3
Enterococcus species (2)			2
Staphylococcus epidermidis (2)		1	1
Nisseria meningitidis (1)		1	
Nisseria gonorrhoeae (1)			1
Salmonella typhimurium (1)		1	
α-*hemolytic streptococcus* (1)		1	
Corynebacterium diphtheriae (1)			1

The most common infecting organism was *Staphylococcus aureus* in all age groups. As previously stated, the group II child is particularly susceptible to *H. influenzae* infection (Nelson and Koontz, 1966). This is thought to be due to the poor antibody response to capsular polysaccharides in this organism. Although adolescent venereal disease has received renewed attention in recent years, only one case of gonorrheal arthritis (hip joint) was encountered.

In the absence of a positive joint culture, diagnosis requires at least two of the following findings in the joint aspirates:

a) a grossly purulent appearance
b) organism identified on Gram stain
c) pus cells identified on Gram stain
d) a significant elevation of the leukocyte count.

If an aspirate is unobtainable (eg, sacroiliac joint sepsis), the diagnosis rests on the accumulated clinical evidence plus the signs of secondary bony involvement by radiographs.

Forty-two aspirates revealed organisms by Gram stain. Pus cells were quantified as "many" or "moderate" in most specimens. Leukocyte counts were performed on 47 aspirates, the counts ranging from $5.0 \times 10^9/l$ to $370 \times 10^9/l$ Thirty-three patients had cell counts above $50.0 \times 10^9/l$. The patient with the count of $5.0 \times 10^9/l$ had gram-positive cocci on the direct smear of the aspirate.

Radionuclide scanning was useful for investigation of suspected sepsis in concealed joints. Currently being studied is femoral head viability in the presence of sepsis using scanning techniques.

Treatment

Treatment goals include the control of the systemic disease, decompression of the affected joint, the expedient removal of the purulent effusion (Morrey et al, 1976), and the prevention of the destructive effects of pus on articular cartilage (Curtiss and Klein, 1965; Salter et al, 1981).

Following appropriate culturing, antibiotics were chosen by patient age groupings and the suspected pathogens (Nade, 1983). Ampicillin and a cephalosporin provided an effective therapeutic combination for hematogenous types of joint sepsis. Suspected *Pseudomonas aeruginosa* infections associated with puncture wounds (Chusid et al, 1979) were managed with gentamicin or tobramycin. The definitive antibiotic selection was eventually dictated by culture sensitivity, respecting the appearance of mutant pathogens and the penetration of the drug. The administration routes included intravenous therapy followed sequentially by oral antibiotics, the intervals related to effective therapeutic serum concentrations and patient response (Nelson et al, 1982).

Local treatment modes were determined by joint accessibility, the response to initial therapy and the particular pathogen. Aspiration or repeated aspirations were the sole method of local treatment of 53 joints (47.7%). Most of these joints were readily accessible and easily observed. On the contrary, five septic hip joints were managed by aspiration alone. One of these, a neonate, had a poor result with this management regimen. Following aspiration, joints were irrigated with Ringer's solution. Because of equivalent serum-joint antibiotic concentration, joint instillation of antibiotics was not indicated.

Arthrotomy with drainage, particularly for concealed joints, is the most reliable method of management (Paterson, 1970). Drainage by closed suction irrigation was used for 54 joints. Four patients had an arthrotomy with open (Penrose drain) drainage. Six patients had no surgical procedure: three with sacroiliac joint involvement, two late diagnosed cases (ankle and shoulder) in neonates with polyarticular involvement, and an open bite injury of the proximal interphalangeal joint of a finger.

Results

In all patients the septic process was eventually eradicated. Seven (5.5%) joints had sufficient residual damage to result in permanent disability

(Table III), all encountered during the first five years of this study. No poor results have been encountered since. This improvement is thought attributable to a more aggressive local treatment approach, a more intelligent use of antibiotic therapy, and careful scrutiny of patient compliance (Howard et al, 1976).

Table III. Permanent disability after joint sepsis

Joint involved (No.)	Microbe	Joint destruction
Metatarsophalangeal (1)	*Pseudomonas*	Epiphyseal plate destroyed
Hip (4)	*Staphylococcus*	Dislocation
	Staphylococcus	Avascular necrotic-arthritic
	Staphylococcus	Fibrous ankylosis
	H. influenzae	Avascular necrotic-arthritic
Knee (1)	*Pseudomonas*	Fibrous ankylosis
Shoulder (1)	*Staphylococcus*	Fibrous ankylosis

Fifteen (13.6%) patients had residual joint effects as manifested by radiographic changes only. Most of these demonstrated evidence of a healed focus of osteomyelitis adjacent to the affected joint. Two patients demonstrated transient narrowing of the hip joint, but no permanent effect was subsequently noted.

Conclusion

There is a definite age-related pattern to septic joints, the most typical being those related to *H. influenzae* infections.

The perpetual availability of new and different antibiotics is reflected in the rapid emergence of new and resistant pathogenic mutants.

The early diagnosis and removal of pus from an infected joint is mandatory.

Hip joint sepsis continues to be a major problem, not only because of difficulties in diagnosis and management, but the disasters associated with a poor result. Arthrotomy with drainage is the recommended treatment for hip joint sepsis.

References

1. Chacha, P.B.: Suppurative arthritis of the hip joint in infancy. J. Bone Joint Surg. 53A, 538, 1971.
2. Chusid, M.J., Jacobs, W.M., and Sty, J.R.: Pseudomonas arthritis following puncture wounds of the foot. J. Pediat. 94, 429, 1979.
3. Curtiss, P.H. and Klein, L.: Destruction of articular cartilage in septic arthritis: II, *In vivo* studies. J. Bone Joint Surg. 47A, 1595, 1965.

4. Fink, C.W., Dich, V.Q., Howard, J., Jr., and Nelson, J.D.: Infections of bones and joints in children. Arthrit. Rheum. 20 (Suppl.), 578, 1977.

5. Howard, J.B., Higgenboten, C.L., and Nelson, J.D.: Residual effects of septic arthritis in infancy and childhood. J.A.M.A. 236, 932, 1976.

6. Jackson, M.A. and Nelson, J.D.: Etiology and medical management of acute suppurative bone and joint infections in pediatric patients. J. Pediat. Orthop. 2, 313, 1982.

7. Lunseth, P.A. and Heiple, K.G.: Prognosis in septic arthritis of the hip in children. Clin. Orthop. Rel. Res. 139, 81, 1979.

8. Morrey, B.F., Bianco, A.J., and Rhodes, K.H.: Suppurative arthritis of the hip in children. J. Bone Joint Surg. 58A, 388, 1976.

9. Nade, S.: Acute septic arthritis in infancy and childhood. J. Bone Joint Surg. 65B, 234, 1983.

10. Nelson, J.D. and Koontz, W.C.: Septic arthritis in infants and children: A review of 117 cases. Pediat. 38, 966, 1966.

11. Nelson, J.D.: The bacterial etiology and antibiotic management of septic arthritis in infants and children. Pediat. 50, 437, 1972.

12. Nelson, J.D., Bucholz, R.W., Kusmiesz, H., and Shalton, S.: Benefits and risks of sequential parenteral-oral cephalosporin therapy for suppurative bone and joint infections. J. Pediat. Orthop. 2, 255, 1982.

13. Paterson, D.C.: Acute suppurative arthritis in infancy and childhood. J. Bone Joint Surg. 52B, 474, 1970.

14. Salter, R.B., Bell, R.S., and Keeley, F.W.: The protective effect of continuous passive motion on living articular cartilage in acute septic arthritis. Clin. Orthop. Rel. Res. 159, 223, 1981.

15. Wall, J.J. and Hunt, D.D.: Acute hematogenous pyarthrosis caused by *Haemophilus influenzae*. J. Bone Joint Surg. 50A, 1657, 1968.

16. Wiley, J.J. and Fraser, G.: Septic arthritis in childhood. Canad. J. Surg. 22, 326, 1979.

Current Concepts in the Management of Infected Fractures

R. B. Gustilo

Our concepts in the management of infected fractures have changed during the last ten years. Handling severe open fractures resulting in a high rate of sepsis has provided us with ample experience in the treatment of infected fractures. Wound sepsis in the Type III open fractures varies from 10-50%.

We are grateful to Louis Pasteur for his sound principle which one can apply to the management of infected fractures. "A germ is nothing. It is the terrain or the environment in which the germ grows that is everything."

The second corollary to this principle is that fracture healing can occur in spite of bone infection, provided we decrease the activity of the microorganisms and there is a viable vascular environment at the fracture site.

One must make an early diagnosis and institute immediate, effective treatment. (Table I)

Table I. Principles of treatment of infected fractures

Problems

1) Eradication of infection in both soft tissue and bone
2) Wound coverage
3) Fracture healing

Treatment

1) Radical debridement of necrotic infected tissues
2) Effective antibiotic therapy
3) Secure fracture stability
4) Leaving the wound open
5) Cancellous bone grafting over early or fully developed granulation tissue
6) Appropriate wound closure

The problem of wound coverage falls into four categories in the treatment of infected fractures.

A. Infected fractures with adequate bone and soft tissue coverage

Case 1. Patient had an infected Type III open fracture due to polytrauma for which a plate was applied with delayed closure. Eight weeks later, the

Current Concepts of Infections in
Orthopaedic Surgery

patient returned with an obviously infected wound. He was immediately taken to the operating room, the wound was debrided, and culture for both aerobic and anaerobic organisms was taken from the depth of the wound. At the time of debridement, the internal fixation was stable and the screws were firm. The fracture was not completely healed; the plate was therefore left in place and the wound packed open. The patient was given intravenous oxacillin, 2 g q 6 h for four weeks for coagulase-positive *Staphylococcus*. The wound gradually closed by secondary intention. Six weeks after discharge, the wound had completely healed and the functional result was good.

Case 2. This patient, visiting Minnesota during one winter season, was struck by a car and suffered a closed femoral fracture. Fifteen years before he had had a femoral fracture which was plated, had become infected, and the plate was removed. The patient had not had any drainage for the last 13 years. This time the patient was placed in traction because of the deformed shape of the healed femur. After five days the patient developed a high fever of 103° with a wbc of 20,000. When we aspirated the fracture hematoma, we found purulent material. The patient was brought immediately to the operating room where the wound was opened, debrided, and the pus at and around the fracture site was completely evacuated. The contraindications to an internal fixation at that time were the florid infection and severe systemic symptoms.

In this particular case, a temporary measure of skeletal traction at the proximal tibia was indicated until the acute symptoms subsided. The patient was returned to the operating room on the second and fourth days for repeat debridement. Cultures grew coagulase-positive staphylococci sensitive to cephalosporins. He was given cefazolin, 1 g, intravenously, q 6 h, for four weeks. On the fifth day, the wound looked clean with early granulation tissue and the fracture was stabilized by plating. The wound was left open, followed three days later by cancellous bone grafting. Four weeks later, the wound was almost closed and the patient was sent home. At 20 months, the fracture had completely healed without sepsis and the function of the extremity was good.

Case 3. A patient came to us from Michigan with an infected femoral shaft fracture. Nine months earlier, the patient had an elective plating of a closed femoral shaft fracture which subsequently became infected. The loose plate and screws had been removed as this fixation was not providing any stability. Fracture stability was then secured by applying a Fischer-Hoffmann External Fixator. The wound was irrigated and debrided daily. The sites around the pins, however, became infected and the pins loosened, at which time the patient was sent to us for treatment. On admission, the three proximal pins were loose with obvious pus formation around the sites; the bone was exposed and the ununited fracture was evident. The patient was first placed temporarily in skeletal traction. The wounds were debrided several times in the operating room and they eventually started to granulate. For stability, the patient was returned to the operating room for intramedullary nailing with reaming, the wound being left open. Cancellous bone grafting was done two weeks later and the wound left to heal by secondary intention. Recently, the roentgenographs sent to us from Michigan showed that the fracture had completely healed. There is still minimal drainage, but the patient has returned to work.

Case 4. This patient had a Type III open fracture, treated with delayed intramedullary nailing two weeks after the injury. The patient returned three months later with a swollen thigh, pain, and high fever. The nail was removed as it was loose and an external fixator was applied for stability. Cancellous bone grafting was done two weeks later to fill the gap. The problem with external fixation of the femur is a high incidence of sepsis at the pin sites, causing loosening. The fixator was removed and the femur debrided. Again, to obtain stability, the patient was returned to the operating room and the femur was plated. The wound was secondarily closed five days later with a suction device in place. At two years follow-up, the fracture was completely healed but the leg was two inches short.

Case 5. This patient was a schoolteacher who was sent to us for a femoral fracture after two years of repeated debridement, irrigation, skeletal traction, spica cast and hospitalization for 20 out of 24 months. I believe that everything was done correctly except that stability was not achieved completely. A sinogram was done to determine the extent of the sinus tract. The entire proximal femur was very osteoporotic. The patient was taken to the operating room, the wound completely debrided, irrigated, and left open. After the fourth debridement, the fracture was stabilized with a Zickel nail and cancellous bone graft was done 48 hours later with closure over suction.

The success of the Papineau procedure, as in this case, depends on radical excision of infected tissue and bone. When granulation tissue developed, massive cancellous grafting was done with daily lavage and avoidance of weight bearing until the fracture was healed. This patient was given parenteral antibiotics for four weeks. At six months, the fracture was completely healed. At 19 months, after hospital discharge, the fracture remains healed without drainage and with good function, but a residual 3/4 shortening of the femur.

The principles in these cases of adequate repeated surgical debridement, securing fracture stability, antibiotic therapy, leaving the wound open, and cancellous bone grafting over granulation are important in dealing successfully with infected nonunion.

B. Infected fracture with inadequate soft tissue coverage and without bone loss

Case 6. This report concerns a malunion of a tibia where we did an open nailing to correct the malunion. At the end of three months, the patient returned with an obviously infected wound. The wound was opened, thoroughly debrided, and irrigated. The nail was removed. Stability was secured with external fixation. There was not enough soft tissue coverage over the exposed bone. The wound was treated locally by irrigation and wet dressing 3-4 times daily. The cavity was packed with cancellous bone over healthy granulation tissue three weeks later. Several weeks later, split thickness skin graft was done. At 16 months after the Papineau procedure, the fracture was completely healed with good bone coverage and the patient returned to normal activity.

C. Infected fracture with inadequate soft tissue coverage and loss of bone continuity or partial defect

Case 7. This situation presents two problems: inadequate soft tissue coverage and bone loss. The patient had a Type III segmental fracture that became infected in spite of repeated adequate debridement and irrigation, and massive antibiotic therapy. The wound became infected with *Pseudomonas aeruginosa*. Eight inches of bone was left exposed, and only a narrow cortical bone in the midportion of the tibia remained. We achieved stability by applying pins and plaster, followed by repeated debridement and irrigation and repeated split thickness skin graft. Daily cleansing of the wound in the room was done over the bone until good coverage of the entire wound was obtained, when a circular cast was applied. We were planning at that time to have the patient return at a later date for cancellous bone grafting. To our surprise, however, at 11 months after the fracture, we observed abundant callus formation. There must be a periosteal envelope left posteriorly to initiate bone formation. After ten years, one can see that the entire bone has reconstituted without bone grafting and the patient has relatively good function.

Case 8. We had a second patient with an infected fracture following plating. I am convinced that when dealing with an infection in the presence of a loose plate we could save time by removing the plate early and by installing an external fixator. This was done in this case, and the dead bone at the fracture site was removed leaving a gap. After good granulation tissue had developed, massive cancellous bone grafting and repeated split thickness skin grafting were carried out. This is an area where the muscle flap transfer, such as the gastrocnemius or the gastrocsoleus, would have been applicable except for the fact that these muscles were debrided during the initial injury. After having removed the fixator, we were still left with a nonunion but a healed wound without sepsis. A closed tibia nailing with reaming was done with eventual complete healing of the fracture.

D. Infected fracture with exposed metal.

In our institution, we have sent patients home with exposed metal and have not encountered any particular problems. We simply instruct the patient on how to clean the wound and metal three to four times daily.

Case 9. This was a patient with a Type III-B tibia fracture. He had a massive soft tissue injury and plating was done to secure stability. The patient was sent home with instructions on how to irrigate the wound on a daily basis. The patient returned six weeks later with a loose plate which was removed at that time. In seven to ten days, good granulation tissue developed and split thickness skin graft was done. Cancellous bone grafting was performed in the lower part of the leg where bone was still exposed Fracture stability was achieved by applying a half pin external fixator.

The incidence of chronic osteomyelitis in infected Type III open fractures is only 2.2% in spite of a high incidence of wound sepsis of 24% (1975-1979 study). Our success with Papineau procedures is about 89% at one year follow-up.

Summary

In spite of the high incidence of sepsis in Type III open fractures, one must learn how to deal effectively with infected fractures by aggressive surgical debridement and repeated debridement of infected wounds, and by achieving stability of the fracture, leaving the wound open. For stabilization of an infected femur, our choices would be:

1) Plate
2) Intramedullary nail
3) External fixator

For the tibia:

1) External fixator, including tibiofibular synostosis if required
2) Plate
3) Intramedullary nail

Parenteral antibiotics are administered for 4 to 6 weeks. There is no question of the importance of antibiotics as adjuncts to the surgical procedure. They should be administered from 2 to 6 weeks, depending on whether one is confronted with an acute or chronic wound infection. Exposed bone or metal is not an indication for continuing antibiotic therapy. One cannot sterilize an open wound indefinitely. We further recommend performing cancellous bone grafting over a granulating wound (Papineau procedure) and appropriate and timely wound closure.

Infected Pseudarthrosis - Treat the Infection First

A. HÄRLE

Infected pseudarthrosis represents a combination of problems due to various and mostly serious pathologic conditions that act in a vicious circle. Functional and permanent healing can hardly be achieved without controlling all aspects (Waldvogel and Vasey, 1980). To escape this dilemma, a secondary healing with the development of chronic osteomyelitis is often accepted or amputation is even suggested as an unavoidable final solution.

The pathogenesis of infected pseudarthrosis is mostly generated by two or three factors, singly or concurrently: infection, soft tissue damage, and instability of bone fragments (Table I).

Table I. Pathogenesis of infected pseudarthrosis

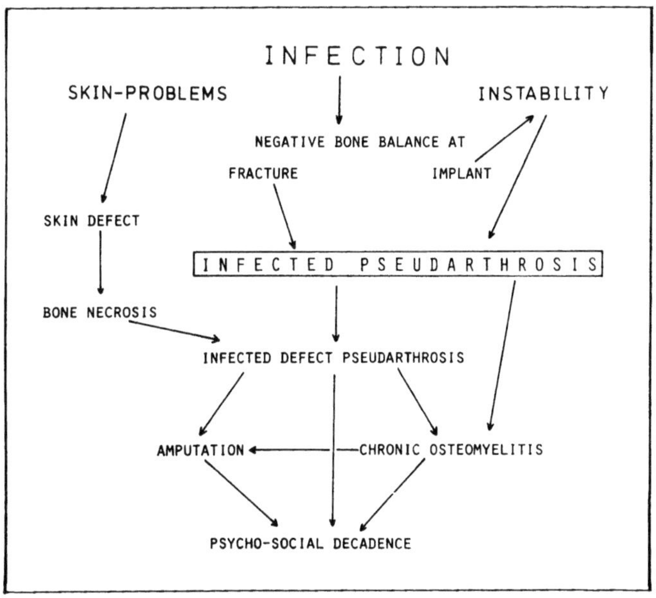

In our view, the infection is of primary importance; bone instability does not initiate this disease. The instability is a consequence rather than the origin of bone infection, which may lead to a negative bone balance. If the instability was not already established, it can be caused or augmented secondarily by an infection-related bone resorption in the vicinity of implant material or at the fracture site.

Current Concepts of Infections in
Orthopaedic Surgery

In planning the course of treatment, the pathogenesis has to be taken into account. As it is often impossible to do all in one operation, a stepwise treatment narrowing down the disease to less complex conditions is indicated. The sequence of the treatment steps should be developed logically based on the pathogenic conditions, and the infection should be eliminated first. We therefore divide the therapy of infected pseudarthrosis into three stages as shown in Table II.

Table II. Stages in treatment of infected pseudarthrosis

Stage 1	Elimination of bone and soft tissue infections with temporary wound coverage.
Stage 2	Establishing a functional and durable soft tissue coverage.
Stage 3	Osseous consolidation by autologous bone grafting and definite fixation of bone fragments.

In stage 1, a careful debridement of the wound is carried out with the removal of all bone fragments that are loose, avital, or surrounded by a pyogenous membrane. The cortical part of long bones is saved as much as possible. The medullary canal within the area of the pseudarthrosis, however, is opened and reamed. Areas of inflamed cancellous bone are also removed as much as possible. In cases where the medullary cavity cannot be reached through the gap of the pseudarthrosis, we cut a lateral cortical window suitable for reaming. Intramedullary sclerotic areas are removed under direct vision. The cortical bone is thinned down to a thickness less than 5 mm with a burr and flexible reamers. Subperiosteal bone exposure should be limited to reduce possible interference with blood supply. The edges of the pseudarthrosis are cleaned carefully and inspected. The completion of medullary reaming is checked by an Ossoscope®. This easy-to-handle optical aid permits a true color and topographic assessment of the canal of long bones for a distance about 25 cm in looking around the corner by means of a cold light mirror (Fig. 1). Inflamed bone tissue, diagnosed by its dark red color that cannot be rinsed off, requires precise excision. If possible, the surgery is done under a tourniquet to obtain a true color assessment and to avoid major blood losses.

The debridement completed, the medullary cavity is packed with Septopal® chains, providing a high local concentration of gentamicin in the infected tissue (Klemm, 1979). To avoid knotting of the chains, we insert them in a spiral-like manner. In view of the low gentamicin diffusion rate of about 1 cm from the beads' surface, a complete filling of the cavity is absolutely necessary (Härle, 1981). Additional Septopal chains are applied within the area of both cortical and soft tissue defects. This allows a levelling for wound closure and avoids crater formation. If primary wound closure is impossible, we use Epigard® (Bohmert et al, 1974) for cover as an interim solution. This synthetic skin is sutured to the wound edges, covering the defect like a tailor-made closure. A description of this technique follows.

Wound drainage plays an important role in these procedures. If primary wound closure is possible, we apply a passive drainage for 24 hours, fol-

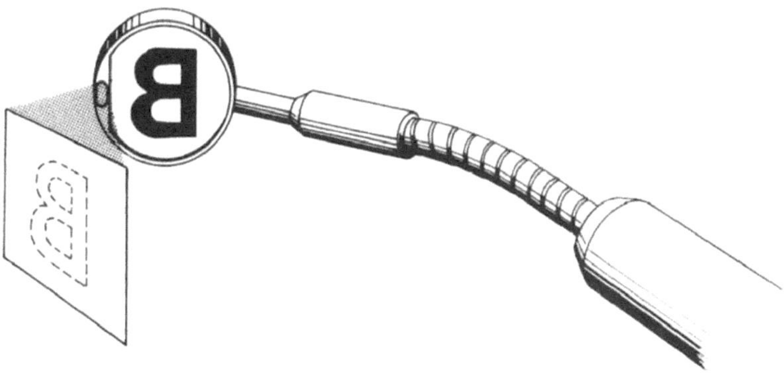

Fig. 1. By means of the cold-light mirror, sections can be assessed which was formerly not possible. This example shows the letter B on the reverse side

lowed by a high vacuum suction drainage (Redon, 1955) aiming at three goals as outlined in Table III. However, in cases of Epigard coverage of the wound, a passive drainage is applied all the time since the artificial skin is permeable to air.

Table III. Goals of high vacuum drainage in treatment of infections

1) No secretion through the wound; otherwise, this would always risk retrograde bacterial contamination.

2) The strong action of high negative pressure approximates the soft tissues close to the gentamicin containing beads, thus reducing the diffusion distance.

3) By the strong vacuum a stabilization of the wound area is achieved comparable to osteosynthesis, thus promoting fast wound healing.

In cases where stage 2 of our treatment principles cannot be completed during the first surgical procedure, adequate soft tissue grafts and procedures have to be applied (Stern et al, 1983). The techniques we use are summarized in Table IV. In our view, only after completion of stage 2 should the autologous bone graft be done. Our aim is not only a stable bone consolidation but also healing of the pseudarthrosis without overt or dormant bone infection. To reach this goal, a prerequisite is a sterile graft bed and avoidance of reinfection via open or secondary healing of soft tissue wounds.

Another aim is to give reconstructed bone defects the best biomechanical properties. This means for long bones to reach the architectural principles of tubes with a differentiation into cortical bone and medullary cav-

Table IV. Reconstruction of skin defects

Local rotational flaps
Skin-mobilization with multiple skin incisions
Myocutaneous gastrocnemius flap
Fasciocutaneous flaps
Contralateral myocutaneous gastrocnemius flap
Vascularized dorsalis pedis flap
Tumbler flap

ity. In stage 3, we therefore reconstruct bone defects using thin, plate-like corticocancellous splints from the iliac crest. The cavity is filled with small cancellous chips for quicker revitalization of the cortical elements. Consequently, during debridement, we are particularly carful when resecting cortical segments.

The stabilization of bone fragments using osteosynthetic material has, in our opinion, no positive influence on the control of the infection. Plates and nails are always to be removed in cases of well established infected pseudarthroses. Certain factors guide us to decide whether immobilization of the fragments by external fixator is indicated during the first operation. If a residual stability is provided by soft tissues and/or the fibula, we decide against external fixation. Likewise, when extensive soft tissue grafts are necessary we avoid an early application of external fixators whenever possible. Instead, we apply plaster of Paris in the presence of instability since an early use of the external fixator interferes with the removal of Septopal chains due to the perforating pins.

After the infection has cleared up, reosteosynthesis may be carried out simultaneously with bone grafting. Our criteria for this step are undisturbed, primary wound healing and normalization of the erythrocyte sedimentation rate (ESR). In the course of aseptic wound healing, the ESR values increase quickly during days 2-5 postoperatively. From days 5-8 on, a normalization in a straight line is observed using a semilogarithmic graph (Härle, 1978; Fig. 2). ESR courses different from that indicate persistence of infection. In such cases we carry out a surgical revision even when there are no signs of inflammation on the wound surface.

Stabilization of bone fragments in stage 3 is done on the arm and lower leg using the external fixator. For the upper leg a replating is applied with special osteosynthesis plates containing Septopal particles providing a very high gentamicin concentration in the vicinity of the implant.

The following case reports will demonstrate our treatment principles.

Case 1.

A 56-year old man was transferred to our hospital with a draining pseudarthrosis nine months after a proximal tibial varus osteotomy. During the first surgical procedure, we removed all implant material. At the level of

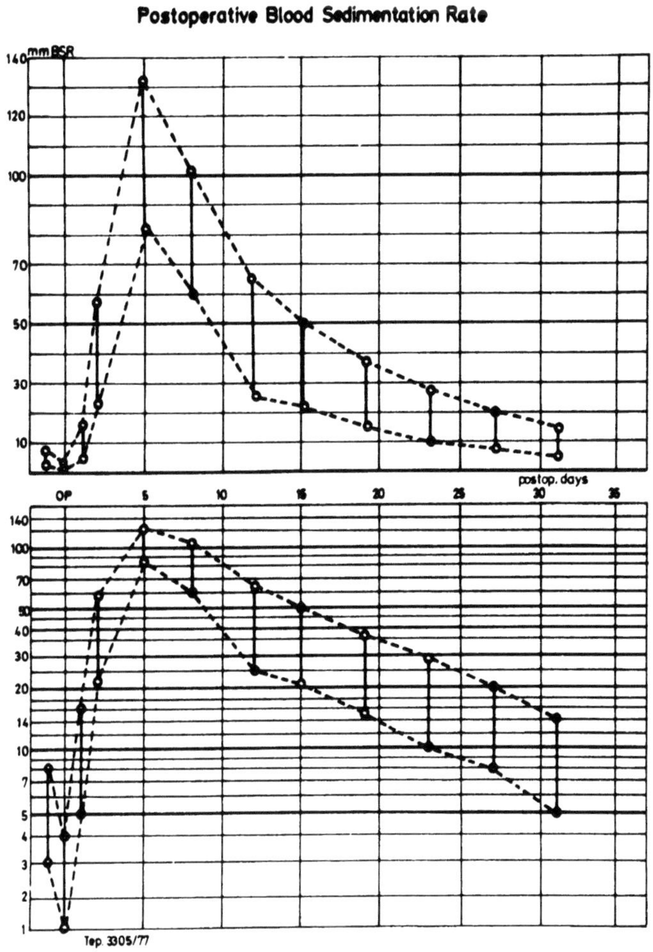

Fig. 2. The ESR rises quickly during the first postoperative days, reaches a peak about the 6th day and decreases progressively. By a semilogarithmic graph, this decrease is to be transformed in a straight line course as demonstrated on the lower part of the figure

nonunion, the tibia was fenestrated and the inflamed cancellous bone was removed from both fragments. We filled the defect with Septopal chains. Immobilization was achieved using a plaster of Paris. Three weeks later, after normalization of ESR, we removed the chains and made a fibular osteotomy, grafting with corticocancellous chips from the iliac crest and compression of the pseudarthrosis by external fixator. Four months later, a stable union was achieved and the fixator could be removed. The patient had already been partially weight bearing during the past six weeks. Further follow-up showed an increasing consolidation of the former pseudarthrosis, ready for full weight bearing and a subsequent remodelling of the cortical and cancellous bone (Fig. 3).

Case 2.

In a 30-year old man, eight operations had led to a distal infected defect pseudarthrosis and severe soft tissue damage with draining sinuses. Since an amputation was suggested, the patient came to our hospital. From an anterolateral approach we removed all bone sequestrae, reamed the medullary canal proximally and distally, and applied Septopal chains. The medial

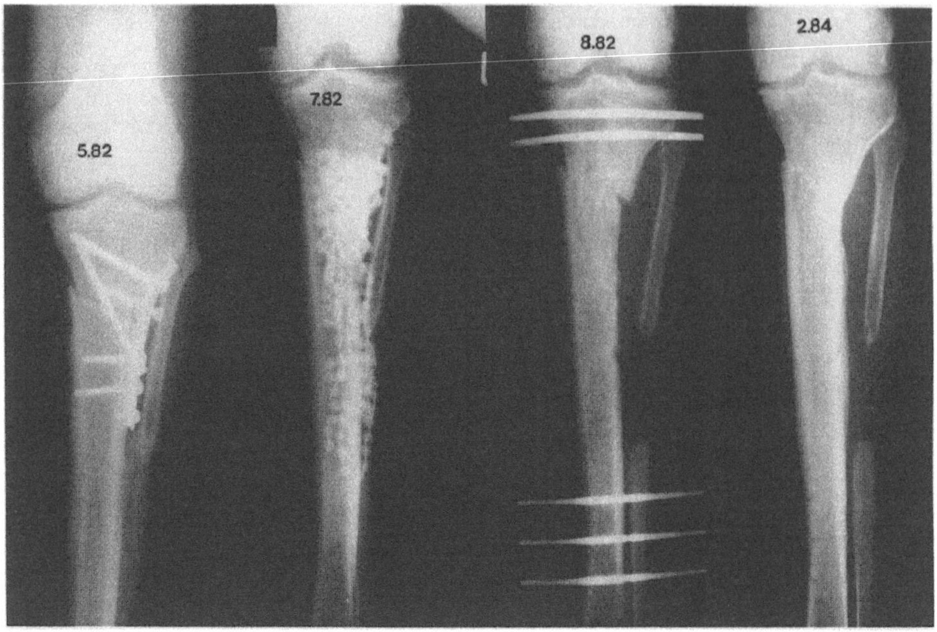

Fig. 3. Infected tibial pseudarthrosis after varus osteotomy. After debride ment, insertion of Septopal chains for infection control. The bone transpla tation and external fixator stabilization produced a stress-resistant consolidation

fistulae were debrided and minichains inserted. After stabilization of the soft tissue conditions and normalization of the ESR, the Septopal chains were removed; 2.5 cm long blocks of corticocancellous bone from the iliac crest were then inserted into the defect for the reconstruction of the medullary canal, and an external fixator was applied. During the course of four months, ossification of the defect pseudarthrosis was observed (Fig. 4) We left the fixation for a total of six months, allowing partial weight bearing in the last four weeks. Further follow-up showed good integration of the bone grafts.

Case 3.

A 22-year old man had a motorcycle accident that had caused severe soft tissue contusion of the lower leg and tibial fracture. Seven months later he was admitted to our hospital for amputation of the lower leg. The previous 13 operations had led to a very large ventral soft tissue and tibial defect. After thorough debridement, we covered the large soft tissue defect with Epigard for control of the infection. A fast abatement of the inflammation was observed. Nevertheless, it took 4-1/2 months to obtain sufficient soft tissue coverage. This was possible by the combined use of a Tumbler (Stenström, 1976) and of a medial gastrocnemius flap (Mathes et al, 1974). Bridging of the 13 cm long bone defect was achieved by using corticocancellous chips from the iliac crest and an internal splinting with the contralateral fibula (Fig. 5). Despite the atrophic tibial bone, good stability was obtained because the pins of the external fixator were guided through the fibular bone graft. Half a year later, when the fibula seemed

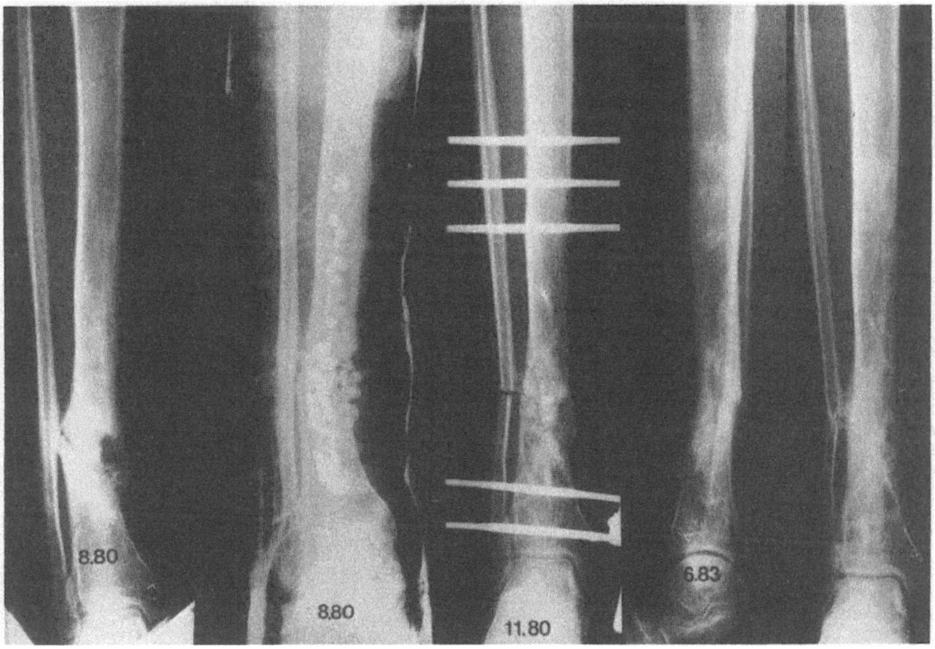

Fig. 4. This infected distal tibial pseudarthrosis was first treated by Septopal insertion. Afterwards, solid iliac crest chips were interposed that became completely integrated

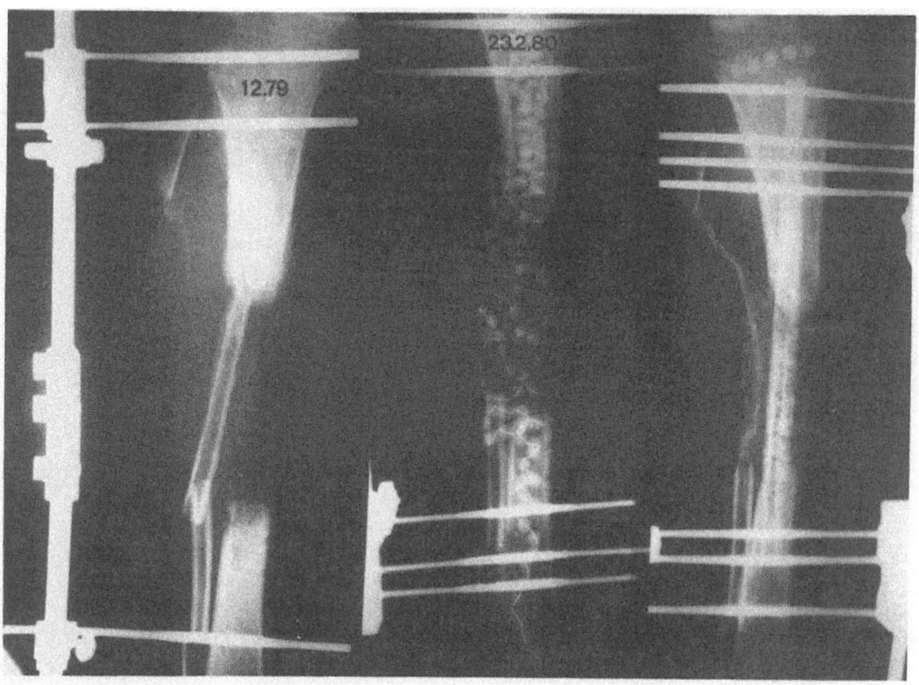

Fig. 5. This extensive bone and soft tissue infection could be controlled by Septopal insertion. For bony bridging we transplanted the contralateral fibula with iliac crest chips

to have consolidated proximally and distally, the patient fell through a glass door and fractured the implanted fibula. An additional bone grafting had no effect on the consolidation of the pseudarthrosis. As the patient did not accept the external fixator any longer, we stabilized dorsally with a plate containing Septopal particles and made a third bone grafting. Twelve weeks later, the patient was allowed to bear partial weight with the aid of a brace. In the following four months, a bony consolidation could be seen and the union improved further in time (Fig. 6).

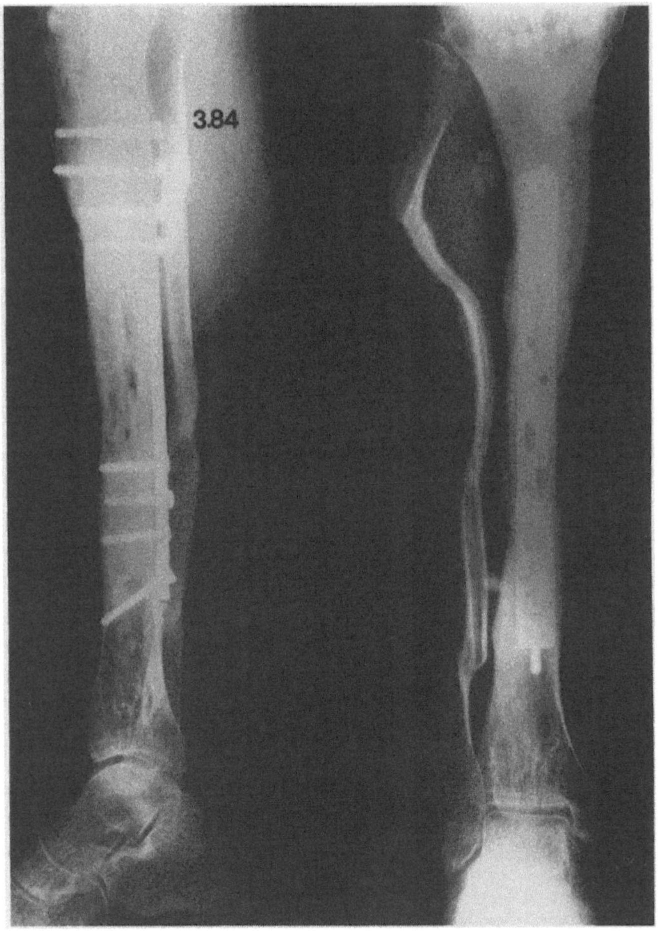

Fig. 6. Because of the pseudarthrosis in the transplanted fibular se ment, a dorsal stabilization was performed by an osteosynthesis plate containing Septopal particles

During the past six years, we have treated in this way 40 infected pseudarthroses, mostly with defects of either the soft tissues or the bones or both. The first step in the course of treatment was always the Septopal application for the elimination of infection subsequent to surgical debridement. In two patients, a relapse of the bone infection occurred during the osseous consolidation period. A further surgical intervention led to definite elimination of infection in these patients as well. Bony consolidation was achieved in all patients, although two have not achieved full weight bearing (Table V).

Table V. Treatment of infected pseudarthrosis (n = 40)

Recurrence of infection during treatment	2	5%
Infection controlled primarily or secondarily	40	100%
Refractures during treatment	2	5%
Bony consolidation of nonunions and refractures	40	100%
Full weight bearing	38	95%
Stress fracture after consolidation	1	2.5%

The osseous consolidation showed, usually after two years, a differentiation between cortical bone and medullary cavity, ie, long bones with good biomechanical properties. In this group of patients, we had two refractures during treatment. In one patient, an asymmetric support of the tibial axis led to increased remodelling and weakening of bone. This was treated again by cancellous bone grafting with subsequent medial plating. Up to now, we have had no recurrence of infection when bone consolidation has occurred, and amputation could be avoided also in very severe cases with extensive soft and bony tissue defects.

Our therapeutic concept concentrates on controlling the infection as the first step of treatment. In our view, this procedure is at least equally effective if not superior with respect to duration of treatment and rate of success compared with other therapeutic regimens.

I therefore conclude by reiterating our basic concept: Treat the infection first and assure its permanent control.

References

1. Bohmert, H., Petzold, D., Schmidtler, F., Simon, R., and Schleuter, B.: Experimentelle und klinische Testung von Polyurethanschaumstoff (EPIGARD) bei Verbrennungen. Langenb. Arch. Suppl. Chir. Forum, 1974, pp 257-259.
2. Härle, A.: Die Bedeutung des postoperativen Verlaufes der Blutsenkungsgeschwindigkeit. Orthop. Praxis 15, 695, 1979.
3. Härle, A.: Treatment of haematogenous osteomyelitis in children by application of gentamicin-PMMA beads. In, Rens, Th.J.G. and Kayser, F.: Local Antibiotic Treatment in Osteomyelitis and Soft Tissue Infections, Int. Congr. Series No. 556, Excerpta Medica Amsterdam, 1981, pp 62-81.
4. Klemm, K.: Indikation und Technik zur Einlage von Gentamicin-PMMA-Kugeln bei Knochen- und Weichteilinfektionen. Aktuel, Probl. Chir. Orthop. 12, 121, 1979.
5. Mathes, S., McCraw, J.B., and Vasconez, L.D.: Muscle transposition flaps for coverage of lower extremity defects. Surg. Clin. North Amer. 54, 1337, 1974.
6. Redon, H.: La fermature sous dépression des plaies étendues. Presse Méd. 63, 1034, 1955.

7. Stenström, S.J.: The tumbler flap. Chir. plastica 3, 211, 1976.

8. Stern, P.J., Neale, H.W., Gregory, R.O., and McDonough, J.J.: Functional reconstruction of an extremity by free tissue transfer of the latissimus dorsi. J. Bone Joint Surg. 65A, 729, 1983.

9. Waldvogel, F.A. and Vasey, H.: Osteomyelitis: The past decade. New Engl. J. Med. 303, 360, 1980.

Infection in Total Joint Replacement: One-Stage Exchange Arthroplasty

H. W. BUCHHOLZ

The title "one-stage exchange arthroplasty" refers to an operation for deep infection in which a meticulous excision of necrotic and infected tissue is performed together with removal of the implant and all cement, following which a new implant is inserted. A review of 583 deep infections so treated was published by Buchholz et al in 1981, but a further review was made in 1983 of a more selected group of these patients and these results are submitted later in this paper.

In general, it is accepted that for the management of chronic deep infection a total excision is necessary, but much discussion continues as to the wisdom of proceeding to immediate reinsertion. In Europe, there has been increasing acceptance of the one-stage exchange procedure but in North America a more cautious approach has been adopted, largely, I suspect, because of the unavailability of antibiotic-loaded cement. A planned two-stage procedure is therefore commonly advocated. It is generally agreed that an excision arthroplasty while usually controlling the infective process yields poor functional results.

At the present time, I firmly believe that a one-stage exchange is most advantageous but it depends for its success on the use of heavily antibiotic-loaded acrylic cement. This has the obvious advantage of sparing the patient a second procedure. I admit that, in some instances, a two-stage plan would give a surer long-term result, but I find that such cases are rare. It is usually impossible to predict which one-stage operations are going to fail and, in view of the relative infrequency of failure, an unnecessary number of patients would be subjected to two major procedures if a two-stage operation were advocated routinely.

During the years of experience which have led to my current view, one of the problems has been the evaluation of the increasingly severe cases which have been referred to us. We have felt it necessary to increase the amount of antibiotic and the mixtures, causing us to vary the technique we have employed. Nevertheless, the relatively large numbers of patients so treated successfully compensates for the variations within the series. We have been perfectly aware of the potential dangers of crude mixing of various combinations of antibiotics in the operating theatre. The mixing process cannot compare with that offered by commercial preparations. Certainly, cement strength characteristics are altered and the cement is weaker. This, together with the impaired bone bed, all contribute to the likelihood of subsequent mechanical failure. Surprising as it may seem, mechanical failure has not occurred as much as one would expect. In fact, we see no difference in the rate of mechanical failure compared with that for operations performed for sterile mechanical loosening. Radiolucent lines occur in

Current Concepts of Infections in
Orthopaedic Surgery

each with about the same frequency. It seems that our follow-up is now sufficiently long to be confident that we can use cement in this way without evidence of subsequent mechanical failure. Obviously it is not an ideal method, but the overriding considerations are the control of infection and the avoidance of two major operations.

Our experience now includes management of 1,386 infected implants; 329 were our own patients and 1,057 were referrals. To obtain a minimum follow-up of two years, 869 one-stage exchange procedures performed between 1972 and 1981 were reviewed in 1983. Patients who died or were lost to follow-up after one year have been included because an actuarial assessment method of presentation has been used (Buchholz et al, 1984). Failure has been defined as recurrence of infection or mechanical loosening. The time from operation to failure or last follow-up when nonfailure was confirmed was recorded for each patient. From these data, life tables were constructed which can be presented graphically. (In future, we intend presenting all our results in this manner.)

Surgical Technique

In the space available only a few general recommendations can be made. A wide range of implants should be available and a large model not only helps to reduce the likelihood of subluxation but also to fill dead space.

The surgical approach should give full access to the field. If a trochanteric osteotomy is performed, section of the bone should not separate a large fragment because of the risk of devascularization. Complete excision of the capsule and related scar tissue must be performed. It may be difficult to decide on the extent of bone resection but, on balance, it is better to preserve bone whenever possible in the knowledge that it will be permeated by adequate antibiotic concentrations with the use of antibiotic-loaded cement. The removal of both components of the prosthesis and cement must be complete even in the absence of loosening of one component. When possible, the femur should not be fenestrated. Usually, removal is possible through the open upper end thereof. Chisels are preferred to mechanical reaming.

The damaged bone bed does not present the rugose cancellous textures seen with an original arthroplasty and it is necessary to key the hard glossy surface so often found. This is time-consuming but now regarded as essential. Careful compressive technique in cementing is necessary. At the close of the operation, copious suction drainage should be employed to bring healthy raw tissues together and obliterate dead space. Sinuses present at the time of operation are no contraindication to a one-stage procedure and can be excised with the whole septic focus.

The amount of antibiotic added to the cement may seem excessive but, as explained above, despite some degradation, mechanical failure does not appear to be a problem. The following examples of our current usage may be offered.

Results

In conventional terms, a 77.4% success rate in the prevention of recurrence of infection and mechanical loosening appears to have been achieved. This is similar to the results published in 1981.

When the survival curves are examined for these cases, they show that after 11 years' follow-up, 50% of the implants will have failed. These results may appear disappointing in comparison with the continued 77% success rate reported in conventional terms but the survival curve takes into consideration the time of failure and also displays the annual failure rate. It is in the light of survival curves that the true state of our results becomes apparent and it is for this reason that in future statistics of this type have to be presented in such cold terms.

The survival terms shown in Fig. 1 relate to the nature of the primary bacterial infecting agent. There appears to be no significant difference in outcome of infections caused by *Staphylococcus* species, anaerobic *Corynebacteria*, *Staphylococcus aureus*, and those cases where no organism could be cultured. The results from the *Pseudomonas* species are significantly inferior. Other organisms known to produce poor results (eg, group D streptococci, *Proteus* and *Klebsiella* species) were rare and therefore their effects become statistically uncertain for the purposes of survival curves. For this reason they have not been included. *S. aureus* has been responsible in 32% of the cases and caused significantly the highest incidence. Accordingly, curve D in Fig. 2 relates to *S. aureus* and is the main determinant in producing the overall survival curve.

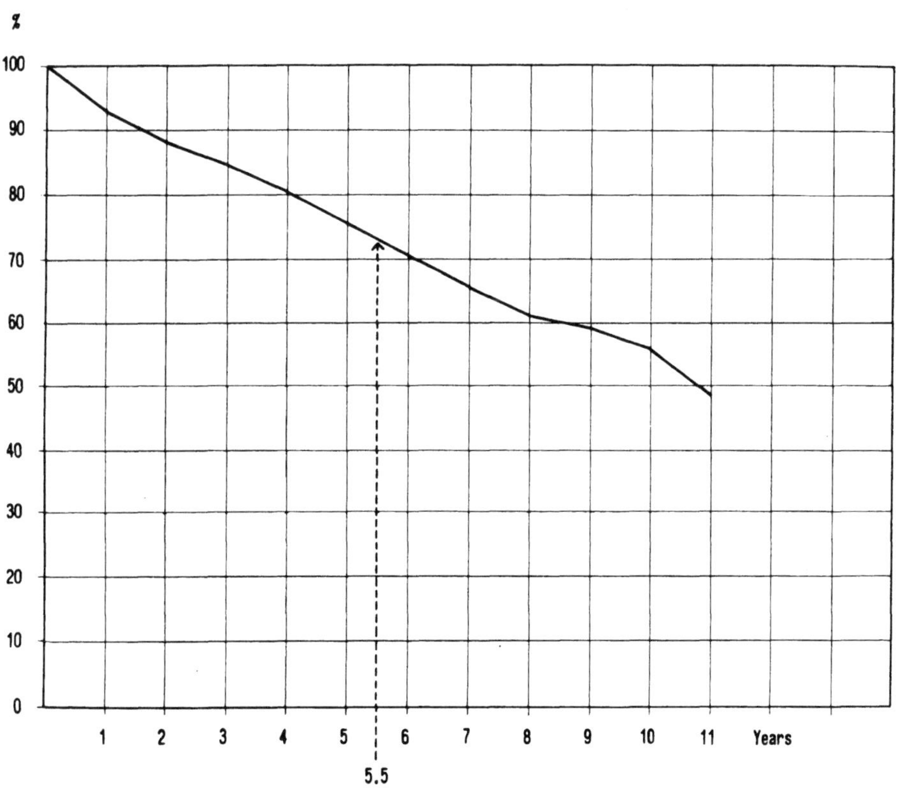

Fig. 1. Failures of one-stage exchange arthroplasties. Percentage survival with respect to time. End point reinfection and/or loosening. Survival function in 825 hip implants (1972-1981)

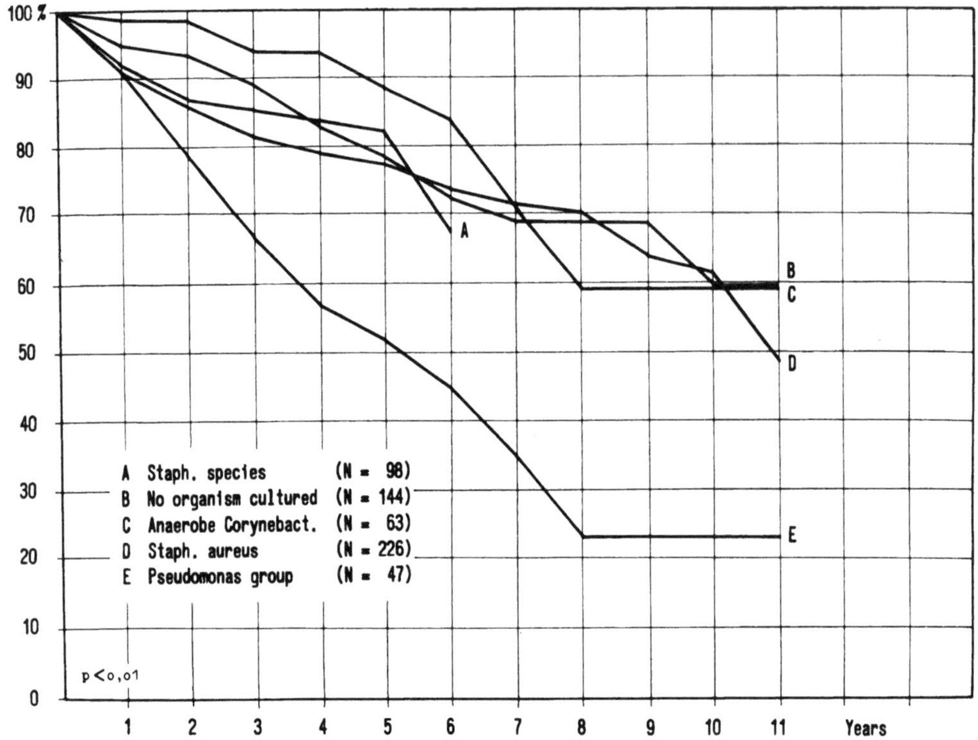

Fig. 2. Survival function of one-stage exchange hip arthroplasties with respect to causative organisms (1972-1981)

The final comparison of these results with those from other centres must be speculative. How uncemented prostheses and future developments will affect the picture is uncertain. In the immediate future, there is no doubt that we must be prepared to treat a large number of patients requiring revision surgery and many of these will be infected.

References

1. Buchholz, H.W., Engelbrecht, E., Lodenkämper, H., Röttger, J., Siegel, A., and Elson, R.A.: Management of deep infection of total hip replacement. J. Bone Joint Surg. 63B, 342, 1981.

2. Buchholz, H.W., Elson, R.A., and Heinert, K.: Antibiotic-loaded acrylic cement (ALAC) - current concepts. Clin. Orthop. Rel. Res. 1984 (in press).

Deep Infection of Total Joint Replacement: Principles of Treatment

R. A. ELSON

In 1977, I worked at the Endo-Klinik in Hamburg and participated in the management of many infected joint arthroplasties treated according to the principles established by Buchholz and his colleagues (1981). Inevitably, I am orientated towards a specific line of treatment but maintain an open mind as to achieving the ideal choice of therapy. At present, I am of the opinion that the basic surgical principle of excision of necrotic or inert material, the administration of systemic antibiotics, and the insertion of a local depot of antibiotics by means of antibiotic-loaded acrylic cement (ALAC) form the basis of best available treatment. My personal series of operations is summarized in Table I. Follow-up is still too short to permit a statement of definitive opinion, but as yet I have had no reason to change my choice of management. Most deep infections occur in conventionally cemented prostheses with loosening of one or both components; consequently, and especially in advanced cases, the mechanical problems associated with a damaged bone bed and loss of gross bone stock are significant. When the appearance of radiolucent zones at the bone/cement interface is alarming, I anticipate mechanical failures in the future apart from the possibilities of recrudescent infection. Nevertheless, the incidence of confirmed reinfection is low and this is the prime consideration in these patients.

Table I. Results of deep infection in total joint replacement*
Follow-up period 0.5-6.25 years

	No. (%)	Results† No. (%)
Infected hip arthroplasties	106	
Positive bacteriologic diagnosis	88 (83%)	
Exchange arthroplasties		
One-stage	97	87/97 (89.7%)
Two-stage	9	8/9 (89%)
Surgical mortality	0	

* Adjunctive treatment: ALAC according to antibiogram; systemic antibiotics since 1979.
† No sign of infection; useful function

Current Concepts of Infections in
Orthopaedic Surgery

My personal experience and that published by other investigators (Buchholz et al, 1981; Carlsson et al, 1978; Eftakhar, 1984) persuade me to summarize the practical management according to the predominant mode of presentation, as follows:

Postoperative Superficial Inflammation

In the roughly 7% incidence of disturbed wound healing, the overwhelming consideration must be prevention of inward spread of infection. Clearly, deep contamination may be present already but there is usually no way of ascertaining it. The area of inflammation lies between two vulnerable suture lines: the skin and the deep fascia. In his appraisal of superficial infections, Eftakhar (1984) gives the impression that it is a self-limiting process provided it is not secondary to a deep infection. I feel the evidence suggests that a superficial infection that apparently resolves must be regarded as a high risk of developing a subsequent deep infection. I have reported elsewhere that tissue necrosis due to strangulation, rough surgical technique or fat sutures are likely sources of superficial inflammation, providing a provident environment for contaminating microorganisms, whatever their source. When observing rising tension it must be relieved by opening the wound and allowing free outward drainage. Systemic antibiotics and a bismuth iodoform paraffin paste dressing are essential adjuncts.

Postoperative Fulminating Toxic Deep Infection

Fortunately, these types of infections occur rarely (two examples in 1,890 hip replacements, one from superficial infection probably, and the other from a hematoma). In such cases, the wound must again be opened and debrided down to bleeding tissue under massive systemic antibiotic cover. An attempt should be made to salvage the implants because their removal is difficult and there is a chance of preserving them. One should consider instilling local antibiotics or, preferably, temporary ALAC pellets. Once control of the cellulitic phase is achieved, the wound may be freshly excised and closed.

Late Acute Toxic Deep Infection

The arthroplasty may be the source or target of a hematogenous process. Obviously, a source should be sought and the bloodstream flooded with appropriate antibiotics. The joint is often remarkably pain-free and diagnosis uncertain unless the joint is superficial like the knee. As soon as diagnosed, even when in doubt, aspiration should be performed just before starting antibiotics and a fine drainage tube inserted through the wide bore aspirating needle whereby intra-articular antibiotics can be instilled regularly at 6-hourly intervals. I have treated three such patients, two with apparent success but the other required a subsequent exchange. Failure to control toxemia emanating from the joint may demand implant excision, occasionally as a matter of urgency.

Late Chronic Deep Infection

This is by far the commonest presentation either with pain, loosening, or sinus formation. In the absence of toxemia, systemic antibiotics have no place until a definite diagnosis has been attempted by aspiration and closed cannular tissue biopsy.

Once the infecting organism has been identified, a complete excision down to healthy tissue should be conducted, erring on preserving bone stock (even if necrotic but provided it has a vascular soft tissue mantle). A sinus is not to be feared since it is a manifestation of something deep and can be excised at the same time unless inaccessible. Systemic antibiotics are now effective and augmented by a depot source afforded by ALAC which will permeate residual necrotic tissue, especially bone; the field can thus be sterilized. A meticulous reimplantation can be performed in most cases as a one-stage exchange and avoids two major operations. The long-term merits of a one- or two-stage procedure are not yet known but I would always advocate the first with confidence. Provided the merits of ALAC are accepted, why not use it for reimplantation?

Undiagnosed Infection

A group of patients exists with unexplained pain which always causes anxiety. The erythrocyte sedimentation rate may be equivocal. Scintimetry and arthrography are usually not helpful in my experience. Even biopsy may be negative in cases where the infection has localized in an inaccessible area of the bone/cement interface; I have fenestrated and biopsied one localized infected area in the femoral shaft with a positive microbial culture. A useful scheme of evaluation has been proposed by van Rens and Sloof (1984). Serial radiographs are probably the most valuable single diagnostic tool. A retrospective study of late deep infections often reveals a history of pain earlier, and these patients must be reviewed repeatedly.

References

1. Buchholz, H.W., Elson, R.A., Engelbrecht, E., Lodenkamper, H., Rottger, J., and Siegel, A.: Management of deep infection of total hip replacement. J. Bone Joint Surg. 63B, 342, 1981.

2. Carlsson, A.S., Josefsson, G., and Lindberg, L.: Revision with gentamicin-impregnated cement for deep infections in total hip arthroplasties. J. Bone Joint Surg. 60A, 1059, 1978.

3. Eftakhar, N.S.: Infection in Joint Replacement Surgery. C.V. Mosby Co., St. Louis, Toronto, 1984.

4. van Rens, Th.J.G., and Sloof, T.J.J.: The investigation of the painful total hip. In, Ling, R.S.M. (Ed.): Complications of Total Hip Replacement 1984.

Revision of Infected Total Joint Replacement: Swedish Experiences

L. LINDBERG

In 1978, our group reported in the Journal of Bone and Joint Surgery (Carlsson et al, 1978) on the result of revisions with gentamicin containing bone cement of 77 infected total hip arthroplasties. We still follow these patients and in 1983 a new review of their situation was made. In this report the results of the last review will be described and some other experiences discussed.

Materials and Methods

The original series consisted of 77 deep infections around total hip arthroplasties, consecutively revised with gentamicin-containing bone cemment during 1974-1977. After a dropout of seven patients (all rated healed from the infection), the present patient material consists of 70 total hip revisions in 70 patients. Included in the series are 15 patients who have died 16 months or more after the revision.

Fifty-two patients were operated in one stage and 18 in two stages. In the two-stage procedure, the prosthesis and the cement were extracted, systemic antibiotics were given, and the new prosthesis was inserted with gentamicin cement an average of 12 months after the extraction (range 2-41). To extract the cement from the femur, we cut a longitudinal slot in the femoral diaphysis with an oscillating saw. A femoral component with a stem long enough to reach below the distal end of the slot was then used. The definite diagnosis of an infection was made by bacterial culture from tissue biopsies taken during the operation (Kamme and Lindberg, 1981). The new prosthesis was fastened with a bone cement containg 0.5 g gentamicin per package, and all patients were given a systemic antibiotic for six months after the revision. The patients have been followed up with clinical and radiologic examination and erythrocyte sedimentation rate (ESR) determinations each or every other year.

Healing of the Infection

Healing results of the infections after one revision are shown in Table I, the 1978 figures shown in brackets.

The average observation time for the surviving 55 patients is 85 months (range 40-120). The remaining 15 patients died on an average of 54 months after the revision (range 16-94). The average observation time for the whole group of healed patients is 43 months (16-120).

Current Concepts of Infections in
Orthopaedic Surgery

Table I. Healing of infections after one revision*

	Healed	Infected	Doubtful
One stage	43 (39)	9 (5)	0 (8)
Two stage	14 (14)	4 (3)	0 (1)
Total	57 (53)	13 (8)	0 (9)

*1978 figures in brackets

As can be seen from the table, in 1978 it was not possible to determine whether the infection was healed or not in nine patients. In four patients, the infection proved to be healed whereas in the remaining five the infection persisted. Thus, the healing rate after the first revision was 57 of 70 (81%). Of the 13 infected patients, seven were revised a second time with a short-term, two-stage revision with gentamicin cement beads (Hovelius and Josefsson, 1979). After this second revision, all seven patients are rated as healed. The total healing rate after the second revision is, therefore, as of now, 64 of 70 patients (91%). It is to be noted that the patient population was not selected, but consists of 70 consecutively operated cases. In this series it is not possible to establish any difference as to the healing rate between the one-stage and the two-stage group.

Noninfectious Loosening

As the bone stock in hips which have been infected probably is of inferior quality, a comparatively high rate of noninfectious loosening may be expected. To determine the rate of noninfectious loosening, the radiograms were examined in the group of surviving patients in 1983 who had undergone only one revision. This group consisted of 46 patients; one was living abroad and could not be reached. The group investigated consisted of 45 healed cases (32 one-stage and 13 two-stage). Standardized radiograms had been taken prospectively in every patient under investigation, and in each case the whole series of radiograms after the revision was examined for progressing resorption of the bone surrounding the cement and for any change of position of the components.

In 21 patients observed for an average of 89 months (63-112), no change of the position or bone resorption could be seen, except the discrete formation of a maximum of 1 mm bone cement radiolucency that normally often develops during the first 6-12 months after revision. In 24 patients, different degrees of progressing bone resorption was seen outside the cement, indicating an actual or potential loosening -- in five around the acetabular component after an average of 93 months (75-101); in eight around the femoral component after an average of 78 months (40-93); and in 11 around both components after an average of 84 months (48-124). In eight of these 24 patients, a second revision was carried out and in all bacterial cultures from tissues adjacent to the prosthesis were negative (Kamme and Lindberg, 1981). There seems to be a difference in the rate of noninfectious loosening between the one-stage and the two-stage groups. In the one-stage group radiographic signs of loosening were found in 22 of the 32 cases: in four patients around the acetabular, in seven around the femoral, and in 11 around both components. In the two-stage group, no signs of loosening could be seen in 11 of the 13 patients. In the remaining two, the acetabular and the femoral component respectively seem to be loose, 101 and 93 months after the revision.

Discussion

At an early stage of the investigation, it was obvious that the revisions should be done as early as possible. Conservative treatment does not lead to healing of the infection but only to a larger infectious lesion and more destruction of the bone stock. This means lessened chances of healing and of a stable fixation of the new prosthesis (Lidgren et al, 1977).

A most important prerequisite for a good functional result is to have a large set of different types and sizes of prosthetic components on hand. Formerly, we recommended a slot in the femoral diaphysis to enable us to remove all the cement and infected tissue from the marrow cavity. In most cases we now avoid making a slot in the femur since, in most cases, it is possible to remove cement and tissue from the proximal end of the femur with the use of special chisels, cement drills and other tools especially designed for this purpose. Avoiding the slot means that the new cementing technique can be used, such as plugging of the femur, cement gun, and proximal seal. Naturally, pressurizing of the acetabulum, high pressure lavage, and low blood pressure anesthesia should be used whenever possible.

A new, low viscosity gentamicin cement is now under clinical investigation in Sweden. The comparatively high rate of noninfectious loosening makes a good cementing technique imperative. The commercially available gentamicin cement only contains 0.5 g gentamicin per package. As it is possible to mix at least up to 2 g antibiotic in the cement without too much impairment of the mechanical strength, it is desirable to admix another 1.5 g of gentamicin or another suitable antibiotic to the cement in the infected cases.

Summary

No statistically significant difference in healing of the infections could be found between the one- and two-stage groups in our patient series. During the last four to five years, we have, however, made increasing use of the short-term, two-stage method with gentamicin containing polymethylmethacrylate beads, attempting to improve our results (Lindberg, 1984). The method implies that the old prosthesis with all the cement and infectious tissue is removed. Instead of the immediate insertion of a new prosthesis, however, the wound cavity is filled with gentamicin cement beads, the wound primarily sutured, and a drainage used for a maximum of 24 hours. The beads are left in the wound cavity for three or four weeks after which a second operation is performed during which the beads are removed and the new prosthesis inserted with gentamicin cement in the usual manner. During this time the microbes have been identified, their resistance pattern determined, and an adequate systemic antibiotic therapy started. The method has considerable advantages compared with the earlier two-stage method. The delay until the patient has a new hip is only a few weeks compared with an average of 12 months in our earlier series and the treatment of the infection is certainly more effective. About 25 patients are being treated in this manner by our group but the observation time is still too short to come to any conclusions.

Our experience indicates that these operations should be centralized in certain departments with special interest and experience. The infection rate in our department is now mostly beyond 1%. This means that even large departments performing 200-300 primary total hip arthroplasties per year will not have to revise more than two or three infections a year. These are too few cases for a general surgical department to obtain sufficient experience to manage severe infections.

References

1. Carlsson, A.S., Josefsson, G., and Lindberg, L.: Revision with gentamicin-impregnated cement for deep infections in total hip arthroplasties. J. Bone Joint Surg. 60A, 1,059, 1978.

2. Hovelius, L., and Josefsson, G.: An alternative method for exchange operation of infected arthroplasties. Acta Orthop. Scand. 50, 93, 1979.

3. Kamme, C., and Lindberg, L.: Aerobic and anaerobic bacteria in deep infections after total hip arthroplasties. Clin. Orthop. 154, 201, 1981.

4. Lidgren, L., Carlsson, A.S., and Lindberg, L.: Antibiotikabehandlung bei infizierten totalen Gelenkplastiken. Orthopädische Praxis 13, 344, 1977.

5. Lindberg, L.: Replacement operation for infected total hip arthroplasties. In, Eftekhar, N. (Ed.) Infection in Total Joint Replacement. C.V. Mosby Co., 1984, pp 283-301.

Reimplantation of Infected Joint Replacements: Elution Studies of Gentamicin from Cement and Beads

E. A. SALVATI, J. J. CALLAGHAN, B. D. BRAUSE, R. F. KLEIN, and R. D. SMALL

Introduction

Approximately 120 infected prosthetic joint replacements have been reimplanted since 1968 at The Hospital for Special Surgery in New York. The earlier experience included primarily one-stage reimplantations, the antibiotic therapy being selected by the treating orthopedic surgeon. Reimplantations after 1975 were performed primarily in two stages, including a standardized six-week intravenous antibiotic regimen. Minimal 1:8 peak bactericidal serum levels were the objective, monitored by a consultant in infectious diseases.

A 90% success rate has been achieved in eradicating infection in patients reimplanted after 1975, with a minimum follow-up of two years. Inability to obtain a 1:8 peak bactericidal serum level, immunologic deficiency, frailty of the patient, inadequate soft tissues, severe bone loss, and poor potential for rehabilitation were considered contraindications for reimplantation (Salvati et al, 1982).

Since mid-1982, the use of Palacos®-gentamicin impregnated cement (PG) was included in the reimplantation procedure, based on European experiences reporting 77 to 90% success with one-stage reimplantation, despite extending the indications to all infections (Buchholz et al, 1981; Carlsson et al, 1978). In addition, PG was used in patients undergoing joint replacement who were at higher risk of infection due to complicated revision surgery, previous multiple operations, suspicion of sepsis, infections at other body sites, previously irradiated joints, immunodeficient and immunosuppressed patients.

Beads of antibiotic-impregnated cement (Palacos-gentamicin; Septopal®) (Hovelius and Josefsson, 1979) were also incorporated in the treatment of infected joints. The beads were introduced after thorough debridement and removal of prosthetic components and acrylic cement (Fig. 1a, 1b). To maintain local gentamicin levels, no closed suction-irrigation was used in these cases (only suction for 24 hours).

The current prospective study was initiated to analyze gentamicin concentrations in joint fluid, serum and urine of patients having received PG and impregnated beads and to monitor any toxic side effects.

Materials

Palacos-gentamicin cement consisting of 0.5 g gentamicin per 40 g cement pack was used for total joint replacement. In hip replacements, one packet

Current Concepts of Infections in
Orthopaedic Surgery

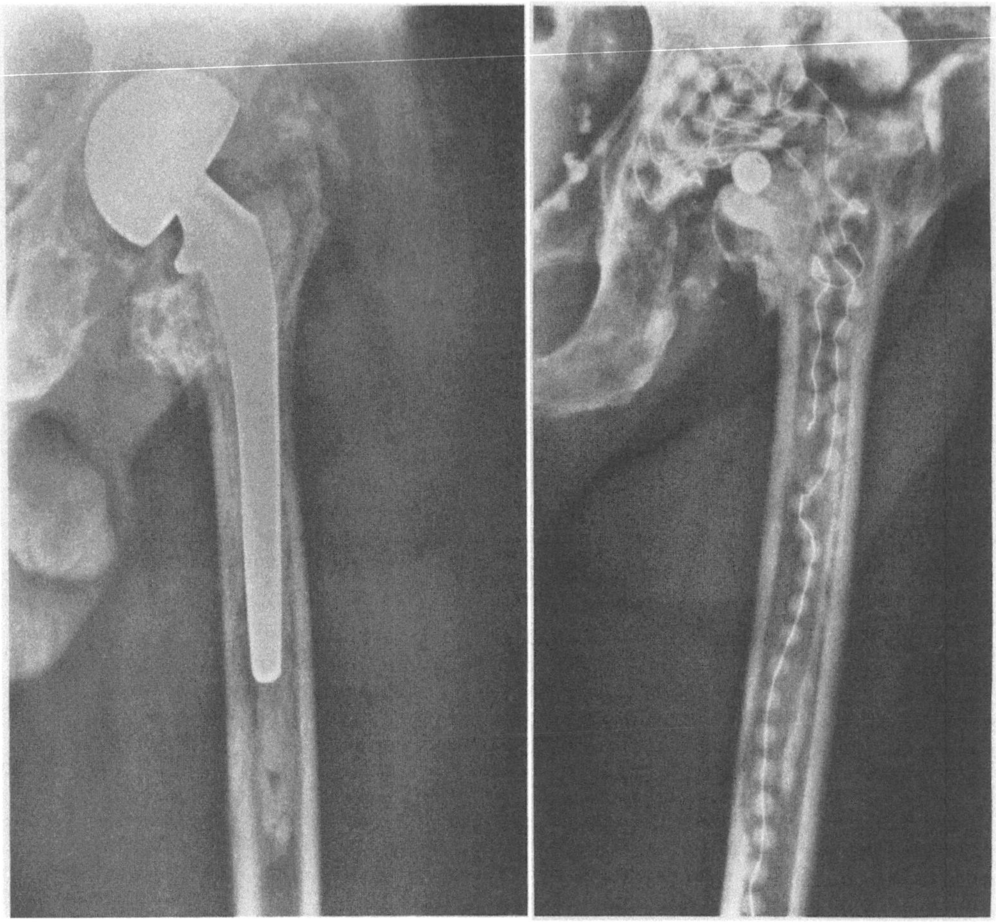

a b

Fig. 1. a) Radiograph of an infected cement bipolar implant. b) Radiograp after removal of prosthetic components and acrylic cement, and introduction of gentamicin-impregnated beads

was used for the acetabulum and two packets for the femoral canal; in knee replacements, one packet was used for the femur and one for the tibia. Two to five chains of Palacos-gentamicin beads were inserted in the acetabulum and femoral canal during the first stage of a two-stage reimplantation. Each bead is 7 mm in diameter and contains 4.5 mg gentamicin base. The beads are strung on a chromium-nickel multistranded thread with 30 beads to a chain.

Method

Radioimmune assays, using ^{125}I-labeled gentamicin "Coat a Count" (Diagnosti Products Corporation, Los Angeles, California) assay, were performed on the joint fluid drainage and aspirate, serum, and urine of patients implanted with PG or beads. This assay is specific for gentamicin and precise to within 7 to 10%, depending on the concentration of the sample. The low end sensitivity is 0.1 µg/mL.

Joint fluid levels were obtained from the suction drainage at 24 hours, occasionally at 48 hours, when possible by joint aspirate at 2 to 6 weeks and at the time of surgical removal of the beads. Serum levels were assessed 1 hour and 24 hours postoperatively, and weekly thereafter during hospitalization. Urine levels were assessed by 24-hour collections, taking 5 mL aliquots. These samples were obtained on day 1 and weekly thereafter during hospitalization.

In a control group, ten patients undergoing total joint replacement received intravenous gentamicin (1.5 - 2.0 mg/kg loading dose and 1.5 mg/kg every 8 hours) for 48 hours as part of their antibiotic prophylaxis. Twenty-four hour wound drainage samples, peak and trough serum levels, and 24 hour day 1 urine collection were assayed.

To confirm bioactivity of the molecular gentamicin measured by radioimmune assay, five samples were analyzed simultaneously by bioassay and radioimmune assays. The tube dilution bioassay was employed with twofold fluid dilutions using a selected *Staphylococcus epidermidis* isolate as test organism (minimal inhibitory concentration = 0.2 µg/mL (Table I).

Table I. Radioimmunoassay (RIA) versus bioassay

Substrate	Time	Range of accuracy	
		RIA	Bioassay
Cement	24 h	5.8 (5.6-6.1 µg/mL)	16 (8-32 µg/mL)
Cement	24 h	10.5 (10.1-10.9 µg/mL)	16 (8-32 µg/mL)
Beads	48 h	24.6 (23.4-25.8 µg/mL)	16 (8-32 µg/mL)
Beads	3 mo	21.0 (19.8-22.2 µg/mL)	16 (8-32 µg/mL)
Beads	3 mo	1.9 (1.6-2.2 µg/mL)	3.2 (1.6-6.4µg/mL)

Serial BUN, creatinine levels and bedside audiograms were obtained to evaluate nephrotoxicity and ototoxicity.

Results

Thirty patients were implanted with PG (21 hips and nine knees) and 15 with beads (all hip joints). Day 1 wound drainage levels in the control patients receiving intravenous gentamicin averaged 2.1 µg/mL (range 0.9 to 5.2 µg/mL). Day 1 wound drainage gentamicin levels in the PG group ranged from 2.7 to 38.9 µg/mL (mean 15.1), approximately 7 times the control; and at day 2, 2.1 to 32.1 µg/mL (mean 11.0). At day 1, levels in patients with beads were 19.6 to 69.5 µg/mL (mean 36.1), approximately 18 times the control; and at day 2, 24.6 to 47.9 µg/mL (mean 35.5). Joint fluid aspirates were as high as 5.0 µg/mL at four weeks in PG and 22.3 µg/mL at 6 weeks in beads (Fig. 2 and 3).

Control peak serum levels (20 min post dose) in the parenterally-administered group averaged 4.0 µg/mL (range 1.7 to 6.7 µg/mL). Gentamicin serum levels of patients implanted with PG at 1 hour ranged from 0 to 3.8 µg/mL (mean 0.3); at 24 hours 0 to 1.0 µg/mL (mean 0.4); and at day 7 all were 0 µg/mL. Trace

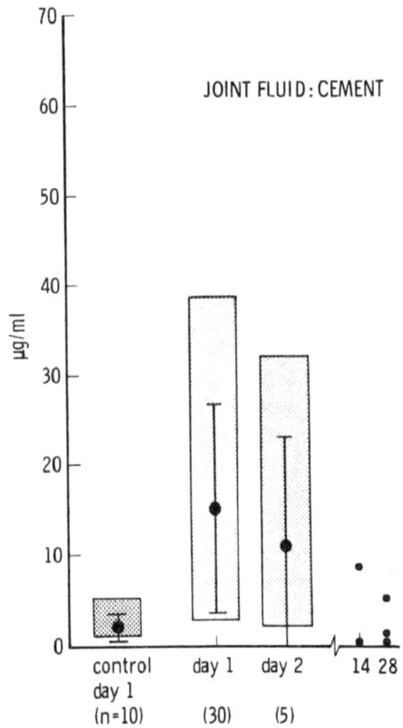

Fig. 2

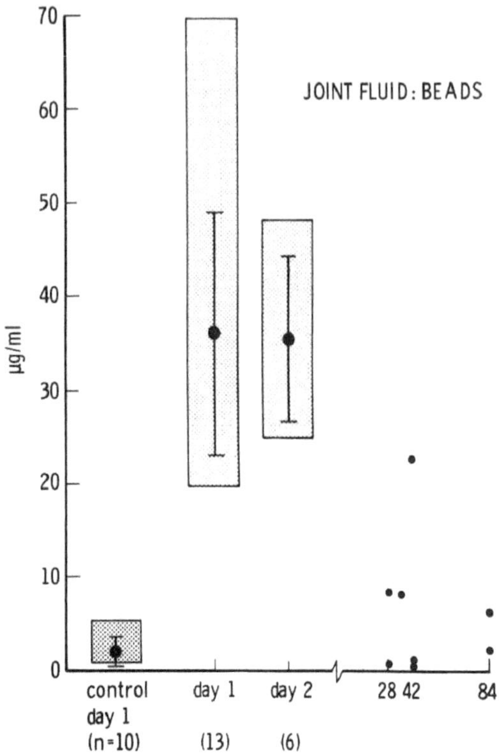

Fig. 3

Fig. 2. Gentamicin joint fluid levels in patients implanted with gentamicin cement. Dots represent single joint aspirates. Control represents joint fluid levels obtained after intravenous gentamicin administration

Fig. 3. Joint fluid levels in patients implanted with gentamicin-impregnated beads

levels were occasionally measurable over the next 4 weeks (Fig. 4). In the patients implanted with beads, serum gentamicin levels at 1 hour ranged from 0 to 1.0 μg/mL (mean 0.2). Twenty-four hour levels ranged from 0 to .08 μg/mL (mean .02); and day 7 levels were 0 to .07 μg/mL (mean .01). Trace levels were detectable at 42 days in one specimen (Fig. 5).

Control patient day 1, 24-hour urine collection levels averaged 22.8 μg/mL (range 5.2 to 53.2 μg/mL). Urine levels in patients with PG at 24 hours were 0 to 3.1 μg/mL (mean 0.8); at day 7, 0 to 2.4 μg/mL (mean 0.4); and at day 14, 0 to 1.0 μg/mL (mean 0.2). Trace levels were detectable at 28 days (Fig. 6). Urine levels in patients with beads were 0.1 to 4.9 μg/mL (mean 1.6) at day 1; 0 to 4.7 μg/mL (mean 1.7) at day 7; .06 to 2.8 μg/mL (mean 1.1) at day 14; with trace levels still detectable at day 63 (Fig. 7).

Seven samples of beads were obtained from hip joints 6 to 12 weeks after their initial insertion. Each bead was immersed in 1 mL of saline for 24 hours. Elution rates were 34, 32, and 25 mg/bead/24 hours from the beads

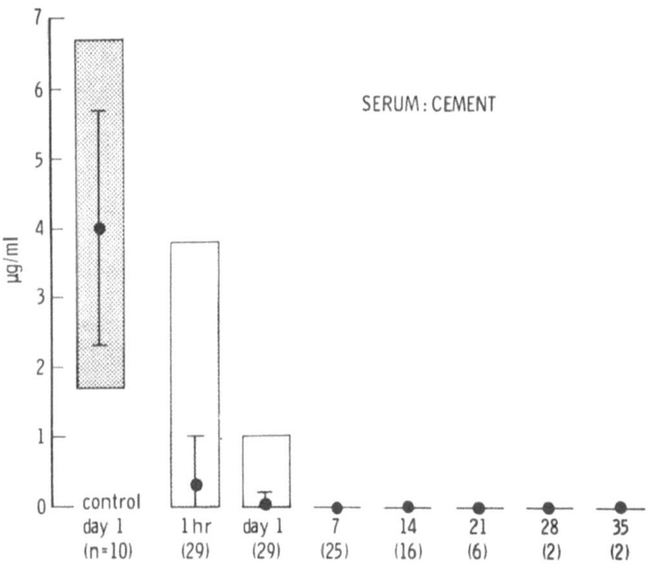

Fig. 4. Serum levels in patients implanted with gentamicin cement

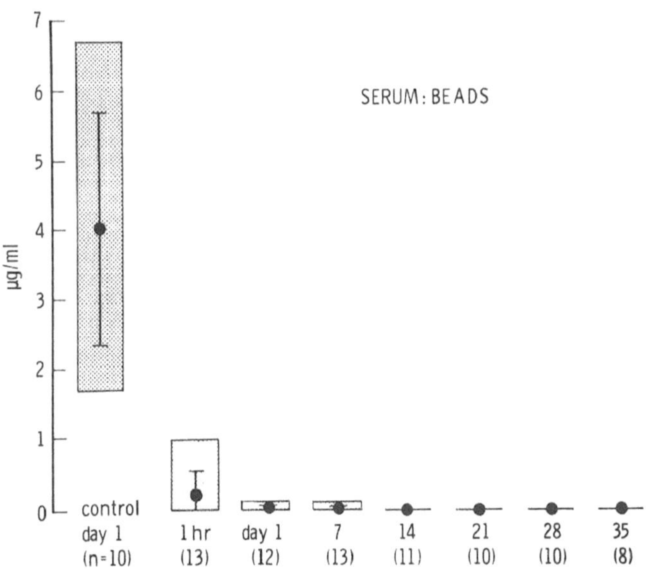

Fig. 5. Serum levels in patients implanted with gentamicin-impregnated beads

which had been implanted for six weeks and 18, 17, 16, and 12 mg/bead/24 hours from the beads which had been implanted for 12 weeks (Fig. 8).

As illustrated in Table I, bioassays are not as precise as radioimmune assays. However, the radioimmune assay measures molecular gentamicin, and confirmation of bioactivity of the specimen is important. Simultaneous bioassay and radioimmune assay of five specimens, both of beads and PG taken at various times after implantation, confirmed bioactivity. In addi-

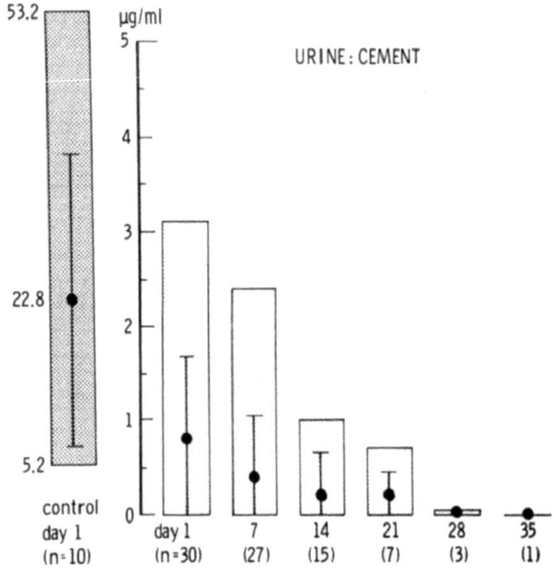

Fig. 6. Urine levels in patient
implanted with gentamicin cemen

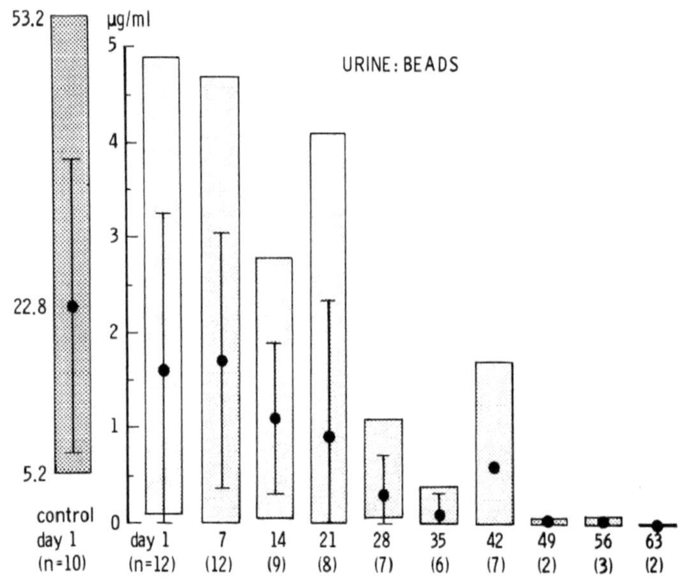

Fig. 7. Urine levels
patients implanted wi
gentamicin-impregnate
beads

tion, concentrations of gentamicin determined by the radioimmune assay correlated with the levels of bioactive antibiotic within the range of accuracy afforded by each test.

No persistent elevations in BUN and creatinine assays were observed. No symptoms of eighth nerve toxicity were noted, and serial audiograms showed no changes greater than 15 decibels.

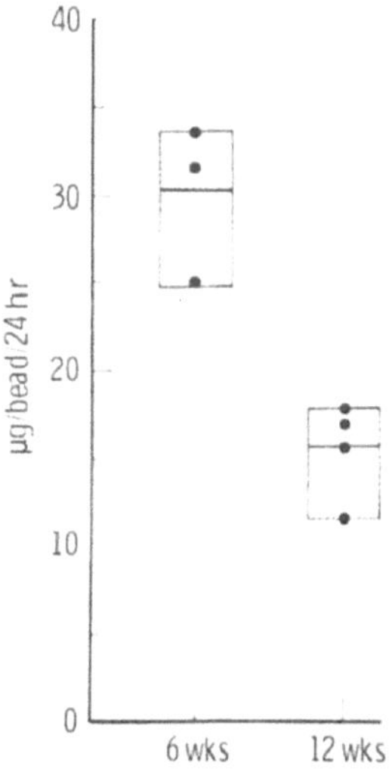

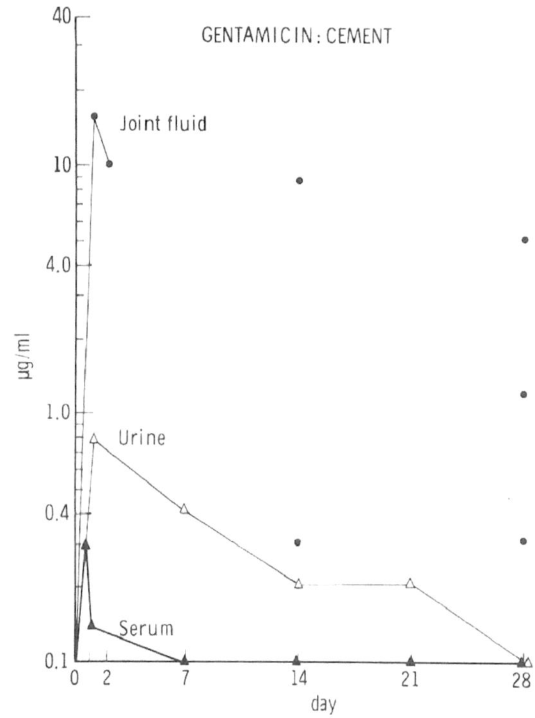

Fig. 9. Summary of levels obtained in patients implanted with gentamicin cement (logarithmic scale)

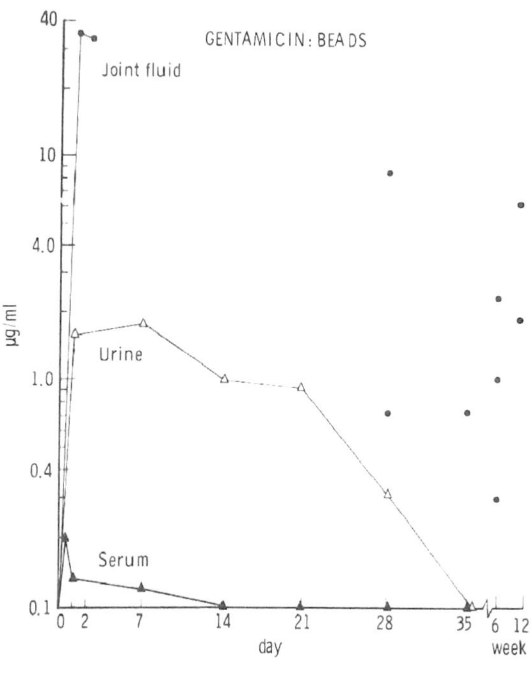

Fig. 10. Summary of levels obtained in patients implanted with gentamicin-impregnated beads (logarithmic scale)

Discussion

This study confirms previous reports concerning joint fluid, serum, and urine levels of gentamicin obtained in humans implanted with gentamicin-impregnated cement (Buchholz et al, 1981; Carlsson et al, 1978; Torholm et al, 1983; Wahlig et al, 1978; 1984). Most previous studies of gentamicin-impregnated beads were undertaken in patients with chronic osteomyelitis rather than with infected prosthetic joints, using bioassays to analyze the various specimens. In the current study we used radioimmune assays (a more sensitive and accurate technique) with confirmation by bioassay. The bioassay also proved the biologic activity of the eluted gentamicin, even in the samples obtained several months after implantation.

High gentamicin levels in joint fluid were obtained (mean 36.1 µg/mL in patients with beads and 15.1 µg/mL in patients with PG)(Fig. 9 and 10). In view of the high local levels of gentamicin documented in this study, the concept of sensitive and resistant microorganisms will have to be redefined Microbial sensitivity is currently based on peak serum levels. Most microb defined as resistant by this criterium might be sensitive when exposed to levels 10 to 20 times higher than those obtained with intravenous administration.

Low serum and urine concentrations of gentamicin were found (Fig. 9 and 10). Trace urine concentrations were detected at day 28 in one PG-implanted patient, and at day 63 in one bead-implanted patient. No nephrotoxicity or ototoxicity was observed; none would be expected considering the low serum and urine levels determined in this study.

This report supports the safety and efficacy of the use of impregnated bead and PG in the treatment of infected joints and in reimplantation of prosthe tic joints.

References

1. Buchholz, H.W., Elson, R.A., Engelbrecht, E., Lodenkamper, H., Rottger, J., and Siegel, A.: Management of deep infection of total hip replacement. J. Bone Joint Surg. 63B, 342, 1981.
2. Carlsson, A.S., Josefsson, G., and Lindberg, L.: Revision with gentamicin-impregnated cement for deep infections in total hip arthroplasties. J. Bone Joint Surg. 60A, 1059, 1978.
3. Hovelius, L. and Josefsson, G.: An alternative method for exchange operation of infected arthroplasty. Acta Orthop. Scand. 50, 93, 1979.
4. Salvati, E.A., Chekofsky, K.M., Brause, B.D., and Wilson, P.D., Jr.: Reimplantation in infection: a 12-year experience. Clin. Orthop. 170, 62, 1982.
5. Torholm, C., Lidgren, L., Lindberg, L., and Kahlmeter, G.: Total hip joint arthroplasty with gentamicin-impregnated cement. A clinical study of gentamicin excretion kinetics. Clin. Orthop. 181, 99, 1983.
6. Wahlig, H., Dingeldein, E., Bergmann, R., and Reuss, K.: The release of gentamicin from polymethylmethacrylate beads: An experimental and pharmacokinetic study. J. Bone Joint Surg. 60B, 270, 1978.
7. Wahlig, H., Dingeldein, E., Buchholz, H.W., and Bachmann, F.: Pharmacokinetic study of gentamicin-loaded cement in total hip replacement. Com parative effects of varying dosage. J. Bone Joint Surg. 66B, 175, 1984.

Septic and Aseptic Hip and Knee Replacements: Results of Revision

J. P. McElwain and G. A. Hunter

The Hip

The results of revision for septic and aseptic hip replacement have been well documented by James et al (1982). From a review of the current literature, they showed a 71% success rate of revised hip arthroplasty in cases of past or current sepsis, compared with 54% excellent or good results in hips without evidence of infection (Tables I and II). The reinfection rate in the septic group was 17%; in the aseptic group the infection rate was 12%. The best results in the aseptic group were recorded in the revisions of the uncemented Ring prosthesis compared with a similar type of prosthesis or with a conventional cemented type. The most successful results in the septic group were recorded by Fitzgerald and Bryan (1981) using parenteral antibiotics only. They conceded that most of the patients in the septic group were heterogenous, and therefore better results would be expected following total hip arthroplasty after sepsis than after revision of cemented total hip arthroplasty. They emphasized the organism should be identified, and antibiotic sensitivity obtained before surgery. Infections due to *Pseudomonas aeruginosa*, *Proteus* species, Group D *Streptococcus*, and *Escherichia coli* were associated with a higher incidence of failure, and if infected with these organisms, the patients would be better advised to accept excision arthroplasty.

The Knee

Revision in the absence of sepsis (Table III)

In an early report from the Mayo Clinic by Wertzberger and Bryan (1979) on 100 aseptic knee revisions, 22 required a second revision and two further patients required a third revision. Overall, 39 patients had mild or moderate pain. They concluded that lucent lines were significant only in the painful knee.

Dupont et al (1980) reported on 103 revisions with a follow-up of six months to seven years, and demonstrated that 15% were failures due to pain and 20% were motion failures. There was a 3% incidence of infection and 7% required a second revision. The overall success rate was 70%. They outlined that failures due to pain were five times more common, motion failures twice as common, and infection rates six times higher than after primary total knee replacement. Obese osteoarthritic patients who had multiple procedures constituted an especially high risk category. The highest incidence of failure was in revision from one unconstrained to another unconstrained prosthesis.

Current Concepts of Infections in
Orthopaedic Surgery

Table I. Total hip revision in the absence of sepsis

Series	No.of hips	Follow-up period	Mean follow-up	Rating	Percent good results	Percent failure	Percent infection
Dandy and Theodorou, 1975[10]	73	Not stated		Not stated	Satisfactory: 40	60	17
Hoagland et al, 1979[15]	65	2 - 6 y		Harris	Excellent-Good: 60	40	17
Hunter et al, 1979[17]	140	6 mo-10 y	3 y	Harris	Excellent-Good: 24	76	35
Jones, 1979[22]	68	3 y	3 y	Ring's criteria	Excellent-Good: 81	19	4.4
Stillwell et al, 1980[29]	79	3 y	3 y	Modified Harris	Excellent-Good: 83	17	Not stated
Anderson and Murray, 1981[1]	55	1 - 9 y	3 y	Harris	Excellent-Good: 55	45	2
Cameron and Fedorkow, 1981[6]	15	1 - 4 y	2 y	Harris	Excellent-Good: 33	67	5
Pellici et al, 1981[26]	110	2 - 9 y	3.4 y	Chart review and radiographic analysis	Excellent-Good: 60	40	4
Welch, 1981[32]	56	Not stated		Charnley	Good: 50	50	16

In 661 hip revisions in the apparent absence of sepsis, results were overall:
Harris, excellent-good and successful" results, 54%; failure, 46%; infection 12%.

(Reproduced by kind permission of the Editor, Clin. Orthop. Rel. Res. 170, 88, 1982.)

Table II. Total hip revision after current or quiescent sepsis

Series	No.of hips	Follow-up period	Mean follow-up	Rating	Antibiotics	Percent good results	Percent failure	Percent reinfection
Carlsson et al, 1978[8]	77	6 mo-1 y	1 y	Charnley	Parenteral + in cement	Success: 78	22	22
Elson, 1979[12]	48	1 3/4 y		Success	In cement	Success: 86	14	Not stated
Wilson et al, 1978[34]	51	1 - 5 y	1 y	Not stated	Parenteral	Success: 82	18	12
Hughes et al, 1979[16]	26	6 - 9 y	8 y	Hospital for special surgery	Parenteral	Excellent-Good: 73	27	15
Hunter, 1979[18]	65	1 mo-6 y	2 y	Harris	Mixed group: parenteral + in cement	Excellent-Good: 25	75	35
Lautenbach and Weber, 1980[25]	20	6 - 42 mo		Not stated	In cement	Success: 80	20	5
Buchholz et al, 1981[5]	583	1-131 m	41 mo	Success	In cement	Success: 77	23	Not stated
Cherney and Amstutz, 1981[9]	76	2 y min		Not stated	Not stated	Not stated	14	14
Fitzgerald and Bryan, 1981[13]	111	2-11 y		Not stated	Parenteral	Success: 90	10	10
James et al, 1981[21]	65	3-10 y	5 y	Harris	Mixed group: parenteral + in cement	Excellent-Good: 8	76	Not stated
Jupiter et al, 1981[24]	57	35-43 mo	42 mo	Harris	Parenteral	Excellent-Good: 77	23	7

In 1063 hip revisions associated with sepsis, results were overall:
Harris, excellent-good and "successful", 71%; failure, 29%; reinfection, 17%.

(Reproduced by kind permission of the Editor, Clin. Orthop. Rel. Res. 170, 88, 1982.)

Table III. Total knee revision in the absence of sepsis

Series	No. of knees	Follow-up	Rating	Percent good result (1st revision)	Comments
Dupont et al, 1980[11]	103	6 mo - 7 y	Points system	Success 70%	Infection rate 3% Further revision 7%
Samuelson et al,[28] 1980	13	6 - 26 mo	N.A.	Success 100%	Short follow-up period
Cameron et al, 1981[7]	73	3.3 y	Modified B.O.A.	Excellent-Good 30%	Infection rate 11%
Ahlberg and Lunden, 1981[2]	21	N.A.	N.A.	Good 40%	-
Bryan and Rand, 1982[4]	227	Mean 5.5 y	N.A.	Satisfactory 67%	Further revision 22%
Insall and Dethmers, 1982[19]	72	Minimum 2 y	Hospital for Special Surgery	Good-Excellent 89%	Pain relief not comparable to primary replacement
Thornhill et al, 1982[30]	65	24 - 60 mo	Robert B. Brigham Hosp.	Improved 81%	Failure 12%
Goldberg and Sachs, 1983[14]	67	2 - 8.5 y	N.A.	Good 40%	Further revisions 7% Infection 2% Failures 21%
Kim and Finerman, 1983[24]	100	1 - 8.9 y	N.A.	Improved 78%	Marginal improvement in function

In 741 knee revisions in the absence of sepsis, results were:
Good-excellent, "successful", "improved", and "satisfactory" in 66% of cases; infection rate 5%

N.A.: not available

Salvage of a nonhinged failed total knee replacement, where loss of bone from the proximal tibia is considerable, has been demonstrated successfully by Samuelson et al (1980) in 13 patients using a special cast cobalt alloy implant in conjunction with the standard ICLH tibial implant. The follow-up ranged from six to 26 months. They showed that it is always possible to reestablish good stability to the knee by simply applying proper tension to the soft tissues. No failures during this short follow-up period were observed.

Despite the use of parenteral and local antibiotics, Cameron et al (1981) reported an 11% infection rate after revision of 73 aseptic knees. Only 30% were considered good or excellent results, the highest failure rate being in the hinged and constrained type prosthesis. Perhaps the lower incidence of success was based on a more critical appraisal of the results and their longer average follow-up.

Insall and Dethmers (1982) point out that revision surgery should be performed as soon as failure is diagnosed since delay only results in progressive bone destruction. Eighty-nine percent of patients in their series were rated excellent or good, despite the fact that the level of pain relief was not comparable with those undergoing primary knee replacement. They reported a higher incidence of extensor mechanism problems and radiolucent lines which were nonprogressive.

Nonprogressive radiolucent lines were reported in 65% of revised knees by Thornhill et al (1982). They concluded, based on their study, that the many causes of loosening could now be prevented with careful patient selection and a proper surgical technique.

Goldberg and Sachs (1983) reviewed the results of revision of 67 knees in which a partially constrained prosthesis was used in most of the first arthroplasties. Five were revised again for loosening with occurrence of one deep infection. Overall, only 40% were excellent or good results. Two-thirds of the knees had significant radiolucent lines while only one-third had normal alignment. Because of the high failure rate, they concluded that a better effort must be made to obtain the best results possible at the initial replacement.

Revision after sepsis (Table IV)

A small series from Cameron et al (1981), using a modified BOA rating system, reported success rates in 25% of patients for one-stage reimplantation despite the use of antibiotic loaded cement. Pain, bone loss, instability and reinfection were the main factors accounting for failure.

Walker and Schurman (1983) documented success in 10 delayed exchange total knee replacements. Absence of infection after at least two years' follow-up was reported in all patients. Gram-positive organisms were cultured in 86% of cases. After surgery, their patients were better off in respect to joint pain, slightly worse off as to overall function, and unchanged as to joint movement before total knee replacement. Relevant information as to the type of prosthesis used for both the initial and exchange replacement, the use of local or systemic antibiotics, and the amount of bone loss and ligamentous instability were omitted from this report. Delayed exchange was not defined.

Table IV. Total knee revision in the presence of sepsis

Series	No. of knees	Follow-up	Rating	Antibiotics	Percent good result (1st revision)		Comments	
Cameron et al, 1981[7]	5	Mean 2 y	Modified B.O.A.	Parenteral + in cement	Good	20%	Failures	80%
Walker and Schurman, 1983[31]	10	N.A.	N.A.	N.A.	Success	90%	Amputation in one patient	
Rand and Bryan, 1983[27]	14	Mean 3.3 y	N.A.	Parenteral	Success	28%	Further revision Arthrodesis	42% 28%
Insall, et al, 1983[20]	11	Mean 34 mo	Hospital for Special Surgery	Parenteral	Excellent-Good	81%	Mild-moderate pain	36%
Borden and Gearen, 1984[3]	8	Mean 34 mo	N.A.	Parenteral	Success	88%	Reinfection	12%

In 48 knee revisions in the presence of sepsis, results were: Good-excellent, "successful" 63%

N.A.: not available

From three reports in the recent literature, the stated time interval between removal of the prosthesis and delayed reimplantation appears to be directly related to the success or failure of this procedure. Rand and Bryan (1983), reporting on 14 infected knee replacements where reimplantation of a new prosthesis was performed within two weeks of removal of the infected one, had an overall success rate of only 35%. Success was expressed in terms of pain relief, motion and stability. Fifty-seven percent of knees were infection free with an average follow-up of 3.3 years. After the first revision, 28% had functional arthroplasties, 28% required arthrodesis for sepsis, and 42% were revised again. Salvage was more successful when low virulent organisms were isolated. Antibiotics were administered parenterally for 7-90 days after reimplantation. They recommended that reimplantation within two weeks should not be done unless under unusual clinical circumstances, such as infection caused by a low virulent organism.

Insall et al (1983) reported 81% excellent-good results with a mean follow-up of 34 months following delayed reimplantation in 11 knees. The procedure included removal of prosthesis and all the cement, six weeks intravenous antibiotics, and reimplantation with a total condylar type prosthesis. Infection was eradicated in all but one of the knees before reimplantation. All antibiotics were discontinued three to eight days after reimplantation. The dosage and selection of antibiotic depend on the cultured organisms, and the antibiotic therapy should be monitored by an infectious disease consultant. Reimplantation is not recommended in elderly patients in poor general health and when mixed organisms are isolated on culture.

Borden and Gearen (1984) reported similar success with two-stage reimplantation in seven out of eight knees. Specific antibiotic therapy was not mentioned and delayed exchange was not defined.

Discussion

When comparing the results of both these groups, the average chance of success in the absence of sepsis is 66%, whereas in the presence of sepsis the results show an average 63% excellent-good results. This is not unexpected, considering that some of the revisions were performed to salvage a failed hinge type prosthesis with associated bone and ligamentous destruction.

The best results in the aseptic group were reported by Insall and Dethmers (1982) where early revision from one unconstrained to another unconstrained type of prosthesis was performed. They recommend early intervention to preserve as much bone stock as possible.

When reviewing the long-term results of revision for sterile loosening, where a similar type of prosthesis was used for the initial arthroplasty, the results would appear to deteriorate with time (Bryan and Rand, 1982).

The literature contains few reports on revision for septic loosening. The most successful results were reported by Insall et al (1983), where all foreign material, including the necrotic tissue, was removed. The infection was controlled by the administration of antibiotics for six weeks and a new prosthesis was reimplanted when the knee was infection free. Similar results were confirmed by Borden and Gearen (1984), although the precise details of their procedure were not defined. Long-term follow-up data are inadequate but it would appear that by using this treatment regimen acceptable results can be obtained, albeit in the short term.

Comparison of the different series in both groups is difficult because of the lack of comparable rating systems, the differences in the duration of follow-up, and the method of follow-up, whether it is a personal review, by telephone or by postal questionnaire. The definition of good results and failures are variable. To make valid comparisons, specific rating systems must be used with a minimum of a four to five year follow-up period.

When contemplating revision surgery in the presence or absence of sepsis for hips and knees, consideration should be given to the following points:

- the patient's age and general medical state;
- the condition of the joint to be revised, with specific reference to the amount of bone destruction and the quality of the surrounding soft tissue;
- the skill and experience of the surgical team available to perform the task;
- in the presence of sepsis, revision surgery is not recommended when gram-negative anaerobic or mixed organisms are grown on culture.

References

1. Anderson, M.A. and Murray, W.R.: Revision surgery for failed total hip arthroplasty. Orthop. Transactions 5, 75, 1981.
2. Ahlberg, A. and Lunden, A.: Secondary operations after knee joint replacement. Clin. Orthop. Rel. Res. 156, 170, 1981.
3. Borden, L.S. and Gearen, P.F.: Management of the infected total knee arthroplasty. Presented at The American Academy of Orthopaedic Surgeons, Atlanta 1984.
4. Bryan, R.S. and Rand, J.A.: Revision total knee arthroplasty. Clin. Orthop. Rel. Res. 170, 116, 1982.
5. Buchholz, H.W., Elson, R.A., Engelbrecht, E., Lodenkämper, H., Rotger, J., and Siegel, A.: Management of deep infection of total hip replacement. J. Bone Joint Surg. 63B, 342, 1981.
6. Cameron, H.U. and Federkow, D.M.: The early results of the Bateman single assembly total hip used as a revision prosthesis. Acta Arthop. Belg. 47, 49, 1981.
7. Cameron, H.U., Hunter, G.A., Welsh, R.P., and Bailey, W.H.: Revision of total knee replacement. Can. J. Surg. 24, 418, 1981.
8. Carlsson, A.S., Josefsson, G., and Lindberg, L.: Revision with gentamycin impregnated cement for deep infections in total hip arthroplasties. J. Bone Joint Surg. 60A, 1059, 1978.
9. Cherney, D.L. and Amstutz, H.C.: Total hip replacement in previously septic hips. Presented at the 48th Annual Meeting of the American Academy of Orthopaedic Surgeons, Las Vegas, 1981.
10. Dandy, D.J. and Theodorou, B.C.: The management of local complications of total hip replacement by the McKee-Farrar technique. J. Bone Joint Surg. 57B, 30, 1975.
11. Dupont, J.A., Campbell, E.D., and Lumsden, R.M.: Total knee arthroplasty revisions. Orthop. Transactions 3, 321, 1980.
12. Elson, R.A.: The management of deep infection involving joint implants J. Bone Joint Surg. 61B, 118, 1979.

13. Fitzgerald, R.H. and Bryan, R.S.: Indirect exchange of the infected hip implant. Course in Traumatic and Reconstructive Surgery of the Adult Hip, Harvard Medical School, Boston, September 1981.

14. Goldberg, V.M. and Sachs, B.L.: The results and complications of revision total knee arthroplasty. Orthop. Transactions 7, 547, 1983.

15. Hoagland, T., Razzano, C.D., Marks, K.E., and Wilde, A.H.: Revision of total hip arthroplasties. J. Bone Joint Surg. 61B, 247, 1979.

16. Hughes, P.W., Salvati, E.A., Wilson, P.D., and Blumenfeld, E.L.: Treatment of subacute sepsis of the hip by antibiotics and joint replacement. Criteria for diagnosis with evaluation of 26 cases. Clin. Orthop. Rel. Res. 141, 143, 1979.

17. Hunter, G.A.: The results of re-insertion of a total hip prosthesis after sepsis. J. Bone Joint Surg. 61B, 422, 1979.

18. Hunter, G.A., Welsh, R.P., Cameron, H.U., and Bailey, W.H.: The results of revision of total hip arthroplasty. J. Bone Joint Surg. 61B, 419, 1979.

19. Insall, J.N. and Dethmers, D.A.: Revision of total knee arthroplasty. Clin. Orthop. Rel. Res. 170, 123, 1982.

20. Insall, J.N., Thompson, F.M., and Brause, B.D.: Two stage reimplantation for the salvage of infected total knee arthroplasty. J. Bone Joint Surg. 65A, 1087, 1983.

21. James, E.T.R., Hunter, G.A. and Cameron, H.U.: Total hip revision arthroplasty. Does sepsis influence the results. Clin. Orthop. Rel. Res. 170, 88, 1982.

22. Jones, J.M.: Revisional total hip replacementment for failed Ring arthroplasty. J. Bone Joint Surg. 61A, 1029, 1979.

23. Jupiter, J.B., Carchmer, A.W., Lowell, J.D., and Harris, W.H.: Total hip arthroplasty in the treatment of adult hips with current acquiescent sepsis. J. Bone Joint Surg. 63A, 194, 1981.

24. Kim, L. and Finerman, G.: Results of revisions for aseptic failed total knee arthroplasties. Orthop. Transactions 7, 535, 1983.

25. Lautenbach, E.E.G. and Weber, F.A.: Total hip replacement after chronic hip infection. J. Bone Joint Surg. 62B, 282, 1980.

26. Pellici, P.M., Wilson, P.D., Sledge, C.B., Salvati, E.A., Ranawat, C.S., and Poss, R.: Results of revision total hip replacement. In, The Hip, Proc. 9th Open Scientific Meeting of the Hip Society, C.V. Mosby Co.1981, pp. 57-70.

27. Rand, J.A. and Bryan, R.S.: Reimplantation for the salvage of an infected total knee arthroplasty. J. Bone Joint Surg. 65A, 1081, 1983.

28. Samuelson, K.M., Freeman, M.A.R., and Day, W.H.: Salvage of failed total knee replacements; is a hinge necessary? Orthop. Transactions 4, 98, 1980.

29. Stillwell, W.T., Hamati, Y.I., Drinker, H., and Turner, R.H.: Total hip revision; indications and techniques. Orthop. Transactions 4, 326, 1980.

30. Thornhill, T.S., Dalziel, R.E., and Sledge, C.B.: Alternatives to arthrodesis for the failed total knee arthroplasty. Clin. Orthop. Rel. Res. 170, 131, 1982.

31. Walker, R.H. and Schurman, D.J.: Management of infected total knee replacement. Orthop. Transactions 7, 416, 1983.

32. Welch, R.B.: Femoral Revisions. In, The Hip. Proc. 9th Open Scientific Meeting of the Hip Society, C.V. Mosby Co. 1981, pp 25-36.

33. Wertzberger, K.L. and Bryan, R.S.: Analysis of failed total knee arthroplasty, excluding infection, undergoing reoperation. Orthop. Transactions 3, 265, 1979.

34. Wilson, M.R., Fitzgerald, R.H. and Coventry, M.B.: Reconstruction (delayed) by total hip arthroplasty after resection arthroplasty for infection. In, The Hip. Proc. 6th Open Scientific Meeting of the Hip Society, C.V. Mosby Co. 1978, pp 149-161.

Infection: Occupational Hazard to the Surgeon

N. E. MacDonald

Surgeons and other hospital personnel are often exposed to infectious diseases within and outside the hospital. They may thus be a source of transmission of infections to patients, other employees, and members of their households. Although many of these infections may be minor and of little consequence -- eg, *Staphylococcus aureus* nasal carriage -- others may be serious and even life threatening -- eg, fulminating hepatitis B virus infection. This paper briefly reviews a number of these occupational infectious hazards.

Microbial Infectious Hazards

S. aureus colonization and infection

S. aureus remains an important cause of hospital-acquired infection accounting for 15-20% of all nosocomial infections (Crossley et al, 1979). Due to environmental factors, surgeons and other hospital personnel have a higher staphylococcal colonization rate than the general public and are often the source of these nosocomial infections (Smith, 1979). The anterior nares are a prominent site for colonization and, unfortunately, eradication of nasal carriage is often difficult and frustrating. Recently, rifampin has proven to be effective in the eradication of staphylococcal nasal carriage (Wheat et al, 1981). Although this is usually not a major personal health problem for the surgeon, therapy may be indicated if his patients' wound infection rate is high or if he himself has recurrent furunculosis.

Resistant and miscellaneous microorganisms

Surgeons and other hospital employees may become colonized with multiple drug resistant microbes, such as aminoglycoside-resistant *Pseudomonas aeruginosa*. These organisms rarely cause a problem in normal hosts and thus the healthy surgeon is not at risk. The possibility of transmitting these organisms to patients can be reduced with good handwashing practices. However, physicians as a group are poorly compliant with this procedure (Albert and Condie, 1981).

Hospital personnel are also at risk of contracting tuberculosis from infected patients who have endobronchial disease or cavitary tuberculosis if the tubercle bacilli are present on smear. In general, discharges from draining tuberculous sinuses and urine from patients with genitourinary tuberculosis are much less infectious. Patients with tuberculosis become noninfectious a short time after starting treatment with appropriate antimycobacterial agents, thus reducing the risk to contacts (Glassroth et al,

Current Concepts of Infections in
Orthopaedic Surgery

1980). Skin testing and/or chest roentgenograph surveillance of hospital personnel can improve early detection of tuberculosis and thus reduce the risk of spread to other patients or family members.

Viral Infectious Hazards

Viral hepatitis

Viral hepatitis, particularly hepatitis B virus (HBV), has long been recognized as a major nosocomial hazard both to patients and to hospital employees. Unfortunately, as little as 10^{-7}mL of sera from a human chronic HBV carrier can transmit HBV infection (Gerety, 1981). Infected saliva and semen can also transmit HBV (Scott et al, 1980).

In developed countries, the incidence of HBV in the general population is approximately 3.5 per 10,000 persons per year. Unfortunately, the incidence is ten times higher in hospital personnel (Chaudhary, 1983; Janzen et al, 1978; Maynard, 1983). HBV infection in hospital personnel appears to be associated more often with handling and obtaining clinical specimens than with direct patient contact (Gerety, 1981). However, surgical and dental personnel are at higher risk than medical personnel because of their direct contact with blood.

Infection can be prevented by employing good technique in the operating room or when handling contaminated specimens. Although hepatitis B immunoglobulin and immunoglobulin have both been shown to be relatively effective for postexposure prophylaxis, neither are entirely satisfactory (Seeff and Hoofnagle, 1979). The newly licenced killed hepatitis B virus vaccine has proven to be efficacious for preexposure prophylaxis in controlled clinical trials in high risk populations (Szmuness et al, 1980). Since the vaccine is expensive and not all health care workers are at equal risk, most experts recommend selective immunization and prevaccine screening (Grady, 1982; Krugman, 1982; National Advisory Committee on Immunization, 1982). Surgeons are among the high risk groups and are frequently recommended to receive vaccine. At this time the risks from the vaccine appear to be minimal (Boucher and Fruesz, 1983; Krugman, 1980; Szmuness et al, 1980) and the benefits large.

Other viral agents

Surgeons and other hospital personnel are all at risk when exposed to rubella, varicella-zoster, measles, or mumps viruses unless immune due to prior infection or immunization. This risk is increased for personnel working on pediatric wards. Rubella-susceptible employees including men and women in all age groups who have contact with pregnant patients should be immunized. Although immunization is usually optional for employees who do not work in areas of the hospital serving pregnant patients, it should be encouraged (Klein, 1981). Surgeons who have not had chickenpox should avoid caring for children with acute infection. Since these children rarely have orthopedic problems at the time of infections, this is usually not an issue. Surgeons who have never had measles or mumps should consider immunization if they deal with pediatric patients.

Viruses associated with respiratory tract infections and/or gastroenteritis such as respiratory syncytial virus, parainfluenza virus, and rota virus can all be acquired from patients. Infections are usually self-limited and relatively minor. Surgeons can reduce this risk by practicing good infection control techniques, especially handwashing.

Herpes virus infection

Herpetic whitlow -- herpes simplex virus infection of the fingers -- is a rare event in the general population, but is a recognized hazard of medical practice (Rosato et al, 1970). This infection is usually acquired through exposure to infectious oral or tracheal secretions of affected patients. This risk can be minimized by wearing gloves on both hands when dealing with these patients (Greaves et al, 1980).

Fungal and Parasitic Infection Hazards

In general, fungal and parasitic infections are not major occupational health hazards for surgeons or other personnel. An important exception is *Coccidioides immitis*. This infection has been transmitted from patient to physician via plaster casts and dressings used in the care of a child with *C. immitis* osteomyelitis (Eckman et al, 1964). Since this organism is easily spread by the airborne route, suitable precautions should be taken in dealing with these patients.

Acquired Immune Deficiency Syndrome (AIDS)

Acquired immune deficiency syndrome (AIDS) is a newly recognized disease characterized by deregulation of the cell-mediated immune system and manifested by opportunistic infections, unusual neoplasms, and autoimmune phenomena in previously healthy persons (Landesman and Vieira, 1983). A retrovirus is currently thought to be the putative pathogen. Although AIDS has generated much anxiety, the risks to hospital employees caring for these patients appears to be minimal. A recent report from the Center for Disease Control revealed that of 1,831 cases of AIDS reported as of July 1983, only four cases were health care personnel not known to belong to groups at risk for AIDS (Editorial, 1983). Only one of these four patients had any contact with an AIDS patient and this was only indirectly. Transmission of AIDS within hospitals has not been reported. Thus, surgeons and other health care personnel appear to be at no greater risk for developing AIDS than members of the general population. The Center for Disease Control does recommend, however, that health care personnel take precautions similar to those recommended for HBV carriers when dealing with AIDS patients (Editorial, 1982). Lifestyle seems to be an important factor in preventing AIDS.

In summary, most of the occupational infection hazards for surgeons and other hospital employees can be minimized with good infection control practices and appropriate preemployment immunizations. Physicians must recognize that the simple technique of good handwashing before and after each patient visit can not only reduce the risk of nosocomial infections for the patient but also decrease the risk for themselves.

References

1. Albert, R.K. and Condie, F.: Hand-washing patterns in medical intensive-care units. N. Engl. J. Med. 304, 1465, 1981.

2. Boucher, D.W. and Furesz, J.: Hepatitis B vaccine and acquired immune deficiency syndrome (AIDS). Can. Dis. Weekly Rep. 9, 45, 1983.

3. Chaudhary, R.K.: Prevalence of hepatitis B markers in selected health care personnel from the Canadian forces. Can. Dis. Weekly Rep. 9, 197, 1983.

4. Crossley, K., Loesch, D., Landesman, B., Mead, K., Chern, M., and Strate, R.: An outbreak of infections caused by strains of *Staphylococcus aureus* resistant to methicillin and aminoglycosides. I. Clinical studies. J. Infect. Dis. 139, 273, 1979.

5. Eckmann, B.H., Schaefer, G.L., and Hupper, M.: Bedside interhuman transmission of coccidioidomycosis via growth on fomites. An epidemic involving six persons. Amer. Rev. Resp. Dis. 89, 175, 1964.

6. Editorial: Acquired immune deficiency syndrome (AIDS): Precautions for clinical and laboratory staffs. Morbid. Mortal. Weekly Rep. 31, 577, 1982.

7. Editorial: An evaluation of the acquired immunodeficiency syndrome (AIDS)reported in health-care personnel - United States. Morbid. Mortal. Weekly Rep. 32, 358, 1983.

8. Gerety, R.J.: Hepatitis B transmission between dental or medical workers and patients. Ann. Intern. Med. 95, 229, 1981.

9. Glassroth, J., Robins, A.G., and Snider, D.E.Jr.: Tuberculosis in the 1980s. N. Engl. J. Med. 302, 1441, 1980.

10. Grady, G.F.: Heaptitis B immunity in hospital staff targeted for vaccination. Role of screening tests in immunization programs. J.A.M.A. 248, 2266, 1982.

11. Greaves, W.L., Kaiser, A.B., Alford, R.H., and Schaffner, W.: The problem of herpetic Whitlow among hospital personnel. Infect. Control 1, 381, 1980.

12. Janzen, J., Tripatzis, I., Wagner, U., Schlieter, M., Muller-Dethard, E., and Wolters, E.: Epidemiology of hepatitis B surface antigen (HBsAg) and antibody to HBsAg in hospital personnel. J. Infect. Dis. 137, 261, 1978.

13. Klein, J.O.: Management of infections in hospital employees. Am. J. Med. 70, 919, 1981.

14. Krugman, S.: The newly licensed hepatitis B vaccine. Characteristics and indications for use. J.A.M.A. 247, 2012, 1982.

15. Landesman, S.H. and Vieira, J.: Acquired immune deficiency syndrome (AIDS). A review. Arch. Intern. Med. 143, 2307, 1983.

16. Maynard, J.E.: Nosocomial viral hepatitis. Am. J. Med. 70, 439, 1981.

17. National Advisory Committee on Immunization: Statement on hepatitis B virus vaccine. Can. Dis. Weekly Rep. 8, 221, 1982.

18. Rosato, F.E., Rosato, C.F., and Plotkin, S.A.: Herpetic paronyclia - an occupational hazard of medical personnel. N. Engl. J. Med. 283, 804, 1970.

19. Scott, R.M., Snitbhan, R., Bancroft, W.H., Alter, H.J., and Tingpalapong, M.: Experimental transmission of hepatitis B virus by semen and saliva. J. Infect. Sci. 142, 67, 1980.

20. Seeff, L.B. and Hoofnagle, J.H.: Immunoprophylaxis of viral hepatitis. Gastroent. 77, 161, 1979.

21. Smith, I.M.: *Staphylococcus aureus*. In, Mandell, G.L., Douglass, R.G., and Bennett, J.E. (Eds.): Principles and Practice of Infectious Disease, 1979. pp 1530-1552.

22. Szmuness, W., Stevens, C.E., Harley, E.J., Zang, E.A., Oleszko, W.R., William, D.C., Sadovsky, R., Morrison, J.M., and Kellner, A.: Hepatitis B vaccine. Demonstration of efficacy in a controlled clinical trial in a high-risk population in the United States. N. Engl. J. Med. 303, 833, 1980.

23. Wheat, L.J., Kohler, R.B., White, A.L. and White, A.: Effect of rifampin on nasal carriers of coagulase-positive staphylococci. J. Infect. Dis. 144, 177, 1981.

Isolation of the Infected Patient

J. C. N. WESTWOOD

Introduction

The practice of isolating patients with dangerous diseases is probably as old as Homo sapiens even if the learned medical profession did not accept the "germ theory of disease" before the nineteenth century and with it the possibility that one person might infect another. Certainly, ordinary people had no doubts, at least in respect to certain diseases such as leprosy and bubonic plague -- although they were actually wrong in the latter case. Leper colonies and the practice followed during the Black Death of walling entire families into their houses when a case of plague had occurred amongst them testify clearly to this fact. Nevertheless, isolation as a means of controlling the spread of infectious diseases has usually proved a dismal failure even in modern times. The need for the isolation of infected patients in hospitals is still the subject of dispute and is often resented alike by patient and treating physician. This unfortunate reaction results from a failure to understand the purpose and the limitations of the practice. Consequently, it often results in the closing of the stable door after the horse has gone -- and it is often the wrong stable door and even the wrong horse. Moreover, the true culprit may not even be a horse but rather an inoffensive mouse which comes and goes through a hole in the stable wall unnoticed.

The first step in correcting this misunderstanding should be to forget the term "isolation" with its implication of locking up the patient and throwing away the key. The basic purpose is, of course, to prevent the transfer of a disease from the infected patient to persons who are not infected. Isolation is intended not only to confine the patient but also to limit contamination to a known circumscribed area and consequently entails a complex of technical procedures beyond just the physical segregation of the patient. It may indeed be effective for the purpose intended but may still fail to achieve control if, as is usually the case, the infected patient is not the real danger.

In clean orthopedic surgery, for example, postoperative wound infection is usually the result of the introduction of microbial contamination in the operating room during the operation itself and is not derived from the subsequent proximity of an infected patient. While an infected patient may indeed be a source of infection, the danger is not that of direct transfer of infection to another patient but rather its indirect transfer through one or more contacts -- the inoffensive mice -- who may pick up and carry the causal organism without evidence of the fact. Moreover, while the carrier state may be purely mechanical, as by contaminated hands, its more

Current Concepts of Infections in
Orthopaedic Surgery

serious and threatening form is that of colonization of the carrier which may arise without contact with an infected person. In the case of *Staphylococcus aureus*, for example, the carrier state is already established in over 25% of the normal population and usually reaches still higher levels in hospital staff exposed to patients. Consequently, to prevent the spread of infection it is necessary to concentrate on the agent of infection rather than on infection itself. The disease process is a secondary factor and may be a poor indicator of the spread of the infecting agent and may also be misleading as to the mechanism of transmission.

Poliomyelitis and meningococcal meningitis are both infections of the central nervous system. Obviously, their infectious agents locked into the CNS are no danger to anyone other than the patient. Yet, both are highly infectious diseases not by virtue of the clinical cases but due to the associated subclinical spread, usually undetected, and the long-term carriers seeded through the community. In institutional communities, particularly military recruit barracks, the silent carrier epidemic of meningococcal colonization may involve 95% of the community population while giving rise to only a few apparently sporadic cases of clinical meningitis. Isolation of the clinical cases can do nothing to halt the spread of the epidemic or the occurrence of further cases -- the wrong horse too late.

The spread of poliomyelitis is similar, and even in severe epidemics only about 10% of the infected population develop paralytic symptoms. In their clinical presentation both diseases are CNS infections, but this fact gives no clue as to their modes of transmission which are totally different. Poliomyelitis is primarily an intestinal infection spread by the fecal-oral route while meningococcal infection is respiratory in origin and the carrier state is nasopharyngeal. Even in the isolation of clinical cases, therefore, the same measures would not be appropriate for the two diseases. If such factors are not understood and taken into account in establishing isolation policies, these will not only be ineffective but much time and effort will be wasted on useless procedures.

Epidemiology of Infection

The relevant aspects of infection may be summarized in the form shown in Figure 1, with the understanding that this is a simplification that does not show the underlying chain which keeps the infection going in the human population. It represents only the mechanisms involved in a single transfer of an infectious agent. Three basic elements must be present -- a source, a transfer mechanism, and a recipient. Each of these elements is susceptible to differing approaches in any attempt to halt the transfer process.

The source of the causative agent may be: (Fig.1)

1. *Environmental:* This category would include the general hospital environment which could mediate such diseases as Legionnaires disease or could harbor dust or contamination in which potentially infective organisms can survive. Certain types of equipment may also be included, such as respiratory apparatuses and humidifiers.

2. *Patients:* Patients may shed organisms into the environment from a focus of infection.

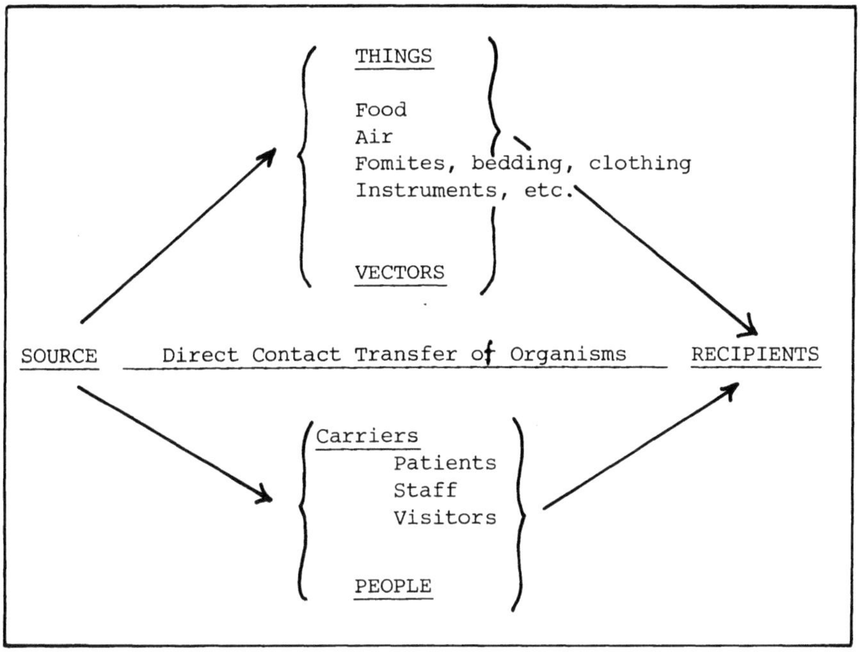

Fig. 1. Basic epidemiology of infection

3. *Carriers:* Patients may carry organisms possibly unrelated to the reason for their admission. Staff or visitors may also be carriers.

Control

Environment. Environmental sources must be identified and eliminated. This may be difficult when a major item such as the water supply is involved. In most hospitals, however, minor sources such as dust, respiratory therapy equipment or humidifiers should not present uncontrollable problems.

Infected patients. Those who are shedding organisms may be treated to eliminate their infective state, or may be segregated with full isolation precautions or appropriate modifications thereof. Discharging wounds may require no more than occlusive dressings.

Carriers. These individuals present a more difficult problem since they cannot readily be identified. Overt infections in staff or visitors are more easily detected but the true carrier state is seldom investigated unless during an outbreak of identifiable infection such as may occur with methicillin-resistant staphylococci. When such carriers are detected, the options are to cure the carrier state or to exclude the carrier from patient contact.

Transmission

Transmission is the most complex issue in the chain of events since so many different factors may be involved. In general, one may consider direct and indirect routes. The direct route represents the transference by physical contact of infective material from one patient to another, usually by the hands of the nursing staff or physicians. This type of transfer should not occur and indicates faulty procedures.

More difficult to control are the indirect routes of which there are many. They may be divided into the three general categories of "Things", "Vectors" and "People".

Except in the tropics or under special circumstances, vectors are not of major importance in the modern hospital setting. Similarly, "Things" should not be major problems in efficiently run hospitals of modern design but may be difficult to control in older establishments. Even in modern settings, however, the requirements of invasive instrumentation require continuous alertness. "People" are again the main problem and the carrier who may become colonized with dangerously pathogenic hospital strains of microorganisms is both difficult to detect and difficult to eliminate. Obviously, such individuals may be regarded as either sources of transmitting agents and have been deliberately included in both categories.

Control measures in this complex area must be tailored to the particular circumstances and no attempt will be made to cover all possibilities in this paper.

Recipient

The final stage is that of the susceptible recipient. This may be another patient but may also be a member of the hospital staff or a visitor. Visitors can be shrouded in minimal protective clothing but can only be effectively protected by exclusion when the hazard is considered severe enough to warrant it. Staff must be protected primarily by effective methods, including the proper use of protective clothing, but they may also require prophylactic vaccination or antimicrobial therapy.

The patient may be protected by reverse isolation at an appropriate level, by vaccination where applicable, or by antimicrobial prophylaxis. In orthopedics, the direct protection of the patient who is to undergo surgery is by far the most effective measure.

It should be noted that the epidemiologic outline in Figure 1 is general and covers more than the type of problem likely to be encountered in the orthopedic field. Nevertheless, it provides a basis on which to devise appropriate measures for the more specific orthopedic situations. What we have endeavored to emphasize and illustrate is that "Isolation" as a method for the prevention of the spread of infection is only a part of what is required. The procedure undoubtedly has merits but if it is applied without an understanding of the entire mechanisms underlying the problem it is likely to be a failure.

Conclusion

Infections in the orthopedic field fall generally into two areas: 1) established osteomyelitis or suppurative arthritis -- which are either closed types of infection or are relatively easily controlled by minimal segregation and good dressing techniques; and 2) postoperative infections following clean surgery, particularly arthroplasty. These latter infections are of the greatest concern and there is general consensus that such infections are initiated by microbial contamination in the operating room itself at the time of surgery. Once the wound is sutured and sealed, there is little likelihood that subsequent infection is derived from ward procedures. If this is indeed the case, then the only danger from the ward is before the patient reaches the operating room -- the patient acquiring an induced carrier state which will increase the likelihood of contamination of the wound at the time of surgery. It is at this stage that isolation is likely to be of most value -- but it is not isolation of the infected patient which will achieve this result but isolation of the candidate for surgery. This is the patient who should be protected by segregation.

Isolation Ward (Septic Ward) for Infected Patients

I. Kempf, M. A. Sittler, L. Lecocq, and M. Klem

Introduction

The Centre de Traumatologie et d'Orthopédie de Strasbourg, which opened in 1975, contains 250 beds and has an isolation ward of 16 beds for infected patients. In the old hospital, a unit consisting of eight beds was started in 1968 at a time when surgery of bone and joint infections was recognized as requiring specialized treatment and, therefore, separate wards to take proper care of these patients. The objectives established in 1968 are still valid today: first, to take care of patients with bone, joint or soft tissue infections in a specially designated unit; second to introduce hygienic measures to avoid transmission of microbes to prevent further contamination of other infected patients, and to protect noninfected patients.

Isolation Ward for Septic Patients

The unit

This ward, isolated and separated from the other wards, contains two operating rooms, 16 beds in six double rooms, and one room with four beds. The layout was designed to position the rooms conveniently for patients and staff. The isolation is achieved by a closed door with a bell. The long access corridor is divided in two to create a lock. Here, change rooms for the staff are located (Fig. 1).

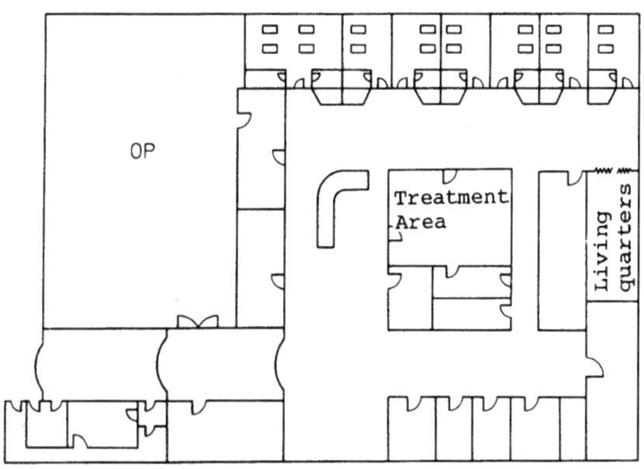

Fig. 1. Architectural design and layout

Current Concepts of Infections in Orthopaedic Surgery

Hospital staff

The medical team includes one staffman in charge of the ward and his chief resident. These two physicians do not work full time on this ward. A full-time resident and a consultant bacteriologist complete this team.

The paramedical team consists of 20 persons: a head nurse, six registered nurses, eight nursing assistants, three housekeepers, one secretary and a half-time physiotherapist.

Patient population

All patients with bone, joint or soft tissue infections, primary or secondary, are admitted to the Isolation Ward.

In 1983, we admitted 216 patients: 170 men and 46 women, an occupancy of 90% compared with 86% occupancy for the entire hospital. The average stay was 25.35 days as compared with 10.5 for the rest of our institution.

Of the patients, 25% had been transferred from the other wards. The rest came from our city and its surroundings and also from other countries. Interestingly, 7% of these patients came to us from psychiatric institutions.

The breakdown of infections is shown in Table I.

Table I.

Infection	No. of patients
Infected pseudarthroses	30
Osteitis after compound fractures	28
Suppurative arthritis	33
Osteomyelitis	4
Deep infections after total hip replacement	2
Wound breakdowns (necrosis, skin slough, infected stumps, etc.)	34
Pin tract infections	2
Abscesses	14
Infected bursitis	3
Infected hematoma	18
Drainage from old osteitis	13
Panaritium, burn, infected cysts	7

Flow and organization of care

The basic principle is the strict separation into clean and dirty areas. The flow must be based on a logical sequence of steps to protect the patient, the staff, and the remaining part of the hospital against any dissemination of microbes. Special measures are taken concerning linen, other material, dressings, diagnostic apparatuses and equipment. Strictest regulations have to be adhered to as to washing of hands.

Linen

Clean linen is stored in special lockers on arrival. Before any linen change, the clean stock is placed on a trolley. The nurse and her assistant put on a plastic apron, and the dirty linen is put into a plastic bag mounted on a special stand. Once the bed is changed, the nurse and her aide put the plastic apron into the plastic bag and wash their hands. The dirty linen is then carried into a holding area and is double bagged. This area has two doors: one toward the unit, the other leading to the outside. The person carrying away the bags is not admitted to the unit.

Materials and clothing

We do not repeat the flow used for the linen, but it should be stressed that individual clothes trolleys are numbered as to room and patient, and the treatment room is divided into a clean and dirty side.

Clothing procedures

The physician and the nurse put on a single-use gown. Dirty clothes are removed with special gloves having a large cuff which permits pulling the glove over the clothes (Fig. 2). Both are put into the plastic bag which will later be incinerated. All the clothes are sterilized in the autoclave of the Isolation Ward.

Hand washing

Before and after any act, hand washing is obligatory. This also helps to separate clean from dirty areas.

Radiologic equipment

The Isolation Ward has its own mobile roentgen unit which remains in the Ward. Thus, a potential source of contamination is eliminated.

Miscellaneous measures

Other important points:

- For cleaning of the Isolation ward, special agents recommended by the bacteriologist are used as part of our infection control measures.
- All rooms are disinfected twice a month. Moreover, patient rooms and beds are thoroughly cleaned after discharge. The operating rooms are disinfected after the daily schedule is terminated.
- Visitors are admitted daily from 1 pm to 8 pm. Each visitor has to wear a gown and plastic boot-covers.
- The patients can leave the ward to go to the cafeteria or to walk in the park. The dressing, however, will be done before and covered by clean linen. Patients with drains are excluded from these privileges.

Some of the measures outlined above and the rigid discipline carried out in this Ward may seem exaggerated, but we believe they are based on sound bacteriologic and scientific facts relative to hygiene and prevention of infection.

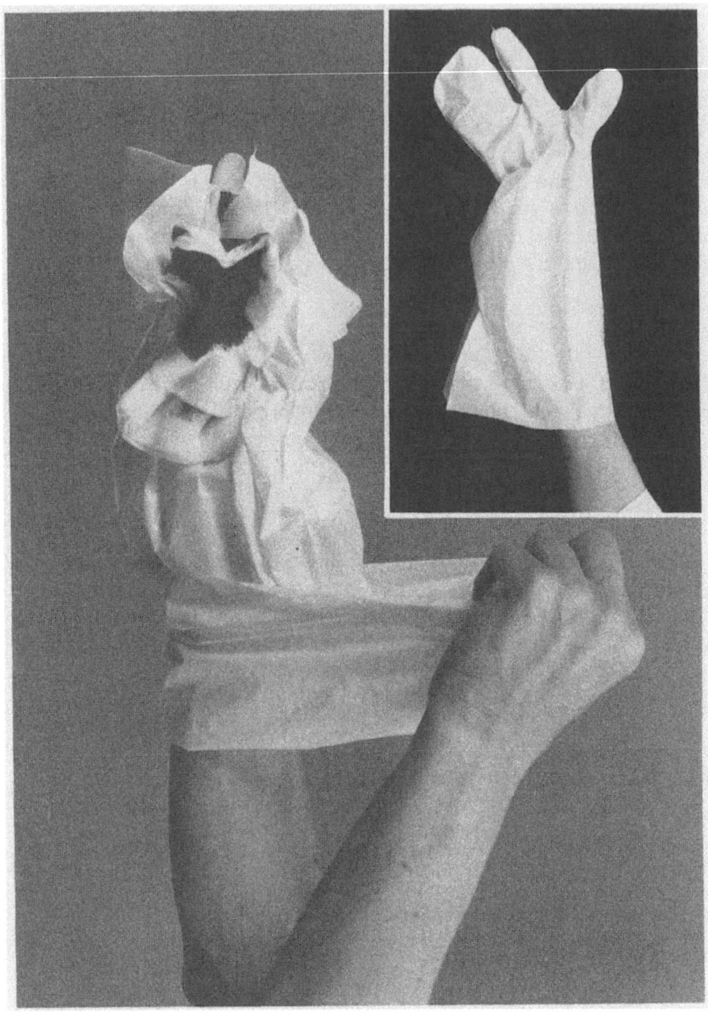

Fig. 2. Double-purpose glove to pick up and bag contaminated materials

Needless to say, such a ward creates problems for personnel and patients. This is how our nurses feel: "We found that most of our patients exhibit a particular psychologic behavior. They often come from homes with unfavorable conditions and their personal hygiene is certainly not optimal. Moreover, it is difficult to keep them occupied.

The isolation in the ward is often perceived as the result of a treatment failure. The rules and regulations of the ward, relative to the rigid precautions against infection, may give the impression that the patient has a plague and is therefore rejected by the others. This impression is especially accentuated by the isolation of the ward and the precautions taken while entering and leaving the ward.

The hospital stay is prolonged for certain patients. Readmissions occur frequently. Besides, patients are uncertain as to the treatment outcome.

After a prolonged stay, anxiety about returning to an active life may affect their will for complete recovery. The ward may thus become a second home. The patients know each other, discuss their problems and their treatment regimens. A case of recurrence is talked about by everybody and the disappointment shared by all. Such a demoralizing situation leads in certain patients to aggressiveness, often expressed as hostility towards the health care team.

This team, on the other hand, has it own problems; for example, the fact that most patients who are admitted to the ward have experienced a treatment failure also reflects on the staff.

Recurrences, despite all precautions, are demoralizing. We are happy when cured patients come back to the Outpatient Clinic to visit and say hello to us. Such success is encouraging for us.

Another problem is that the Isolation Ward is small. All rooms border on the same corridor. This leads to a familiarity among the health care staff and the patients which is sometimes difficult to tolerate. It is preferable that a certain distance be kept between patients and personnel so that the staff can demand strict adherence to the regulation."

Despite some troublesome personal and interpersonal problems that can arise due to the rigid rules and regulations, an isolation ward has definite advantages, such as -

1) grouping of infected patients in a specific setup which permits specialized care;

2) adherence to rigid rules of hygiene helps to avoid or to reduce the transmission of microbes and superinfection;

3) the daily routine imposes on the health care team -- physicians, residents, nurses, and other personnel -- a most rigid discipline. They realize that the rules have to be followed, and that the management of an isolation ward requires full cooperation and devotion to an important task.

Antibiotic-Resistant Microorganisms

A. M. R. MacKenzie

Microorganisms may be resistant to antibiotics by one of four basic mechanisms:

1) they may synthesize enzymes that inactivate antibiotics;
2) target sites on the microorganisms may be resistant to antibiotic binding;
3) they may become resistant to particular antibiotics by the development of metabolic pathways which bypass the site of the antibiotic's action;
4) they may modify their inner or outer membrane to prevent the penetration of the antibiotic to the microbial target site.

It must be emphasized that antibiotic susceptibility is a measurement and not a qualitative definition. For logistic reasons, most laboratories report microorganisms as being "sensitive" or "resistant" to a particular antibiotic. In addition, some laboratories also report a category of "intermediate sensitivity". Even within the range of "sensitive" the actual degree of susceptibility can vary widely. For instance, in the case of *Pseudomonas aeruginosa*, a minimal inhibitory concentration of less than 4 mg/L for tobramycin is regarded as being sensitive according to internationally recognized criteria. A "sensitive" organism can therefore have a minimal inhibitory concentration as high as 4 mg/L or as low as 0.4 mg/L, and either of these would be regarded as sensitive to tobramycin. From the practical management point of view, however, these two strains differ widely as to causes of infections. It is much more important in the case of the first rather than the second strain to ensure achievement of adequate antibiotic serum concentrations, and relapse due to inadequate therapy is more likely in the case of the first strain.

In many infectious diseases a wrong choice of antibiotic becomes obvious by early failure of clinical response. In certain circumstances, however, failure to eradicate the infecting organism is not initially clinically obvious, and will only become manifest as a recrudescence of infection after cessation of therapy. Two examples of this situation are endocarditis and osteomyelitis. It has been established in both that inadequate therapy will only result in temporary improvement and not permanent cure. The management of these situations demands attention to detail in the selection of antibiotic with the best possible antimicrobial activity, and in ensuring that this antibiotic is used optimally to obtain the highest possible antibiotic level at the site of infection. In certain situations *in vitro* sensitivity reports may be correct by the standard laboratory criteria but clinically misleading in that failure of therapy would be likely. These are reviewed below, with particular reference to orthopedic practice.

Current Concepts of Infections in
Orthopaedic Surgery

Tolerant Staphylococci

Some strains of *Staphylococcus aureus*, although apparently sensitive to isoxazolyl penicillins, such as cloxacillin, by the standard laboratory sensitivity criteria, are only inhibited and not killed by these antibiotics. These strains may be reported as sensitive by the laboratory using the standard tests and the antibiotic tolerance will only be apparent when the actual bactericidal action of the antibiotic is examined.

The prevalence of these strains has been estimated to be about 25% to 50% (Lorian, 1980). The clinical significance of this phenomenon is difficult to determine. The relatively high prevalence of these tolerant strains suggests that it is not always clinically significant. There are, however, case reports of pneumonia (Svenungsson et al, 1982) and soft tissue infections (Denny et al, 1979) in which failure of therapy with single antibiotics was attributable to tolerance. There are no controlled observations on the significance of tolerance in the therapy of orthopedic infections, and the variability of response of these patients would make the data difficult to obtain. It is possible that in some patients tolerance may result in delayed clinical response which could be accelerated by the addition of a second drug (an aminoglycoside or rifampin). For a review of this topic, see Kaye (1980).

Cross Resistance of *S. aureus* between Methicillin and Cephalosporins

Methicillin/cloxacillin resistant *S. aureus* strains are frequent in some locations and the prevalence of these strains has increased significantly in the last decade. Detection of this type of resistance is not difficult in the laboratory, although culture conditions have to be carefully controlled. Methicillin-resistant *S. aureus* strains are resistant to all beta-lactam antibiotics, although cephalosporins may give results in the laboratory indicating *in vitro* susceptibility. Therapy with these antibiotics, however, frequently results in failure (Acar et al, 1978; Myers and Linnemann, 1982). Therefore, when methicillin resistance is detected, laboratory reports indicating cephalosporin sensitivity should be disregarded and the organism considered resistant to all beta-lactam antibiotics (Wenzel, 1982).

Strains of *Staphylococcus epidermidis* show methicillin resistance more frequently than strains of *S. aureus*. These strains frequently show *in vitro* sensitivity to cephalosporins (Archer, 1978), but there may be a phenomenon similar to that described for *S. aureus*. In one study, methicillin-resistant *S. epidermidis* showed sensitivity to cephalothin by standard methods, but tests of bactericidal activity showed tolerance to the same agent. The authors of this study recommended that bactericidal as well as standard inhibitory tests be used before a decision is made to treat methicillin-resistant *S. epidermidis* infections with cephalosporins (Laverdière et al, 1978). Cephalosporins should therefore only be used for *S. epidermidis* infections after careful laboratory assessment and after consideration of the use of other possible agents.

The Use of Cefamandole

Cefamandole is, on first examination, an attractive antibiotic for the initial management of many orthopedic infections in children, given its high *in vitro* activity against staphylococci, streptococci, and *Haemophilus influenzae*. This antibiotic does not, however, enter the cerebrospinal fluid (CSF) compartment in therapeutic amounts. Cases have been reported (Marks, 1981) where patients being treated for invasive nonmeningitic *H. influenzae* type B disease developed meningitis on therapy, despite the *in vitro* sensitivity of the organism. Two such cases have also been seen by the author (unpublished). These occurrences are probably due to the coexistence of unrecognized early meningitis together with the diagnosed infection under treatment. The use of an antibiotic which does not penetrate the CSF allows the development of meningitis during the course of treatment. It is most important, when it is felt necessary to use cefamandole, that the possibility of meningitis be recognized, both initially and later if the patient does not show the expected clinical response.

Emergence of Resistance during Treatment

This has been described for many antibiotics, but two are of particular significance in orthopedic practice.

Fusidic acid

This highly active antistaphylococcal antibiotic has been widely used for the management of staphylococcal osteomyelitis. Development of resistance of strains under treatment has been reported when the antibiotic is used alone, and it is probably advisable that this antibiotic always be used in combination. The possibility that resistance has emerged in this way should be considered in situations where relapse has occurred (Amirak et al, 1981; Patterson and Mansell, 1973).

Rifampin

This antibiotic is being used increasingly in orthopedic practice due to its high activity against *S. aureus*. The antibiotic has a high mutation rate to resistance. The ease with which strains of organisms under treatment become resistant has been well known for many years in the case of tuberculosis. The same phenomenon occurs with *S. aureus*, and for this reason this antibiotic should never be used alone for the therapy of major infections.

Summary

In orthopedic practice, the choice of an antibiotic should be guided by laboratory susceptibility test results. Special considerations are:

1. Antibiotic serum levels should be monitored in treating infections where the causative organism has marginal susceptibility to the antibiotic.
2. Cephalosporins cannot be regarded as a substitute for cloxacillin or methicillin in the treatment of methicillin-resistant *S. aureus* infections, even though *in vitro* tests may indicate cephalosporin sensitivity. The same restriction probably applies to *S. epidermidis*.
3. Resistance can emerge in the course of treatment. This happens easily with rifampin, and, less often, in the case of fusidic acid.

References

1. Acar, J.F., Courvalin, P., and Chabbert, Y.A.: Methicillin resistant staphylococcaemia: Bacteriological failure of treatment with cephalosporins. Antimicrob. Agents Chemother. 14, 280, 1978.

2. Amirak, I.D., Li, A.K.C., Williams, R.J., and Noone, P.: A fatal infection caused by methicillin resistant *Staphylococcus aureus* acquiring resistance to gentamicin and fusidic acid during therapy. J. Infect. 3, 50, 1981.

3. Archer, G.L.: Antimicrobial susceptibility and selection of resistance among *Staphylococcus epidermidis* isolates recovered from patients with infections of indwelling foreign devices. Antimicrob. Agents Chemother. 14, 353, 1978.

4. Denny, A.E., Peterson, L.R., Gerding, D.N., and Hall, W.M.: Serious staphylococcal infections with strains tolerant to bactericidal antibiotics. Arch. Int. Med. 139, 1026, 1979.

5. Kaye, D.: The clinical significance of tolerance to *Staphylococcus aureus*. Ann. Int. Med. 93, 924, 1980.

6. Laverdière, M., Peterson, P.K., Verhoef, J., Williams, D.N., and Sabath, L.D.: *In vitro* activity of cephalosporins against methicillin resistant, coagulase-negative staphylococci. J. Infect. Dis. 137, 245 1978.

7. Lorian, V.: Antibiotics in Laboratory Medicine. Williams & Williams, 1980, p. 451.

8. Marks, M.I.: Antibiotic therapy of serious *Haemophilus* infections: a continuing problem. J. Pediat. 98, 910, 1981.

9. Myers, J.P., and Linnemann, C.C.: Bacteremia due to methicillin resistant *Staphylococcus aureus*. J. Infect. Dis. 145, 532, 1982.

10. Patterson, J.R., and Mansell, P.E.: Fucidin resistant staphylococci in current hospital practice. J. Med. Microbiol. 6, 235, 1973.

11. Svenungsson, B., Kalin, M., and Lingren, L.G.: Therapeutic failure in pneumonia caused by a tolerant strain of *Staphylococcus aureus*. Scand. J. Infect. Dis. 14, 309, 1982.

12. Wenzel, R.P.: The emergence of methicillin resistant *Staphylococcus aureus*. Ann. Int. Med. 97, 440, 1982.

The Use of Antibiotics in Traumatized Patients

R. B. GUSTILO

Serious morbidity and occasionally death may result from wound sepsis in major skeletal trauma. Open reduction and internal fixation of long bone fractures and open fracture treatment are, therefore, the major indications for antibiotic prophylaxis. Currently, wound sepsis rate following joint replacement and major trauma surgery with antibiotic prophylaxis is less than 2%. The consequences, however, are devastating requiring prolonged and repeated hospitalization, repeated extensive surgical debridement, and prolonged antibiotic coverage resulting in an expensive undertaking. The comparative hospital expenses for infected and noninfected total hip replacement, hip nailing, and Type III open fracture reduction at Hennepin County Medical Center and Metropolitan Medical Center in Minneapolis is shown in Table I. Such expenses showed a 5-10 times increase for hospitalization of infected patients. Worse are the consequences of wound sepsis, such as loss of joint function, arthrodesis, and occasionally loss of the extremity or even life.

Table I. Hospital stay and expenses: Infected vs noninfected fractures

	Average hospital stay (days)	Cost ($)
Hip fractures		
noninfected	13	3,250
infected	66	33,000
Open fractures - Type III		
noninfected	19	4,750
infected	108	54,000
Total hip replacement		
noninfected	13	10,000
infected	83	64-92,000

Undoubtedly, the goal to prevent wound sepsis is paramount to all surgeons and the first question is: How effective is antibiotic prophylaxis to prevent wound infection?

Current Concepts of Infections in
Orthopaedic Surgery

Miles et al (1957) demonstrated in laboratory animals that effectiveness of antibiotic prophylaxis depends on adequate drug concentrations in wound tissue or hematoma before bacterial contamination occurs. Introduction of antibiotics after inoculation of a hematoma with microbes did not prevent wound sepsis. Indeed, earlier studies of antibiotic prophylaxis given post-operatively did not prevent wound sepsis. In fact, some investigators have reported higher postoperative wound infections. Boyd et al (1973) were the first to conduct a prospective double-blind study in patients with hip fractures using oxacillin. Their statistical results showed reduced infection with antibiotic prophylaxis. A double-blind prospective study in patients with hip fractures using cefalothin was conducted in our institution by Drs. Burnette, Gustilo and Williams in 1980. The results revealed a 0.6% infection rate in the patient group receiving antibiotic prophylaxis compared with 4.7% infection rate in the placebo group (Burnett et al, 1980). Other subsequent studies showed similar results.

The second question is: What is the best antibiotic for prophylaxis? Cefazolin is our number one choice. It is effective against gram-positive and some gram-negative microorganisms; it is relatively nontoxic and it is inexpensive. Among the cephalosporins, we believe cefazolin is the drug of choice for prophylaxis on the basis of bone penetration, ease of administration, and cost.

The third question is: When do we give the antibiotic, how long, and how much? Several studies clearly indicate that antibiotics diffuse rapidly into the synovial fluid and into bone. Our studies of five different cephalosporins (Table II) showed that peak bone levels occurred within 60 minutes of drug administration. The advantages of a 2 g dose is based on a consistently higher bone level compared with a 1 g dose.

Table II. Bone and serum concentrations of five cephalosporins

Antibiotic	Antibiotic concentration (mean) 1 g dose		2 g dose		Time of bone sampling* (mean)	
	Bone (mg/g)	Serum (mg/mL)	Bone (mg/g)	Serum (mg/mL)	1 g dose	2 g dose
Cephalothin	0.5 (SD = 0.21)	5.3	0.9+ (SD = 0.45)	31.5	91	63†
Cefazolin	5.9	51.7	14.9	98.3	69	51
Cefamandole	--	--	6.7	46.7	--	69
Cefoxitin	3.6	17.5	6.3	39.0	74	69
Ceforanide	9.1	67.8	13.4	144.0	62	82

* In minutes (after completion of intravenous administration)
\+ Statistically significant ($p < 0.01$); 1 g vs 2 g antibiotic concentration
† Statistically significant ($p < 0.01$); timing of 1 g vs 2 g sampling

Postoperative duration of preventive antibiotic administration has undergone a major change. In a recent study of patients undergoing total hip replacement, no differences in infection rate were found between those receiving one day of prophylactic antibiotics and those receiving 7-10 days' prophylaxis postoperatively (Riska, 1980; Schurman et al, 1980). Similarly, Nelson et al (1983) found no difference in infection rate between patients receiving antibiotics for one day prophylactically versus seven days postoperatively. Our practice for the last five years in skeletal trauma surgery has been to give cefazolin, 2 g, in the surgical anteroom immediately before surgery, and to continue with 1 g q 8 h for 24 hours only. Short duration of antibiotic prophylaxis prevents emergence of resistant organisms. The other advantage of giving the antibiotics in the surgical anteroom is that in the rare case of anaphylaxis, it can be treated with resuscitation in a controlled situation.

We chose cefazolin among the cephalosporins at this time based on serum and bone levels, cost, ease of administration, and the sensitivity of the likely infecting organism.

Open Fractures

We believe strongly that antibiotic treatment for open fractures is a therapeutic measure and not prophylactic. Our results (Table III) support the continuous use of a single cephalosporin in Type I and Type II open fractures. However, in Type III open fractures, because of the change of

Table III. Wound sepsis in closed nailing -- femur, tibia, and hip fractures

Type of fracture	Antibiotic*	No. of patients	Days of administration	Wound sepsis rate
Femur (1978-82)	Cefazolin	196	1	0.5%
Tibia (1977-82)	Cefazolin	60	2	3.3%
Hip (1975-78)	Placebo	151	3	4.7% (5)
	Cephalothin	154	3	0.7% (1)
Hip (1979-83)	Cefazolin	478	1	0.4% (2)

* Dosage: 2 g preoperatively and 1 g q 8 h

bacterial pathogens from gram-positive (76%) to gram-negative organisms (87%), our recommendation is a combination of cephalosporins and an aminoglycoside (Table IV). With potential soil contamination, such as farm injuries, we add penicillin G, 10-12 million units daily. Therefore, our current practice for Type I and Type II open fractures is to administer a cephalosporin, 2 g on admission and 1 g q 8 h for three days only. For Type III open fracture, we add an aminoglycoside, either tobramycin or amikacin, for three days only. For farm injuries with potential gas gangrene infection, we use triple antibiotic therapy -- a cephalosporin, an aminoglycoside, and a penicillin. Antibiotics are given again for three days at: 1) wound closure; 2) delayed internal fixation of the open fracture;

Table IV. Bacterial flora of wound infections in Type III open fractures

Culture identification	Study period		
	1980-83	1976-79	1955-75
Gram-positive			
Coagulase-positive	3	4	30
Enterococcus	0	3	0
Total	3	7	30
Gram-negative			
Staphylococcus coagulase-negative	1		3
Escherichia coli	1	5	4
Enterobacter cloacae	0	5	
Enterobacter aerogenes	1	3	
Klebsiella species	1	3	2
Pseudomonas species	2	2	3
Serratia marcescens	1	2	
Morganella morganii		2	
Proteus mirabilis	1	1	3
Proteus vulgaris		1	
Other (G-rod)		0	1
Total	8	27	17
Negative culture	0	0	5

Chi-square for gram-negative vs gram-positive cultures in two time periods is 13.71 with 1 degree of freedom ($p < .01$)

and 3) when cancellous bone grafting is done. Not a single case of gas gangrene has been seen in our institution in over 1500 patients treated for open fracture (Table V).

Summary

Antibiotic prophylaxis is effective in reducing wound sepsis in major elective musculoskeletal surgery. A cephalosporin is the antibiotic of choice, administered at a 2 g dose one hour before surgery and 1 g q 8 h for three days after surgery.

In open fractures, a cephalosporin alone is effective in reducing wound sepsis for Type I and II open fractures and a combination of cephalosporin-aminoglycoside therapy for Type III open fractures is recommended for three days. Penicillin is added for soil contaminated wounds, such as farm injuries.

Table V. Infection rates in 1,537 open fractures -- Hennepin County Medical Center, 1955-1983.

Study period	Fracture types I Inf/N (%)	Fracture types II Inf/N (%)	Fracture types III Inf/N (%)	Total all fracture types Inf/N (%)	Antibiotics used
1955-1960[1]	- Not available -			25/215 (11.6)	Penicillin
1961-1968[2]	- 9/422 - (2.1)		15/36 (44.0)	24/458 (5.2)	Penicillin & chloramphenicol
1969-1975[2]	0/256 (0.0)	2/166 (1.2)	10/98 (10.2)	12/520 (2.3) OXIC	Oxacillin or cephalothin
1976-1979	0/70 (0.0)	2/55 (3.6)	20/82 (24.4)	22/207 (10.6)	Cefazolin
1980-1983	0/53 (0.0)	2/47 (4.2)	4/37 (10.8)	6/137 (4.3)	Cefazolin (I & II) Cefazolin & tobramycin (III)
Total*	0/379* (0.0)	6/268* (2.2)	49/253* (19.3)	89/1537 (5.8)	

* Partial totals which do not include unallocatable data from 1955-1968
[1] Gustilo and Anderson, 1976
[2] Gustilo et al, in press

The overall rate of infections differed significantly across the time periods [chi-square statistic with 3 degrees of freedom = 14.43, ($p<.01$)]. The differences remained statistically significant even with the exclusion of the extremely low rate occurring in the 1969-75 period [chi-square statistic with 2 degrees of freedom = 10.44 ($p<.01$)].

The percentage of infections among the Type III fractures also differed significantly among these periods [chi-square statistic with 2 degrees of freedom = 16.82 ($p<.01$)].

References

1. Boyd, R.J., Burke, J.F., and Colton, T.: A double blind clinical trial of prophylactic antibiotics in hip fracutres. J. Bone Joint Surg. 55A, 1251, 1973.

2. Burnett, J.W., Gustilo, R.B., Williams, D.N., and Kind, A.C.: Prophylactic antibiotics in hip fractures. J. Bone Joint Surg. 62A, 457, 1980.

3. Gustilo, R.B., and Anderson, J.T.: Prevention of infection in the treatment of 1,025 open fractures of long bones. J. Bone Joint Surg. 58A, 453, 1976.

4. Gustilo, R.B., Mendoza, R.M., and Williams, D.N.: Problems in the management of Type III (severe) open fractures. J. Trauma (in press).

5. Miles, A.A., Miles, E.M., and Burke, J.: The value and duration of defense reactions of the skin in the primary lodgement of bacteria. Brit. J. Exp. Pathol. 38, 79, 1957.

6. Nelson, C.L., Green, T.G., Porter, R.A., and Warren, R.D.: One day versus seven days of preventative antibiotic therapy in orthopaedic surgery. Clin. Orthop. Rel. Res. 176, 258, 1983.

7. Riska, E.B.: Are antibiotics necessary in the prevention of infection in total hip replacement. Ann. Chir. Gynecol. 69, 122, 1980.

8. Schurman, D.J., Hirschman, H.P., and Burton, D.S.: Cephalothin and cefamandole penetration into bone, synovial fluid and wound drainage fluid. J. Bone Joint Surg. 62A, 981, 1980.

Parenteral versus Oral Antibiotic Therapy

N. E. MacDonald

Antibiotic therapy for bone and joint infections has virtually eliminated mortality and has significantly decreased deformities and functional disabilities (Dickson, 1945; Waldvogen et al, 1980). Although traditional protocols have stressed the need for prolonged administration of appropriate antibiotics by the parenteral route (McCracken et al, 1978; Rhodes, 1975), this has now been challenged by reports of favorable results with primarily oral antibiotics (Bryson et al, 1979; Feigin et al, 1975; Jackson et al, 1982; Kaplan et al, 1982; Kolyvas et al, 1980; Nelson et al, 1978; 1982; Tetzlaff et al, 1978a; 1978b).

The newer oral antibiotic regimens have many advantages including: 1) lower costs; 2) shortened hospitalization with reduced hospital costs; 3) decreased complications of intravenous lines; and 4) more patient comfort. Despite these distinct advantages, this form of therapy may not always be suitable or possible. In addition, treatment failures may be more frequent with oral therapy if proper monitoring is not carried out (Nelson et al, 1982).

Antibiotic therapy for treatment of any infectious disease is based on three basic principles (Prober, 1982):

1) Adequate antibiotic dosage to kill the offending organism and to reach the site of infection.

2) Antibiotic therapy should be continued until the patient is clinically cured and the risks of relapse and of sequelae are reduced.

3) Therapy must be individualized taking into account any underlying disease, altered pharmacokinetics, presence of a foreign body, and other factors which might hinder successful therapy.

Initial antibiotic therapy for bone and joint infections is usually given intravenously until the acute signs and symptoms of the infection are controlled and necessary surgical procedures have been performed (Jackson et al, 1982; Prober, 1982). Selection of the appropriate antibiotic before culture results from blood, bone or joint fluid are received must be based on knowledge of the pathogens commonly encountered in different age groups and different clinical settings (Table I). Attention must be paid to the patient's drug allergies, liver and kidney function, and other clinical variables. The ability of different antibiotics to penetrate into bone, periosteal tissue and joint spaces must also be considered (Chater et al, 1972; Nelson et al, 1978; Norden et al, 1983; Sattar et al, 1983; Shurman et al, 1980; Tetzlaff et al, 1978). When the patient is afebrile and the

Current Concepts of Infections in
Orthopaedic Surgery

Table I. Most common organisms in acute bone and joint infections

Type of infection		Organism
Osteomyelitis		
Hematogenous -	Neonate	*Staphylococcus aureus* Group B *Streptococcus* gram-negative aerobes (eg, *Escherichia coli*)
	Older infants and children	*S. aureus*
Contiguous -	Postoperative Trauma Soft tissue	Mixed: *S. aureus* gram-negative aerobes
Vascular insufficiency		Mixed: *S. aureus* gram-negative aerobes gram-negative anaerobes gram-positive anaerobes
Sickle cell disease		*S. aureus* *Salmonella* species
Puncture wound		*Pseudomonas aeruginosa*
Immunocompromised		*S. aureus* gram-negative aerobes fungi
Septic arthritis		
Monoarticular -	Children <3 years of age	*Haemophilus influenzae* B *Streptococcus:* Group B, Group A *viridans*, *pneumoniae* *S. aureus*
	3-10 years of age	*S. aureus* *Streptococcus* species *Neisseria gonorrhoeae*
	Older children and adults	*N. gonorrhoeae* *Streptococcus* species *S. aureus*
Polyarticular		*N. gonorrhoeae*

local signs of pain, tenderness, erythema, and immobility have diminished, a switch to oral therapy can be considered.

A number of basic principles should be followed to evaluate a patient's suitability for oral therapy. Ideally, the offending organism should be isolated before switching to oral therapy and antibiotic selection must be based on specific resistance and sensitivity patterns, not just probabilities. For some organisms, such as *Pseudomonas aeruginosa*, no effective oral agents exist and this mode of therapy is not suitable. Where oral agents can be used, the chosen antibiotic should be palatable, especially in the case of children, well absorbed from the gastrointestinal tract, have good penetration into bone and/or joints, and minimal side effects. For example, liquid cloxacillin has a very bitter taste making compliance in young children poor. Liquid cephalexin is much more palatable. Clindamycin, an excellent antistaphylococcal and antianaerobic drug, may cause diarrhea and, more rarely, pseudomembranous colitis. This would make it a poor choice for a patient with underlying bowel disease (eg, neonates recovering from necrotizing enterocolitis who also have staphylococcal osteomyelitis). As a general guideline, a beta-lactam antibiotic such as cloxacillin or cephalexin is given for gram-positive coccal infections. Amoxicillin is recommended for susceptible strains of *Haemophilus influenzae* and chloramphenicol for beta-lactamase producing strains (Jackson et al, 1982). Cefaclor may also be considered but this medication is very expensive and the serum levels may sometimes be inadequate. The recommended oral dosage of the antibiotic is often two to three times that used for minor infections (Table II).

Table II. Dosages of oral antibiotics for bone and joint infections

Antibiotic	Dosage	
Amoxicillin	100 mg/kg/d	q 6 h
Ampicillin	150 mg/kg/d	q 6 h
Cefaclor	150 mg/kg/d	q 6 h
Cephalexin	170 mg/kg/d	q 6 h
Chloramphenicol	75 mg/kg/d	q 6 h
Clindamycin	30 mg/kg/d	q 8 h
Cloxacillin	100 mg/kg/d	q 6 h
Dicloxacillin	75 mg/kg/d	q 6 h
Flucloxacillin	50 mg/kg/d	q 6 h
Fusidic acid	50 mg/kg/d	q 8 h*
Rifampin	20 mg/kg/d (max 600 mg)	q 24 h*

* Not recommended for single drug therapy due to possible emergence of resistant organism. Use in conjunction with another antibiotic

The patient and, in the case of children, the family must also be evaluated. Can the patient swallow and retain the medication? Are intravenous lines difficult to maintain? Could the patient be discharged if oral medication were used? Are the parents sufficiently reliable to trust them to administer the antibiotic in the outpatient setting? Can the family afford the medication? For example, in Ontario, outpatient oral antibiotics are not generally covered by the government insurance program, while inhospital medications are paid. If rifampin or fusidic acid had been chosen along with cephalexin, this may cost $3 to $7 per day, depending on the size of the patient. Many families cannot afford $20 to $50 weekly.

Monitoring of the patient, both clinically and by laboratory measurements, must be done to ensure that oral therapy is effective (Nelson et al, 1982;

Prober and Yeager, 1979). Clinical monitoring involves frequent physical examination during the early part of therapy to assess the suppression and resolution of infection. In addition, long-term follow-up is essential to detect the development of orthopedic abnormalities or chronic osteomyelitis.

Laboratory monitoring to determine whether sufficient antibiotic is being absorbed from the gastrointestinal tract is also vital to the success of oral therapy. Unfortunately, 2% of patients absorb antibiotic slowly from the gastrointestinal tract and never achieve good bactericidal serum concentrations (Jackson and Nelson, 1982). There are two methods of assessing antibiotic absorption (Rosenblatt, 1983). One is to measure antibiotic serum concentrations. Many clinical laboratories do not routinly perform such assays; thus, this method is usually not practical. An important exception is chloramphenicol. Since this drug can cause dose-related bone marrow toxicity, monitoring of levels is important. Peak chloramphenicol concentrations are usually assayed on serum taken 90 minutes after the oral dose. Concentrations of 17-25 µg/mL are efficacious and not toxic (Dajani, 1981). All patients receiving chloramphenicol should have their peak concentrations measured to avoid toxicity.

The second and more frequently used method of assessing absorption is by measuring the minimal inhibitory and bactericidal antibiotic serum concentrations (Rosenblatt, 1983). This is a simple technique available in most microbiology laboratories. This test may be more meaningful clinically since the inhibitory properties of the patient's own serum are also included. It is performed by making serial twofold dilutions of the patient's serum in broth containing a standard inoculum of the patient's own bacterial isolate. The maximum dilution of serum that inhibits growth of the infecting organism is the serum inhibitory titer (SIT), while the maximum dilution that kills over 99% of the organisms is the serum bactericidal titer (SBT). If an organism is not isolated from the patient, a laboratory strain chosen on the basis of being the most probable infecting agent is used in the test. In general, the greater the antibiotic concentration in the serum, the greater the SBT. The peak SIT/SBT are usually assayed. The serum tested has the highest antibiotic concentration which occurs 1-2 hours (90 minutes) after the oral dose has been administered.

Recent uncontrolled studies suggest that peak SBT 1:8 correlated with high cure rates in osteomyelitis (Prober and Yeager, 1979). Low titers have been associated with treatment failure (Nelson et al, 1982). If the titer is 1:8, the clinician must consider several possibilities including poor compliance, improper timing of blood taking, and poor absorption. If the latter is the most probable cause, the dosage may be increased and the titer checked. For beta-lactam antibiotics, probenecid (7 mg/kg/dose) may be added to decrease renal excretion of the antimicrobial and improve serum drug concentrations. Other possibilities include switching to a different antibiotic, eg, from cloxacillin to cephalexin or clindamycin; combination therapy, eg, cephalexin and rifampin; or, if all fails, returning to parenteral administration. Even with intravenous antibiotic administration, home care may be possible (Rehm and Weinstein, 1983; Stiver et al, 1982). SIT/SBT can also be used to monitor intravenous therapy. The peak occurs shortly after the end of the infusion. The SIT/SBT should be followed on a weekly basis to monitor efficacy and compliance of oral or intravenous antibiotics.

The optimal duration of therapy is not clear but most authors agree that it should be based on the patient's clinical response, the roentgenographic changes and the return to normal erythrocyte sedimentation rates (ESR). The usual course of therapy for uncomplicated septic arthritis is three weeks and for osteomyelitis a minimum of four weeks (Jackson and Nelson, 1982). Longer courses are recommended for patients with slow clinical resolution, prolonged elevated ESR, or underlying conditions that may modify the response (eg, chronic granulomatous disease).

There are a number of contraindications to oral outpatient therapy for bone and joint infections. These include 1) unavailability of an effective oral agent (eg, against *P. aeruginosa*); 2) inability of the patient to swallow and/or retain, and/or absorb the medication; 3) poor compliance; 4) inability of the laboratory to perform SIT/SBT; and 5) poor clinical response. When these problems can be avoided, judicious use of oral therapy can significantly improve patient comfort and decrease the cost. However, patients and/or parents must understand that these are not trivial infections. Good compliance and follow-up are vitally important to the successful treatment. If either of these are in doubt, physicians should not hesitate to return the patient to hospital. Failure of therapy may lead to a disabled patient with chronic infection which may not even respond to long-term treatment.

References

1. Bryson, Y.J., Connor, J.D., LeClerc, M. et al: High dose oral dicloxacillin treatment of acute staphylococcal osteomyelitis. J. Pediatr. 94, 673, 1979.
2. Chater, E.H., Flynn, J., and Wilson, A.L.: Fucidin levels in osteomyelitis. J. Irish Med. Assoc. 65, 506, 1972.
3. Dajani, A.S. and Kauffman, R.E.: The renaissance of chloramphenicol. Pediatr. Clin. North Am. 28, 195, 1981.
4. Dickson, F.D.: The clinical diagnosis, prognosis, and treatment of acute hematogenous osteomyelitis. J.A.M.A. 127, 212, 1945.
5. Feigin, E.D., Pickering, L.K., Anderson, D., et al: Clindamycin treatment of osteomyelitis and septic arthritis in children. Pediatr. 55, 213, 1975.
6. Jackson, M.A. and Nelson, J.D.: Etiology and medical management of acute suppurative bone and joint infection in pediatric patients. J. Pediatr. Orthop. 2, 313, 1982.
7. Kaplan, S.L., Masori, E.O., and Feigin, R.D.: Clindamycin versus nafcillin or methicillin in the treatment of *Staphylococcus aureus* osteomyelitis in children. South. Med. J. 75, 138, 1982.
8. Kolyvas, E., Ahronheim, G., Marks, M.I., et al: Oral antibiotic therapy of skeletal infections in children. Pediatr. 65, 867, 1980.
9. McCracken, G.H. and Eichenwald, H.F.: Antimicrobial therapy in infants and children. II. Therapy of infectious conditions. J. Pediatr. 93, 357, 1978.
10. Nelson, J.D., Howard, J.B., and Shelton, S.: Oral antibiotic therapy for skeletal infections of children. I. Antibiotic concentrations in suppurative synovial fluid. J. Pediatr. 92, 131, 1978.
11. Nelson, J.D., Buchholz, R.W., Kusmiesz, H., and Shelton, S.: Benefits and risks of sequential parenteral-oral cephalosporin therapy for suppurative bone and joint infections. J. Pediatr. Orthop. 2, 255, 1982.

12. Norden, C.W. and Shaffer, M.: Treatment of experimental chronic osteomyelitis due to *Staphylococcus aureus*. J. Infect. Dis. 147, 352, 1983.

13. Prober, C.G.: Oral antibiotic therapy for bone and joint infections. Pediatr. Infect. Dis. 1, 8, 1982.

14. Prober, C.G. and Yeager, A.S.: Use of the serum bactericidal titer to assess the adequacy of oral antibiotic therapy in the treatment of acute hematogenous osteomyelitis. J. Pediatr. 95, 131, 1979.

15. Rehm, S.J. and Weinstein, A.J.: Home intravenous antibiotic therapy: A team approach. Ann. Intern. Med. 99, 388, 1983.

16. Rhodes, K.H.: Antibiotic management of acute osteomyelitis and septic arthritis in children. Orthop. Clin. North Am. 6, 915, 1975.

17. Rosenblatt, J.E.: Laboratory tests used to guide antimicrobial therapy. Mayo Clin. Proc. 58, 14, 1983.

18. Sattar, M.A., Barrett, S.P., and Cawley, M.D.: Concentrations of some antibiotics in synovial fluid after oral administration with special reference to antistaphylococcal activity. Ann. Rheum. Dis. 42, 67, 1983.

19. Shurman, D.J., Hirshman, H.P., and Burton, D.S.: Cephalothin and cefamandole penetration into bone, synovial fluid and wound drainage fluid J. Bone Joint Surg. 62A, 981, 1980.

20. Stiver, H.G., Trosky, S.K., Cote, D.D., and Oruck, J.L.: Self-administration of intravenous antibiotics: An efficient, cost effective home care program. Can. Med. Assoc. J. 127, 207, 1982.

21. Tetzlaff, T.R., Howard, J.B., McCracken, G.H., et al: Antibiotic concentration in pus and bone of children with osteomyelitis. J. Pediatr. 92, 135, 1978a.

22. Tetzlaff, T.R., McCracken, G.H., and Nelson, J.D.: Oral antibiotic therapy of skeletal infections in children. II. Therapy of osteomyelitis and suppurative arthrits. J. Pediatr. 92, 485, 1978b.

23. Waldvogen, F.A. and Vasey, H.: Osteomyelitis: The past decade. N. Engl. J. Med. 303, 360, 1980.

Antibiotic-Loaded Acrylic Cement (ALAC)

R. A. Elson

Since the use of antibiotic-loaded acrylic cement (ALAC) was first suggested by Buchholz and Engelbrecht (1970) as a prophylactic measure against infection following joint replacement operations, there has been a remarkable difference in the degree of its acceptance among European and North American surgeons. This was due to the justifiable caution of American colleagues with respect to potential complications (mechanical, allergic, toxic, and antimicrobial resistance). All these risks have been cited in early investigations and all would expose the surgeons using the material casually to serious criticism, if not litigation. However, as the years have gone by, such potential hazards have apparently not occurred. Frankly, I believe that many patients have been unnecessarily deprived of its use and subjected to old-fashioned operations such as resection arthroplasties or multiple-staged revision procedures; unnecessary infections may have followed joint replacements in a previously operated or infected field.

Another factor that has caused doubt is the variability in reported *in vitro* studies. Even allowing for measurement of elution to different media, variable quality of assay techniques, the use of different brands of acrylic cement, the use of different antibiotics, and differently shaped and sized specimens, the first-time reader has difficulty in reconciling some of the conflicting results. Each author has commented as to the clinical application of ALAC and there is also much variance among these reports.

With respect to its prophylactic use, Buchholz and his colleagues while using ALAC were simultaneously improving their surgical expertise of joint replacement procedures (exactly as it happened to Charnley when he developed the clean air technique). Therefore, their early improvements in infection rates (Rottger et al, 1979) cannot be attributed entirely to ALAC, ie, their series were uncontrolled. Unfortunately, as techniques improve in other ways and the undoubted benefits of clean air and systemic administration of antibiotics are accepted, it becomes increasingly difficult to produce controlled data supporting or disproving the additional prophylactic advantages of ALAC. One is therefore obliged to look at past results. Of these, the prospective trial comparing various systemic antibiotics with 0.5 g gentamicin/Palacos© cement conducted by Josefsson, Lindberg and Wiklander (1980), and the results of Wannske and Tscherne (1979), have produced figures suggesting lower infection rates with the use of ALAC.

In the space available, I can list conclusions only from available sources and personal experience. At the present time, these appear to stand continued scrutiny:

Current Concepts of Infections in
Orthopaedic Surgery

1. Without doubt, water-soluble antibiotic substances added in powder form to acrylic cement before polymerization of monomer, elute from the surface of the hardened material into an aqueous environment.

2. Early reports suggest that higher concentrations of antibiotic do not affect the degree of elution but figures published by Wahlig et al (1984) show that the higher the concentration, the greater the elution. The degree of elution, however, is not proportional to the rising concentration of antibiotic added. Solutions of antibiotics admixed to the cement during polymerization are ineffective, cause significant weakening, and should not be used. Water and other molecules enter acrylic cement after implantation by a diffusion process. The elution of antibiotics is a surface phenomenon only because the diffusion/concentration gradient is so steep (Bayston and Milner, 1982). Undoubtedly, the greater the surface area exposed, the greater the elution; thus, a rugose cancellous bone/cement interface will rapidly exhaust the antibiotic content of the protruding beads.

3. Palacos contains polymethylmethacrylate while other brands of cement contain other filler agents. These differences in chemical composition produce different physical properties -- in this instance, elution.

Gentamicin has been most widely studied due to its chemical stability, long-lasting elution (from Palacos), and its broad antimicrobial spectrum. Other antibiotics elute in useful concentrations although sometimes for a relatively short period. Wahlig and Dingeldein (1980) have published controlled comparative figures based on exhaustive *in vitro* tests.

4. Animal studies have, in general, shown that local concentrations of antibiotic are high and that control of infection can be achieved after direct inoculation of the experimental surgical field (Blomgren, 1981; Elson, 1977). Attempts to produce infection by the hematogenous route have shown that an experimental surgical field is vulnerable shortly after the operation but that within a few weeks, presumably as healing advances, it is increasingly difficult to infect the traumatized area. Nevertheless, infection can be produced through a bacteremia in a small proportion of cases. It is disappointing that no experimental proof exists demonstrating that late hematogenous infection can be prevented by ALAC despite the known continued elution of gentamicin from Palacos, albeit in low concentrations (Blomgren, 1981).

5. Of the potential disadvantages, in many thousands of operations using gentamicin/Palacos prophylactically and therapeutically, no allergic reactions have been observed nor emergence of resistant microbial strains. In fact, of the deep infections that have occurred with the use of prophylactic gentamicin/Palacos at the Endo-Klinik in Hamburg, about 50% were caused by strains resistant to gentamicin. Presumably, persistence of gentamicin-sensitive strains is caused by exhaustion of the surface concentrations of gentamicin while the gentamicin-resistant strains may have been resistant from the start; we have no way of proving either contention. We can say, however, that no massive occurrence of gentamicin-resistance in deep infections has been noted.

Mechanical weakening is undoubted. Schurmann et al (1978) showed early that even 0.5 g gentamicin/Palacos exhibited reduced fatigue strength. There is no evidence, however, that gentamicin/Palacos is associated with a higher mechanical failure rate in this low concentration. Of more concern to us is the late effects of adding high concentrations of antibiotic, for here changes in all mechanical variables are easily detected. Thus, those of us who add up to 4 g of antibiotic powder to 40 g of polymer, mixing these two substances relatively crudely, are seriously degrading the cement; the justification in a one-stage exchange procedure for deep infection lies in the essential need to combat the infection. The mechanical results in these exchanges do not seem to be different from the results of revisions for mechanical failure published elsewhere. Only time and careful evaluation will indicate how much this abuse of the cement contributes to late failure.

6. Pharmacokinetic studies in man following the use of ALAC in hip replacement operations confirm that it attains high local tissue concentrations (Wahlig, 1980). Nevertheless, these are variable in bone and soft tissue. I find it difficult to understand how concentrations can be maintained in tissues not immediately adjacent to the bone/cement interface after long periods of time; Schentag (1977) discussed the tissue binding of gentamicin but even this does not explain the persistent tissue levels which are confirmed in current studies. Of undoubted importance is the occurrence of high local concentrations in bone and hematoma after surgery (Elson, 1977). These can be readily confirmed and are vastly above any which can be achieved by systemic nontoxic doses of antibiotic administration. The associated low serum levels and the urinary excretion rate never appear to be toxic.

7. Clinical uses of ALAC:

a) *Prophylactic in first time surgery joint replacements.* As a single prophylactic measure ALAC appears efficacious; combined with other measures (systemic antibiotics and clean air), the additional advantage is probably small. Potential hazards apparently do not exist and at the present time I use all three measures simultaneously. Occasional infection, however, still occurs.

b) *Prophylactic use in joint replacements previously operated.* Following previous surgery or trauma, deep infection rate is usually recorded as being higher. Presumably, microbes reside sometimes in avascular areas; therefore, clean air and systemic antibiotics are obviously less efficacious; ALAC, on the other hand, provides high local antibiotic concentrations which penetrate dead bone and local avascular tissue (Elson, 1977).

c) *Therapeutic use for deep infection.* Despite the most meticulous excision of the infected field, contamination remains. If all tissues are vascular, systemic antibiotics may be effective but especially necrotic bone often remains. A depot source of antibiotic is more efficacious and ALAC fulfills this role. It may be used in pellet form, temporarily, during the interval of a two-stage procedure or definitively during a one-stage revision.

In either case (and also in pellet form for the management of infective osteitis), the basic surgical principle of excision of all dead or inert material is a prerequisite.

References

1. Bayston, R. and Milner, R.D.G.: The sustained release of antimicrobial drugs from bone cement. J. Bone Joint Surg. 64B, 460, 1982.

2. Blomgren, G.: Haematogenous infection of total joint replacement. Acta Orthop. Scand. 52 (Suppl. 18), 1981.

3. Buchholz, H.W. and Engelbrecht, H.: Über die Depotwirkung einiger Antibiotika bei Vermischung mit dem Kunstharz Palacos. Der Chirurg. 41, 511, 1970.

4. Elson, R.A., Jephcott, A.E., McGechie, D.B. and Verettas, D.: Bacterial infection and acrylic cement in the rat. J. Bone Joint Surg. 59B, 452, 1977.

5. Josefsson, G., Lindberg, L., and Wiklander, B.: Systemic antibiotics and gentamicin-containing bone cement in the prophylaxis of postoperative infections in total hip arthroplasty. Clin. Orthop. 159, 194, 1981.

6. Rottger, J., Buccholz, H.W., Engelbrecht, E., and Siegel, A.: Indikation und Technik unter Verwendung von Refobacin-Palacos in der Gelenkprothetik. Akt. Prob. Chirurg. Orthop. 12, 197, 1979.

7. Schentag, J.J., et al: Tissue persistance of gentamicin in man. JAMA 238, 327, 1977.

8. Schurmann, D.J., Swenson, L.W., and Piziali, R.L.: Bone cement with and without antibiotics: a study of mechanical properties. In, The Hip. Proc. Sixth Open Scientific Meeting of The Hip Society, 1978.

9. Wahlig, H. and Dingeldein, E.: Antibiotics and bone cement. Acta Orthop. Scand. 51, 49, 1980.

10. Wahlig, H., Dingeldein, E., Buchholz, H.W., Buchholz, M. and Bachmann, F.: Pharmacokinetic study of gentamicin-loaded cement in total hip replacements. J. Bone Joint Surg. 66B, 175, 1984.

11. Wannske, M. and Tscherne, H.: Ergebnisse prophylaktischer Anwendung von Refobacin-Palacos bei der Implantation von Endoprothesen des Hüftgelenkes in Hannover. Akt. Prob. Chirurg. Orthop. 12, 1979.

Gentamicin-PMMA Beads and Artificial Wound Coverage

A. HÄRLE

Soft tissue damage or loss may be the primary or secondary cause of a microbial infection after injuries of both the lower leg and foot. As long as deeper tissue layers are exposed and thus not protected against environment, the control of infection is never assured. The healthy skin's function is mainly that of a barrier against microbes apart from a temperature balance and the control of protein and fluid losses. Open wounds become contaminated unless the development of blood coagulation or wound scabs build a barrier against microbial invasion (Stern et al, 1983).

Septopal® application needs a closed cavity in which a high antibacterial gentamicin concentration can be built up by diffusion. As the release of gentamicin from the PMMA beads decreases with time (Härle, 1979), it is of advantage that there be no major flow of wound secretion for a few days. Furthermore, leaching of gentamicin is possible only within a wet environment but not from an air-dry surface of beads. The use of Septopal chains in open wounds can cause problems if resistant organisms from the patient's environment contaminate the wound and lead to ·infection.

In infected pseudarthroses or chronic osteomyelitis, the triad of bone infection, soft tissue defect, and soft tissue infection is frequently present. Each component of this triad can initiate or maintain this vicious circle. A prerequisite for the successful treatment of these diseases is the elimination of such infected skin and/or bone defects. Otherwise, the risk of a relapse or a complete reconstruction failure is high. Inflamed soft tissues are predamaged and are easily prone to necrosis, a fact that complicates all therapeutic endeavors. To prevent a later necrosis of the wound edges, major skin tension should be avoided since it hinders primary wound closure. A solution for such a situation is the temporary use of artificial skin to serve as a microbial barrier (Bohmert et al, 1974). When the bone and soft tissue infection is controlled, a solid soft tissue coverage may sometimes be achieved by pedicle and rotation flaps.

In most surgical fields alloplastic material has been successfully used for several decades. No success was achieved, however, until the 1970's with the availability of skin prostheses. Up to that date, fetal calf skin was thought to be the best material. However, fetal calf skin had the disadvantage of lasting a short time only, was difficult to obtain, and had poor resistance, which is characteristic of pig and cadaver skin as well.

PMMA = Polymethylmethacrylate

Current Concepts of Infections in
Orthopaedic Surgery

Wheeler and Alexander (1973) developed and demonstrated in 1973 the temporary artificial skin Epigard®, produced of finely-blistered polyurethane foam with a microporous Teflon® layer. Epigard satisfies the demands expected from a synthetic skin to a high degree and is far superior to all skin prostheses used in the past. Besides providing bacterial resistance, protein and fluid loss is effectively controlled. No significant problems were encountered when Epigard was applied to extensive fresh burns. However, the situation is quite different when a primary bacterial infection of the wound bottom is present. If a microbial contaminated wound funnel is covered with Epigard, an abscess develops under the artificial skin within a few days. Consequently, we combined a temporary prosthetic skin and the potent, locally-acting antibiotic Septopal for the treatment of infected bone and soft tissue defects.

For the past two years, two artificial skin materials have been available in Central Europe: Epigard and Suspurderm® (Betz et al, 1982). Both of these materials, of about 1.6 mm thickness, consist of different cross-linked polyurethane foams (Fig. 1). In Suspurderm, the external boundary layer is formed by a concentrated polyurethane structure; in Epigard by an air-permeable Teflon film. This difference in composition affects fluid absorption and microbial invasion. When the external boundary layer was contaminated with 100 µL of a microbial suspension, this suspension had completely infiltrated Suspurderm, on the average after 220 seconds, whereas no infiltration was observed with Epigard. To find out whether this difference in microbial barrier function is of the same importance in practice, where the environment is always changing from a fluid medium via artificial skin to a gel-like medium, we performed the following test applicable to the clinical situation.

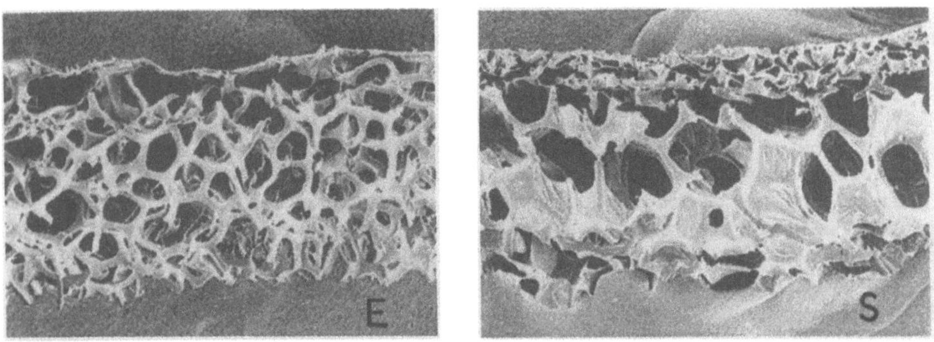

Fig. 1. Two different artificial skin materials: E = Epigard; S = Suspurderm

Petri dishes with a diameter of 57 mm were filled with blood agar to a height of 10 mm and covered with artificial skin (Fig. 2). At the margin, a 4 mm high glass ring was put on the artificial skin and a removable lid was put over the glass ring. The artificial skin was placed with its external side up and then charged with small lobes soaked in microbial suspension, sufficient to contaminate blood coagula or dressing materials.

Microbial isolation was then carried out by impression preparations from the blood agar, not from the lower side of the foam substance. Table I

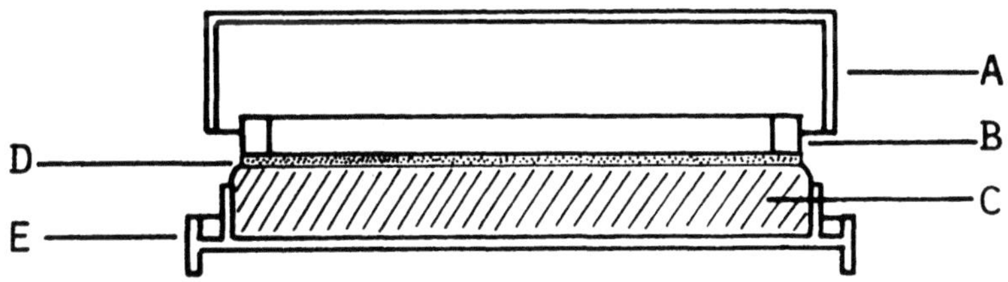

Fig. 2. Test arrangement. A: lid, B: glass ring, C: blood-agar, D: artificial skin, E: Petri dish

Table I. Microbial penetration through artificial skin materials after wet contamination (n = 60)

	Suspurderm 12 hours		Epigard 10 days	
	n	%	n	%
Pseudomonas aeruginosa	12	100	1	8.3
Klebsiella sp.	12	100	-	-
Serratia marcescens	12	100	1	8.3
Staphylococcus aureus	12	100	1	8.3
Escherichia coli	12	100	1	8.3

shows that in all 12 Suspurderm cultures of each microbial type, organisms had penetrated the blood agar after a 12-hour incubation; only 7% of the Epigard cultures were infiltrated after a 10-day contact period.

The synergistic effect of the combination of Septopal and artificial skin is illustrated by the following experiment. We placed a Septopal mini-bead (length 6 mm, width 3 mm, gentamicin content 1.7 mg) in the centre of the Petri dish and covered it with blood agar, which was then covered by Suspurderm. Each plate was then inoculated with 0.1 mL of different microbial suspension, homogenized with a spatula and closed with a lid. Sample preparations were then taken from the blood agar after 12 and 24 hours as well as after 7, 15, 20, and 26 days. The results for Susperderm with and without additional Septopal application are shown in Table II. Whereas all plates showed microbial growth after 12 hours without Septopal, *Pseudomonas* was not cultivated from the blood agar with Septopal before seven days. No *Staphylococcus aureus*, *Klebsiella*, or *Escherichia coli* were isolated during the whole test period.

If Septopal was added to blood agar plates without artificial skin, they were also contaminated by different microbial suspensions; the central inhibition zones were surrounded by an area of clearly visible microbial growth. The diameters of the inhibition zones were practically identical on the 1st and 5th day of the test; they differed considerably, however, as to microbial species. The largest inhibition zones of 5.05 cm on the average were observed for *S. aureus*, followed by *Klebsiella* sp. and *E. coli* with a diameter of 4.8 cm. *Serratia* and *Pseudomonas aeruginosa* showed lower values of 2.25 and 1.65 cm respectively (Table III).

Table II. Microbial penetration through Suspurderm

	12 h		24 h		7 d		15 d		20 d		26 d	
	A	B	A	B	A	B	A	B	A	B	A	B
Pseudomonas	+	0	+	0	+	+	+	+	+	+	+	+
Klebsiella sp.	+	0	+	0	+	0	+	0	+	0	+	0
Staphylococcus aureus	+	0	+	0	+	0	+	0	+	0	+	0
Escherichia coli	+	0	+	0	+	0	+	0	+	0	+	0

A: without Septopal
B: with Septopal

Table III. Inhibition zone in Septopal containing blood agar dishes

	Diameter of inhibition zone at	
	Day 1	Day 5
Pseudomonas aeruginosa	1.65 cm	1.62 cm
Klebsiellae sp.	4.92 cm	4.90 cm
Serratia marcescens	2.25 cm	2.17 cm
Staphylococcus aureus	5.05 cm	5.05 cm
Escherichia coli	4.78 cm	4.77 cm

Summarizing these results we can draw the following conclusions:

1) Both synthetic skin materials show different microbial barrier functions with fluid contamination; with dry (airborne) contamination no differences were observed.

2) Septopal mini-beads produce inhibition zones of 1.6 to 5 cm diameter in blood agar, comparable with postoperative hematoma. Consequently, the bactericidal efficacy necessary for elimination of pathogenic organisms within a cavity filled with hematoma is less than 1.5 cm.

3) The rate of isolated organisms in blood agar is dramatically reduced with the use of artificial skin, Suspurderm combined with Septopal beads.

4) Manipulations, such as removing and replacing the artificial skin, promote the development of superinfections which cannot always be prevented by Septopal beads in blood agar.

The clinical treatment of soft tissue defects approximates the test conditions described above. A dense filling of the hematoma cavity with Septopal is recommended to obtain bactericidal effects. The margins of the prosthetic skin must be fixed to the border of the wound by sutures to prevent superinfections. In the first postoperative days, fibroblasts and blood vessels grow into the polyurethane foam at this contact area, which effects a biologic packing of the hematoma cavity against the environment. By means of the high gentamicin concentration, the hematoma becomes sterile under the skin prosthesis; after approximately 20 days, this hematoma becomes organized and new soft tissue arises around the beads.

Such a treatment was carried out in a patient with an infected ulcer on the back of his foot extending down to the bone, in a dorsalis-pedis-flap procedure. After meticulous removal of the inflamed tissue from the wound funnel and superficial scraping of the bone, Septopal mini-beads were placed into the defect and the cavity appropriately closed with Epigard. Three weeks later, we removed the Epigard and found granulation tissue well vascularized around the Septopal beads, which were then also removed. After another eight days and two Epigard changes, granulation tissue of 3 mm height was present, adequate for skin transplantation (Fig. 3). The full thickness graft taken from a wound gore settled in the back of the foot without any problem.

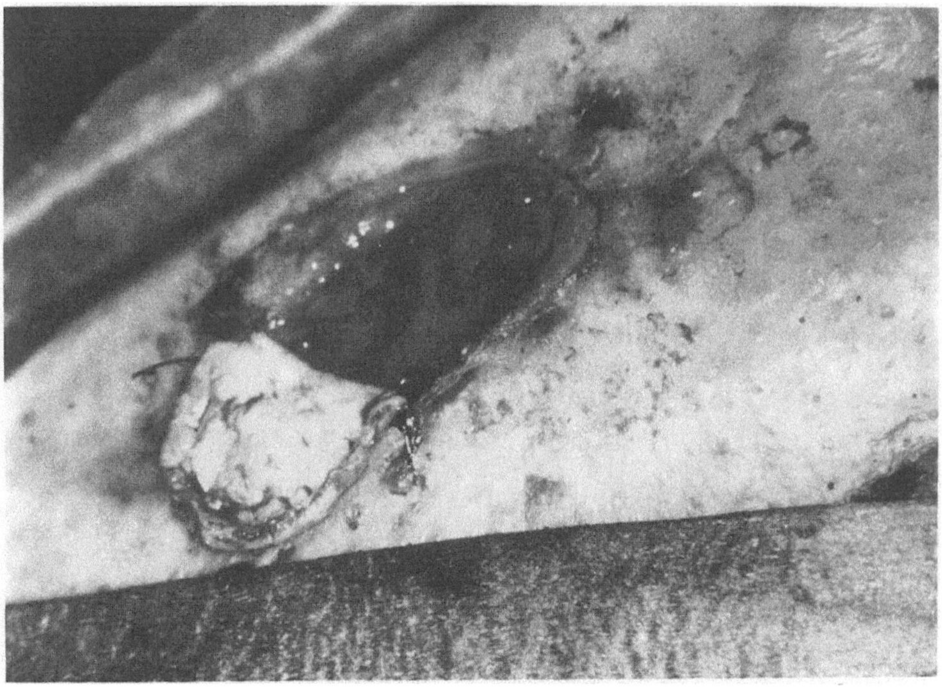

Fig. 3. With the aid of Epigard, well vascularized granulation tissue can be grown for skin transplantation

We have also used the combination of Epigard and Septopal for aseptic operations, when problems arise in wound closure after corrections of foot deformities. As a procedure in a 35-year old man showed, after correcting his foot's maximal equinovarus by 80°, the closure of the resulting large wound gap on the lateral aspect of the ankle was not possible without tension. As prophylaxis against infection, we filled the space with a Septopal chain and closed the defect with Epigard. The Septopal chain which penetrated the skin was pulled out on the sixth postoperative day (Fig. 4).

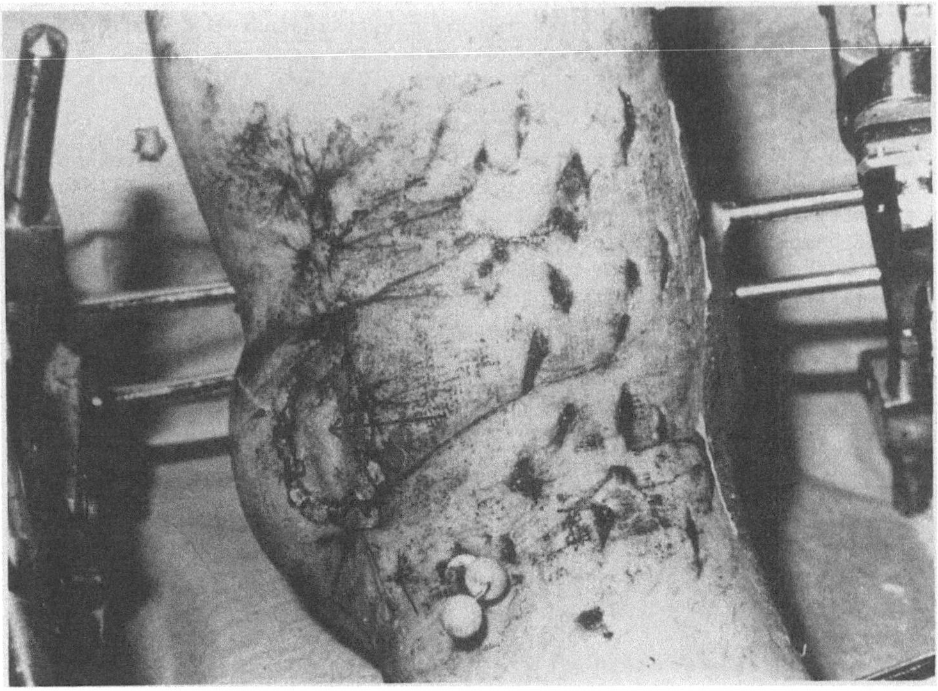

Fig. 4. After extensive operative foot correction the skin at the lateral malleolus could not be closed without tension. We sewed Epigard into the defect (arrow)

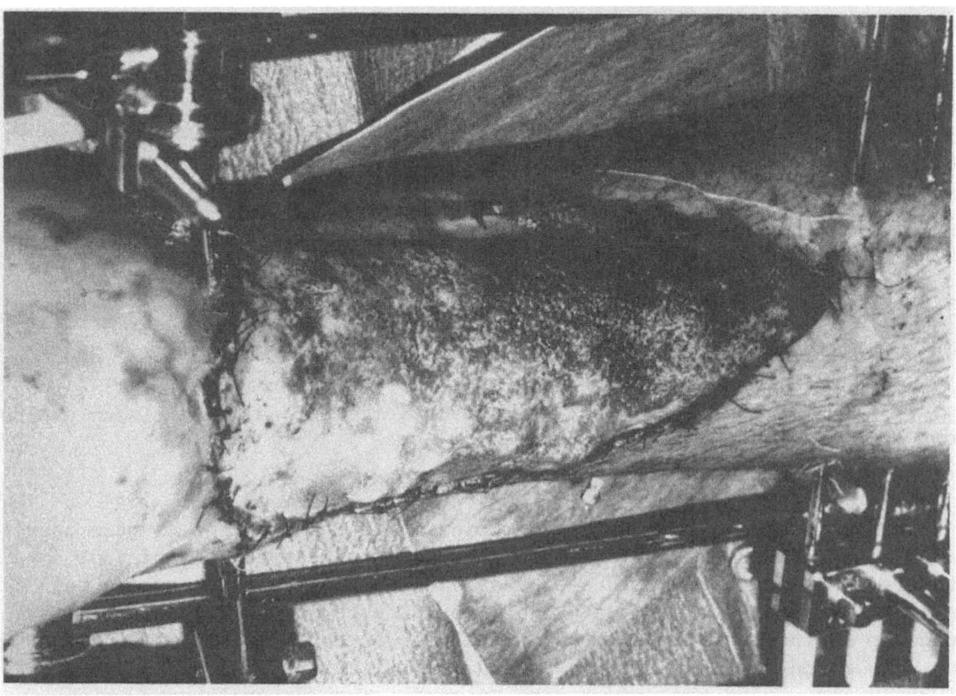

Fig. 5. The extensive soft tissue defect was covered with Epigard; after a few days dry wound conditions had been achieved

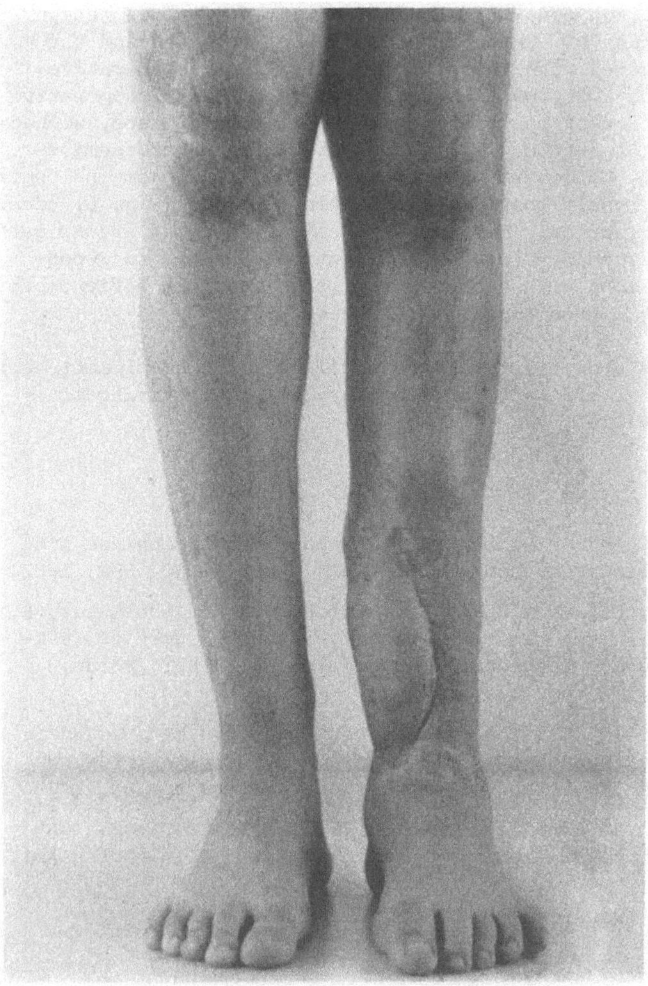

Fig. 6. After several plastic operations a good soft tissue coverage is present at the medial distal lower leg

Three weeks later, the Epigard was removed, and the wound closed over the cavity that was then filled with healthy, fully vascularized granulation tissue. We use the combination of Epigard and Septopal chain commonly for the treatment of soft tissue infections, chronic osteomyelitis, or infected pseudarthroses.

The aim of this first treatment step is to create a sterile environment in soft tissue defects, thereby preparing an aseptic field for the skin grafting operation. If this grafting procedure is not possible without complications, then the combined Epigard/Septopal treatment can be repeated several times as an interim solution. The Septopal chain serves two other purposes besides prophylaxis of infection: first, it keeps the space for the large bone transplant; second, it interposes between the soft tissue and Epigard so that the skin transplant can be done more easily.

A 22-year old motorcyclist with a comminuted distal tibia fracture was transferred to our hospital three months after plating. At the medial side was a large skin defect with an AO-plate totally exposed. The wound was extensively debrided, the medullary canal was reamed, and the metaphyseal cavity cleaned thoroughly. Septopal chains were implanted and the large skin defect was covered with Epigard (Fig. 5). The postoperative course was uneventful with a dry wound margin from the sixth postoperative day on. After normalization of the erythrocyte sedimentation rate, we had to apply a Tumbler flap (Stenström, 1976) and a cross-leg gastrocnemius flap (Mathes et al, 1974) to cover the soft tissue defect, 20 cm in length and 10 cm in width. The result showed a solid skin coverage (Fig. 6) after a successful bony reconstruction. The combined use of Septopal and Epigard enables us to handle infected bone and soft tissue defects and to reconstruct well functioning limbs with a good soft tissue cover in patients for some of whom amputation had been suggested elsewhere.

As our experimental tests show, Septopal and artifical skin complement each other favorably as to their efficacy for temporary aseptic covering of large hematoma-filled cavities.

References

1. Betz, A., Wilker, D., and Schweiberer, L.: Behandlungsergebnisse mit einem neuen Polyurethanweichschaumstoff. Chir. Praxis, 30, 689, 1982.
2. Bohmert, H., Petzold, D., Schmidtler, F., Simon, T., and Schleuter, B.: Experimentelle und klinische Testung von Polyurethanschaumstoff (EPIGARD) bei Verbrennungen. Langenb. Arch. Chir. Suppl. Chir. Forum, 257-259, 1974.
3. Härle, A. and Ritzerfeld, W.: The release of gentamycin into wound secretions from polymethylmethacrylate beads. A study with reference to the animal experiment. Arch. Orthop. Traumat. Surg. 95, 64, 1979.
4. Mathes, S., McCraw, J.B., and Vasconez, L.D.: Muscle transposition flaps for coverage of lower extremity defects. Surg. Clin. North Am. 54, 1337, 1974.
5. Stenström, S.J.: The tumbler flap. Chir. plastica 3, 211, 1976.
6. Stern, P.J., Neale, H.W., Gregory, R.O., and McDonough, J.J.: Functional reconstruction of an extremity by free tissue transfer of the latissimus dorsi. J. Bone Joint Surg. 65A, 729, 1983.
7. Wheeler, L.M., Alexander, J.W.C., Rooney, R.C., McDonald, J.J., and Macmillan, B.G.: Clinical evaluation of EPIGARD®, a new synthetic substitute for homograft and heterograft skin. J. Trauma 13, 374, 1973.

The Use of Gentamicin-PMMA Beads in Chronic Osteomyelitis

J. P. GALEY and H.-K. UHTHOFF

Orthopedic surgeons dread the complications of chronic osteomyelitis. Infection in bone can persist, despite thorough debridement, sequestrectomy, saucerization, and long-term systemic antibiotic therapy.

The concept to use localized antibiotics for the treatment of deep bone infections was first investigated and reported by Buchholz and Gartman in 1972. They demonstrated that antibiotic powder mixed with polymethylmethacrylate (PMMA) could eradicate infections in revisions of total hip arthroplasties. They also tested different antibiotics and found that gentamicin was the antibiotic of choice because of its broad antimicrobial spectrum and best elution properties. Further studies carried out by Marks et al (1976) and Elson et al (1977) revealed that of all tested antibiotics gentamycin eluted best from impregnated cement (Palacos®). Elson also demonstrated *in vitro* that the antibiotic penetrates 7 mm of dead bone. The bactericidal concentration in bone was shown to be from 10 to 100 times that achieved with systemic administration.

The local use of an antibiotic in chronic osteomyelitis was first recommended by Klemm, Wahlig and Jenny in 1972. A PMMA bead containing streptomycin was chosen because of the maximal surface area of the beads and their relative ease of application to the site of infection. The composition of the bead is a homogeneous mixture of 7.5 mg gentamicin sulfate and 20 mg zirconium dioxide as roentgenographic contrast medium in PMMA. The beads have a diameter of 7 mm and are packaged in chains of 30 beads on a surgical wire.

Materials and Methods

The purpose of this paper is to present the Canadian results of the use of gentamicin-PMMA beads, developed by Klemm (1977), as an investigational drug under the control of the senior author between March 1978 and June 1983. During this period, 55 patients were treated with the gentamicin-PMMA beads. Chronic osteomyelitis was diagnosed based on clinical and radiologic evidence of bone infection which had persisted for more than three months from the onset. Five patients were lost to follow-up. One patient died from a brain tumor with less than six months' follow-up and was excluded from the study. Forty-nine patients (34 men, 15 women) were available for review. The mean age at time of surgery was 48.9 years (range: 21-88 years). The mean duration of symptoms before surgery was two years. The patients had an average of two surgical procedures for their osteomyelitis before the procedure using the gentamicin-PMMA beads.

Current Concepts of Infections in
Orthopaedic Surgery

Twenty-five patients developed osteomyelitis after surgery. In 15 patients a compound fracture was the cause of their bone infection. Nine patients had hematogenous, chronic osteomyelitis (Table I).

Table I. Etiology of chronic osteomyelitis (n = 49)

Surgical	25
Compound fractures	15
Hematogenous	9

The sites of infection are outlined in Table II. The lower extremity was involved in 45 of 49 patients. Most of the tibial infections were the result of compound injuries while the hip infections were the sequelae of contaminated total hip arthroplasties or endoprostheses.

Table II. Sites of infection

Sites	No. of patients
Tibia	17
Hip	15
Femur	11
Humerus	3
Knee	1
Calcaneus	1
Lumbar spine (L4-L5 disc space)	1
Total	49

The surgical treatment of osteomyelitis consisted of debridement, sequestrectomy, and curettage of surrounding bone followed by insertion of the gentamicin-PMMA beads to fill the space created. The wound was closed primarily in 43 of 49 patients. Hemovac drainage was used when necessary and was removed 24 to 48 hours after surgery. Systemic antibiotics were not given pre- or postoperatively.

The clinical follow-up was obtained by questionnaires sent to 23 patients in the Ottawa region, to 17 attending orthopedic surgeons, and by personal interview with nine surgeons.

The possibility of gentamicin induced oto- and nephrotoxicity was monitored by pre- and postoperative hearing tests and serum BUN determinations. Serum gentamicin levels were evaluated in all patients postoperatively.

The average time of follow-up was 31.1 months with a range of six to 69 months; 31 of 49 patients had over two years' follow-up.

Success of treatment of the osteomyelitis was determined by complete eradication of wound drainage.

Results

Sixty-seven organisms were isolated from 45 infections (Table III). Four patients had no growth in any cultures, but were included because they fit the criteria as stated above. In 14 patients, more than one organism was isolated. *Staphylococcus aureus* was the single isolate in 17 patients.

Table III. Microbial profile

Microbe	No.
Staphylococcus aureus	24
Pseudomonas aeruginosa	12
Staphylococcus epidermidis	9
Proteus mirabilis	5
Enterobacter sp.	4
Escherichia coli	3
β-hemolytic *Streptococcus*	3
Enterococcus	2
Coliform bacilli	2
Diphtheroid bacilli	1
Streptococcus faecalis	1
Klebsiella	1
Total	67

Serum gentamicin levels were less than 0.5 µg/mL in all patients.

The postoperative drainage from the wound in those patients in whom drainage stopped ranged from 0 to 180 days, with a mean of 19 days.

Twelve patients underwent a second debridement procedure with insertion of more gentamicin-PMMA beads. Seven patients were cured after the second procedure.

Thirty-three of 49 patients had their infection eradicated by this technique , resulting in a 67% success rate. One patient had no drainage at any time.

Table IV. Results of treatment with gentamicin-PMMA beads (n = 49)

Follow-up	No wound drainage
More than 2 years	22/31
1 to 2 years	8/13
Less than 1 year	3/5
Total	33/49

Six wounds were not closed primarily and five of these continued draining.

Twenty-two of the 31 patients with more than two years' follow-up were rated a success. Eight of 13 patients with one or two years' follow-up had stopped draining and three of the five patients with less than one year of follow-up were cured (Table IV).

Discussion

The results of previous studies reported in the literature were used as comparisons with our results in this investigation (Table V).

Table V. Review of three publications on chronic osteomyelitis: treatment techniques and results

Author	Technique	No. of patients	Results
Shannon et al (1973)	Saucerization and primary skin closure	68	68% Satisfactory 43% No draining
Papineau et al (1979)	Sequestrectomy saucerization ± bone grafting ± skin grafting	139	78% no draining
Jenny et al (1980)	Sequestrectomy saucerization gentamicin beads	200	75% Successful

The study by Shannon, published in 1973, was well designed with a minimum of five years' follow-up. The success rate reported was 68% in 68 patients, but only 43% had no draining sinuses at their final follow-up.

The study by Papineau (1979) had incomplete details regarding follow-up and the length of time postoperative antibiotics were used in 139 patients. In this series, 78% of his patients had no wound drainage.

Jenny, one of the original workers using gentamicin-PMMA beads, published a paper in 1980 reporting on the use of the beads in 200 patients with a variety of infections; 125 patients were available for follow-up. Jenny claimed a 75% success rate. However, when he divided the data into subgroups, he had a 68% success rate in infected pseudarthrosis, 58% in infected osteosynthesis, and 73.3% in all other patients with chronic osteomyelitis. Our results compare favorably with those of these investigators.

While gaining experience with the use of the beads, it became evident that extensive debridement and primary closure of the wound were essential. Failure to adhere to the technique resulted in a lower success rate. The fact that five of the six patients with their wounds left open were failures reemphasizes the above points.

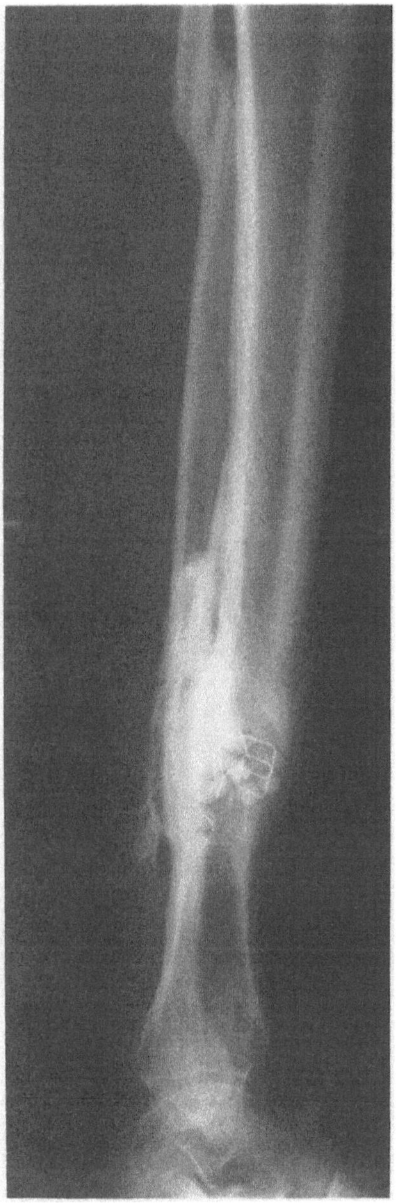

Fig. 1. Radiograph of tibia 9 months after insertion of gentamicin-PMMA beads showing bony overgrowth around the beads preventing their removal

The use of local antibiotics in the treatment of bone infection has advantages over systemic administration. The antibiotic is placed directly at the site of infection. Since the surrounding area may be relatively avascular, this increases the risk of systemic antibiotics not reaching bactericidal levels at the involved site. The antibiotic levels achieved with local therapy, on the other hand, are much higher than levels tolerated systemically. The concerns about using antibiotics for a prolonged period, often intravenously, are no longer a problem.

The use of gentamicin-PMMA beads has some disadvantages. The most obvious is that it requires a second procedure to remove the beads. This problem is being dealt with in two ways. The first is by removing one end of the beads through a separate track, thereby obviating further surgery. The second way is to use a biodegradable medium to transport the antibiotic, which will be discussed in another paper in this book. Another difficulty is bony overgrowth on the beads (Fig. 1), making the removal of the beads difficult. This can be avoided by removing the beads before bony overgrowth can occur.

The use of the antibiotic-impregnated cement beads should not replace good surgical techniques. It is meant as adjuvant therapy only.

Primary wound closure is important when the beads are used. Only one patient's outcome was satisfactory with secondary wound closure. We believe that the beads should not be used when the wound has to be left open.

We observed no adverse effects due to local antibiotic therapy. None of the patients had any allergic reactions to gentamicin.

Our assessement, to date, based on this small series, may be summarized as follows:

1. Wound closure is essential when local antibiotic coverage with gentamycin-PMMA beads is being used.
2. No adverse effects from the gentamicin-PMMA beads were encountered in this study.
3. Gentamicin-PMMA beads are a valuable adjuvant in the treatment of chronic osteomyelitis but do not obviate complete removal of all dead and infected bone and soft tissue before their insertion.

References

1. Buchholz, H.W. and Gartman, H.D.: Infektionsprophylaxe und operative Behandlung der schleichenden tiefen Infektion bei der totalen Endoprothese. Chirurg. 43, 446, 1972.
2. Elson, R.A., Jephcott, A.E., McGechie, D.B., and Verettas, D.: Antibiotic-loaded acrylic cement. J. Bone Joint Surg. 59B, 200, 1977.
3. Jenny, Von G., and Taglang, G.: Lokale Knocheninfektionsbechandlung mit Gentamycin PMMA-Kugelkette. Bertr. Orthop. u. Traumatol. 27, 442, 1980.
4. Klemm, K.: Die Behandlung chronischer Knockeninfektionen mit Gentamycin PMMA Kugeln. Z Unfallchir Rehabilitat Sonderheft, VLE Verlag-GmbH Erlangen, S 1977, pp 20-27.
5. Marks, K.E., Nelson, C.L., and Lautenschlager, E.P.: Antibiotic impregnated acrylic bone cement. J. Bone Joint Surg. 58A, 358, 1976.
6. Papineau, L.J., Alfagene, A., Dalcourt, J.P., and Pilon, L.: Ostéomyelite chronique, excision et greffe de spongieux à l'air après mise à plate extensive. Int. Orthop. (SICOT) 3, 165, 1979.
7. Shannon, J.G., Woolhouse, F.M., and Eisinber, P.J.: The treatment of chronic osteomyelitis by saucerization and immediate skin grafting. Clin. Orthop. Rel. Res. 96, 98, 1973.
8. Wahlig, H., Dingeldein, E., Bergmann, R., and Reuss, K.: The release of gentamicin from polymethylmethacrylate beads. J. Bone Joint Surg. 60B, 270, 1978.

Fibrin-Antibiotic Complex: Laboratory Investigation and Clinical Results

A. BRAUN, A. GÜSSBACHER, W.-D. HEINE, and E. DINGELDEIN

Introduction

Wound debridement, immobilization, and antibiotics are the most important principles in bone and joint surgery for the treatment of sepsis. Antibiotics can be applied systemically or locally.

In 1951, Winter first described the antibiotic-impregnated autologous blood clot for local therapy of a chronic osteomyelitis. Further investigations were carried out with this technique by Bagdy et al (1963), Bikfali et al (1963), Bikfali and Ecke (1960), and Ecke (1962). In 1974, Ecke et al reported 112 patients followed for up to 19 years, treated with the antibiotic-impregnated autologous blood clot, and found a recurrent infection rate of 33.9%. Their results and rate of recurrence of infection were good compared with other techniques such as suction irrigation drainage (43.7%), skin flaps (80%) and muscle flaps (58%).

Autologous cancellous bone grafting is a well established technique to fill infected bone defects (Burri, 1979; Burri and Henkemeyer, 1971; Coleman et al, 1946; De Grood, 1947; Hogeman, 1949; Matti, 1932; Mowlem, 1944; Papineau, 1973; and Popkirov, 1977). Heinemann (1959) recommended, after broad surgical exposure, sequestrectomy and saucerization, closing the bony cavity with a mixture of cancellous bone and tetracycline-impregnated autologous blood.

Histologically, the autologous blood clot showed a rapid migration of fibroblasts and lamellar new bone formation from the edge of the cavity (Beneke et al, 1964). Heiss et al (1963) measured the *in vitro* and *in vivo* elution of streptomycin from an impregnated blood clot. They found a high elution within the first 24 hours, sufficient bacteriostasis over six days in the area of surgery, and sufficient antibacterial coverage in the peripheral blood.

Winter (1951) recommended the use of penicillin powder and a certain ratio of thrombin to blood, or a combination of penicillin, powdered streptomycin, thrombin and powdered fibrin to produce prompt coagulation.

The investigation into antibiotic-impregnated bone cement (Buchholz and Engelbrecht, 1970; Klemm, 1974, 1977) was a further development in local antibiotic therapy (Marks et al, 1976; van Rens and Kayser, 1981).

Pharmacokinetic studies of the release of gentamicin out of Refobacin-Palacos® and PMMA-beads (Septopal®) showed a high local concentration and the advantage of low serum and urine concentrations (Wahlig and Buchholz,

Current Concepts of Infections in
Orthopaedic Surgery

1972; Wahlig et al, 1979). The disadvantages of the PMMA-beads are that they have to be removed within the first two weeks and the necessity of further surgery for reconstructive procedures.

The concept of using a biologic carrier for antibiotics and the subsequent development of the "Fibrin-Antibiotic Complex" was first proposed by Bösch et al (1977a) and was experimentally and clinically developed in the Department of Orthopaedic Surgery in Heidelberg (Braun et al, 1979; Braun et al, 1981; Braun et al, 1982a-d; Braun et al, 1984; Kratzat et al, 1981; Kratzat et al, 1982; Schumacher et al, 1982). Ulatowski et al (1979, 1980, 1981, 1982) also described an antibiotic-impregnated fibrin. Their dry, prepared fibrin-antibiotic technique, however, has disadvantages compared with the intrasurgical clotting technique as to workability, especially with combined cancellous bone grafting.

Highly concentrated fibrinogen coagulated by a thrombin solution and calcium ions into fibrin acts as a biologic tissue adhesive (Matras et al, 1972). This procedure allows new surgical techniques for tissue adhesion (Cotta and Braun, 1982; Spängler and Braun, 1983). Fibrin promotes tissue regeneration with the proliferation of fibroblasts, early capillarization and granulation (Dinges et al, 1982; Heine et al, 1982; Scheele and Pesche, 1982). The physiologic process of fibrin formation can be compared with the final stage of blood clotting.

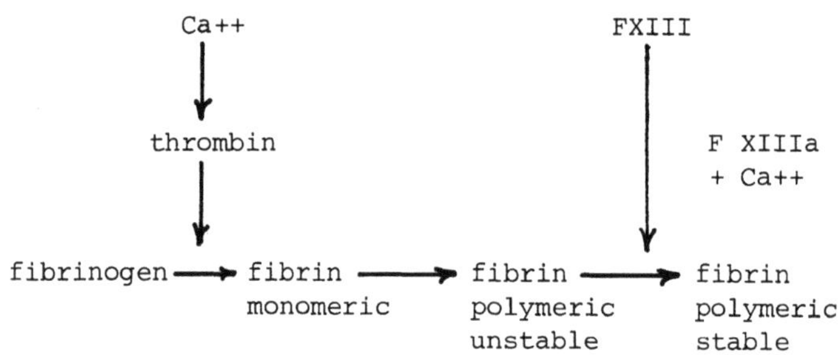

Mixtures of fibrin-sealant and various antibiotics [doxycycline, azlocillin, cefoxitin, fosfomycin, gentamicin, G4 (a gentamicin derivative), tobramycin, cefazedon, cefotaxim and clindamycin] have been studied *in vitro* with regard to coagulation rate, dosage, and release rate of the antibiotic (Redl et al, 1982; Wahlig et al, 1982). Redl et al (1983) observed a prolonged coagulation rate under the effects of local antibiotics, reduced clot formation and a release of antibiotics over a maximum period of four days. Wahlig et al (1982) measured the elution into phosphate buffer at pH 7.4 and into active, pooled human serum. Following high initial concentrations after one hour, all antibiotics showed a rapid decline to subtherapeutic concentrations within two to five days. G4 was the only exception and showed a marked long action. *In vivo* studies with amicain (Bösch et al, 1982), cefotaxim (Zilch et al, 1982), gentamicin, G4, and cefazedon (Wahlig et al, 1982) also showed high initial serum concentrations within the first 24 hours. The gentamicin derivative G4, with its clear long-action is probably more in agreement with clinical and therapeutic requirements. In none of the experiments was a septic sclerotic bony cavity present.

Pharmacokinetic studies, after clinical application of the fibrin-gentamicin complex, have been described by Braun et al (1982b and 1984). Clinical results using the Fibrin-Antibiotic Complex in bone and soft tissue infections are reported with Polybactrin® and Nebacetin® (Bösch et al, 1977a), Nebacetin® (Goudarzi, 1983) and gentamicin (Braun et al, 1982d; Kratzat et al, 1981, 1982).

The interaction of *Staphylococcus aureus* with the fibrin-polymer is not yet known. Hawinger et al (1978) found a clumping activity of staphylococci with fibrinogen and its derivatives. This might be an advantage of the antibiotic-impregnated fibrin in *S. aureus* infections which are common in bone and soft tissue.

Animal Studies

Our own animal studies with the Fibrin-Antibiotic Complex were first published in 1979 (Braun et al).

In 60 rabbits the distal femoral metaphysis was saucerized and the medullary canal was closed by bone wax. The bony cavity was contaminated with a 0.05 mL suspension of 5-20 x 10^6 of a highly virulent strain of *S. aureus* on a collagenic swab. The *Staphylococcus* was sensitive to tobramycin (MIC <0.125 µg/mL). In a random study, the cavity was closed with the fibrin-antibiotic complex in group A and with fibrin alone in the control group B (Fig. 1).

A: 0.45 mL Fibrin-Antibiotic Complex composed of:

- 0.25 mL highly concentrated human fibrinogen
- 0.10 mL distilled water containing 15 mL tobramycin (≈5 mg/kg)
- 0.10 mL thrombin solution (≈300 NIH/mL) and calcium ions (40 mmol/L).

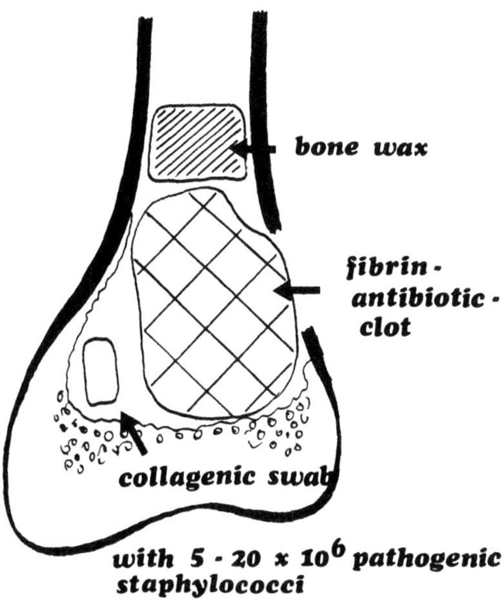

Fig. 1. The distal femoral metaphysis contaminated with 5 x 20 x 10^6 pathogenic staphylococci on a collagenic swab. The defect closed by fibrin-antibiotic clot (group A) and fibrin alone (group B)

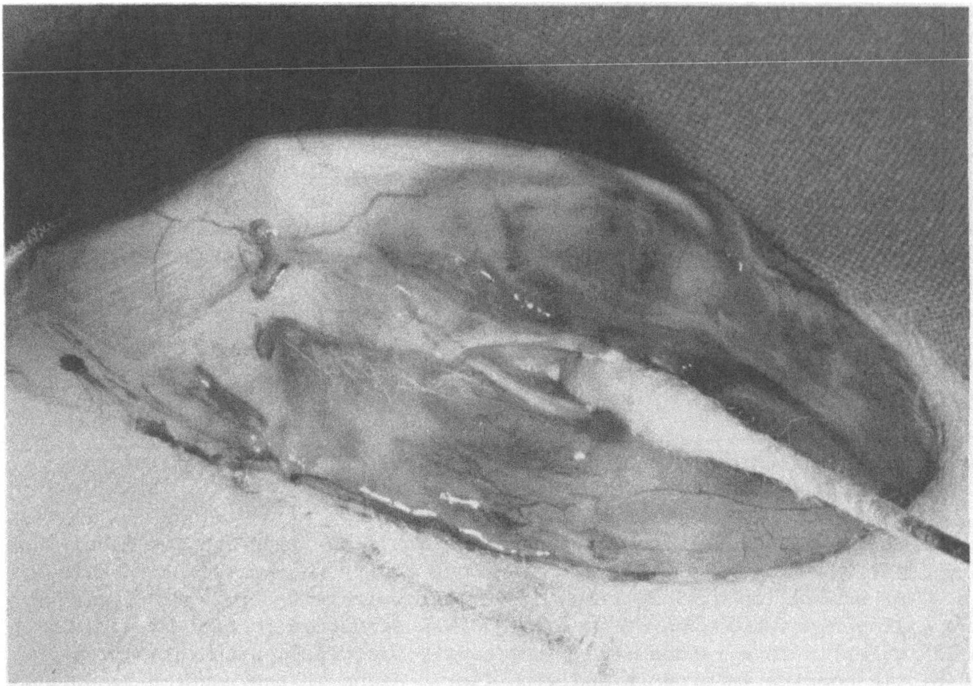

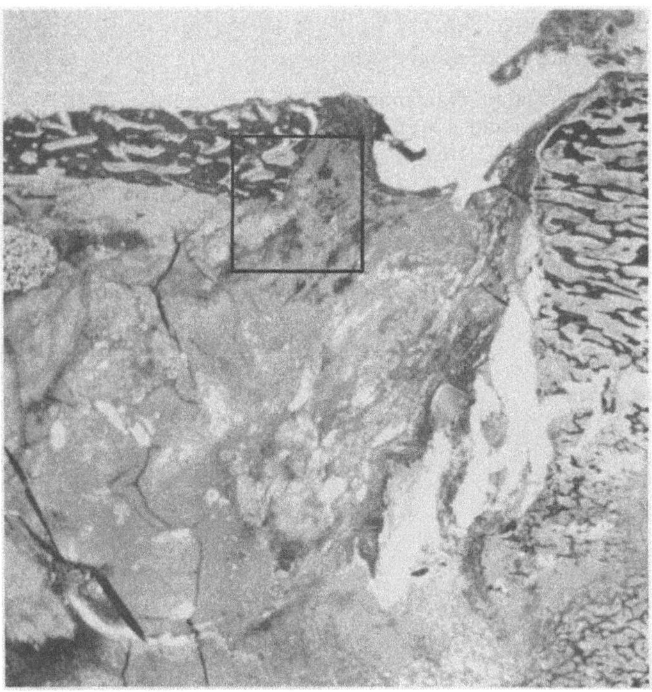

b

Fig. 2. a) No infection after closing of the defect with the fibrin-antibiotic complex (group A). b) Distal femur with Fibrin-Antibiotic Complex 7 days after inoculation with *S. aureus*. Well preserved fibrin clot, surrounded by granulation tissue (Ladewig staining). c) Section of b) Granulation reaction around the fibrin clot with lamellar new bone formation

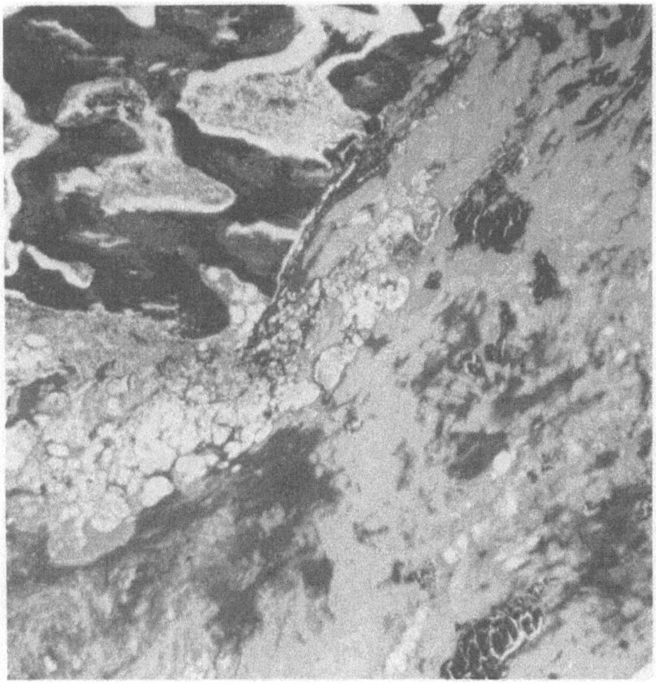

Fig. 2c

B: 0.45 mL fibrin composed of:

- 0.25 mL highly concentrated human fibrinogen
- 0.10 mL distilled water
- 0.10 mL thrombin sol. (≈300 NIH/mL) and calcium ions (40 mmol/L).

Results

The animals -- 30 in each group -- were killed after seven days. Fifteen rabbits of group B died between the second and seventh day due to sepsis. Loss of body weight averaged 560 g. In the group treated locally with the fibrin-tobramycin complex (A), no animal died within the seven days and the loss of body weight averaged 136 g.

Group A: No signs of infection were observed in 22 animals (Fig. 2a); in six animals, the result was not clear, and two animals had obvious infections. All animals except two showed microscopically low grade inflammatory reactions. Exogenous fibrin was still present (Fig. 2b), surrounded by granulation tissue (Fig. 2c) with granulocytes and macrophages. New lamellar bone formation was occasionally seen. The mild local inflammatory reaction did not infiltrate surrounding bone and soft tissue.

Group B: Obvious signs of infection were seen in all animals (Fig. 3a). Seven femurs were fractured at the level of saucerization. Signs of severe infection were found on histologic examination with partly necrotic cortical and cancellous bone (Fig. 3b). The exogenous fibrin clot fragmented and partly disappeared under the influence of high local fibrinolytic activity in the septic area. Surrounding bone and soft tissue were infiltrated by septic inflammation (Fig. 3c).

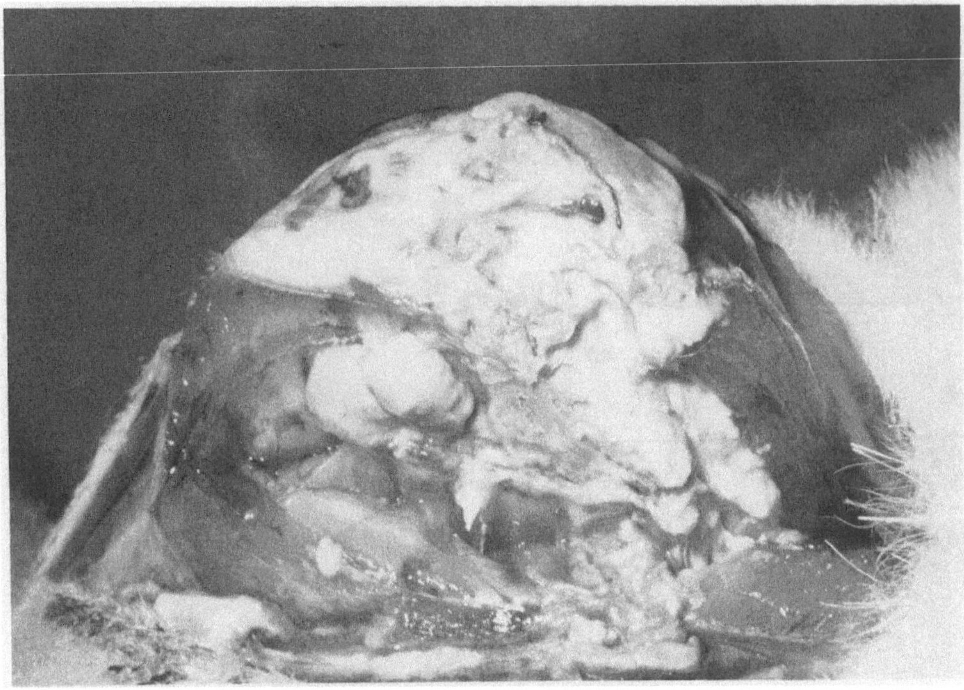

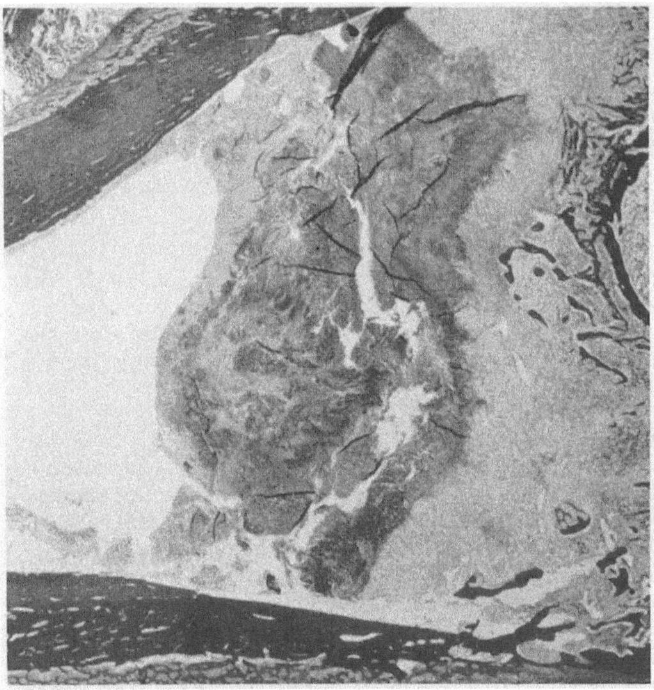

b

Fig. 3. a) Severe infection after closing the defect with fibrin alone (group B). b) Distal femur with fibrin 7 days after inoculation with *S. aureus*. Partly necrotic cortical and cancellous bone. Fibrin clot fragmented. c) Periosteal abscess (arrow). Phlegmonous inflammation in the surrounding muscle

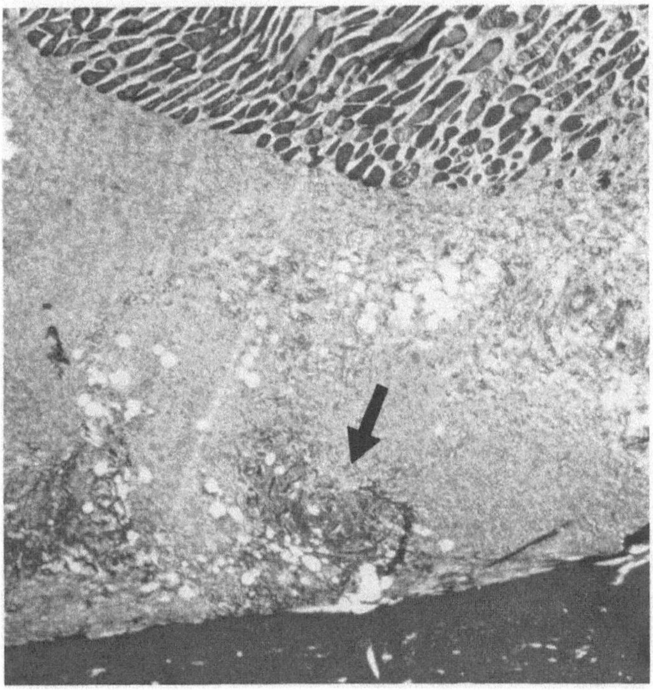

Fig. 3c

Comparing macro- and microscopic results of both groups, the local fibrin-antibiotic treatment showed qualitatively, by the degree of inflammatory reaction, proof of antibiotic release out of the impregnated fibrin-complex.

Smears from the extra-articular soft tissue and from the medullary canal of the distal femur from Group A showed three animals with residual *S. aureus*. In Group B, all smears were positive. The bacteriologic result was highly significant ($p = 0.01$) for an effective discharge of tobramycin out of the fibrin clot.

Table I.

	Sterile	Nonsterile	Total
Group A - fibrin-tobramycin complex	27	3	30
Group B - fibrin	0	30	30
Total	27	33	60

Clinical Studies

Preliminary results *in vitro* and *in vivo* justified the clinical application of the Fibrin-Antibiotic Complex for supplementary local treatment in infected surgical wounds. The advantages are:

1) the physiologic matrix of fibrin compared with polymethylmethacrylate beads (Fig. 4a, 4b);

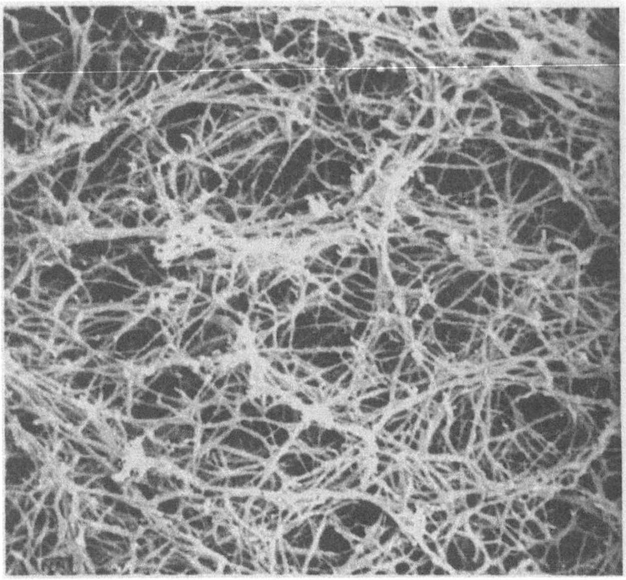

a

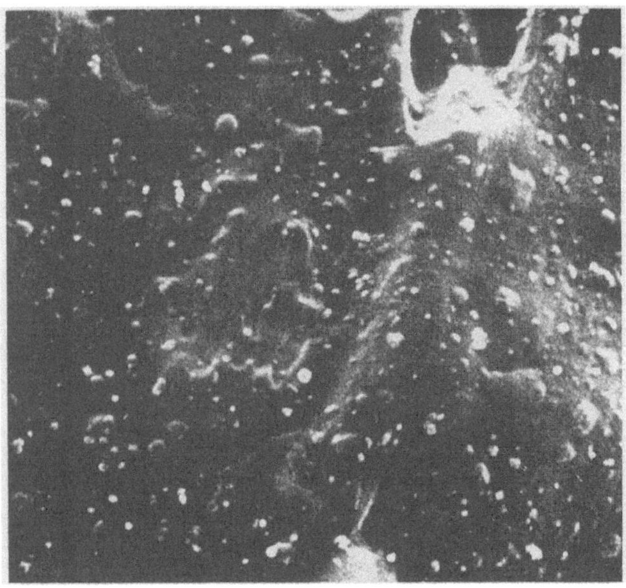

b

Fig. 4. a) Fibrin-Antibiotic Complex. b) Gentamicin-PMMA beads. Surface on scanning electron microscope (5000:1)

2) the plasticity during the transition from fibrinogen into fibrin;
3) the possibility of primary cancellous bone grafting;
4) replacement of granulation tissue with early capillarization;
5) the initially high elution, extending over 2-3 days, of the antibiotics; and
6) the possibility of primary wound closure.

In April 1979, the first antibiotic-impregnated fibrin clot was applied in a ten-year old girl with osteomyelitis of the medial end of the clavicle (Fig. 5a). The infected bone was debrided (Fig. 5b) and filled with fibrin

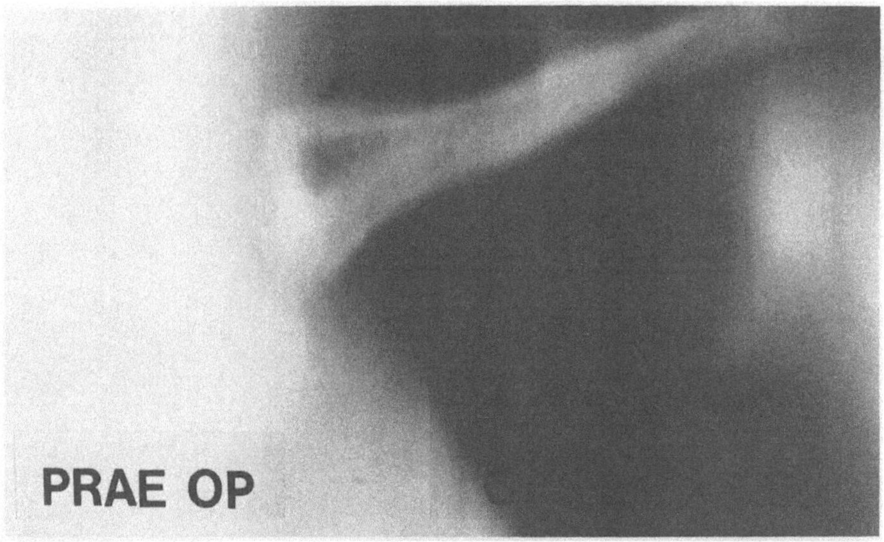

a

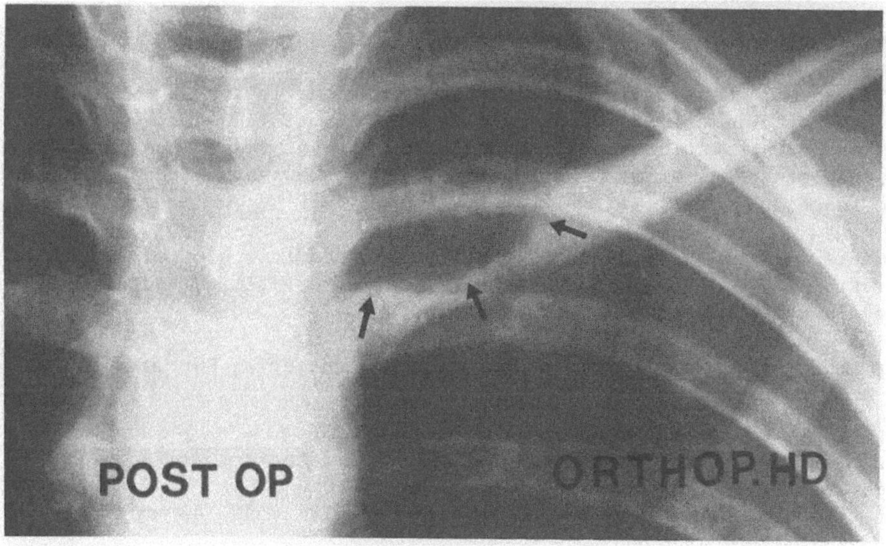

b

Fig. 5. G.Sch., 14-year old girl. a)Osteomyelitis in medial left clavicle. b) Debridement and Fibrin-Antibiotic Complex; primary wound closure and healing April 1979. c) Remodelling of the clavicle 10 months postoperatively. No recurrent infection

containing tobramycin. The wound healed by primary intention, and complete bone remodeling was achieved 10 months postoperatively (Fig. 5c).

Based on our initial good results, we standardized the technique, first without cancellous bone grafting. Tobramycin powder was not available for local application and the antibiotic activity of the commercially available dosage (80 mg) is not sufficient for long-acting local elution, especially in small bone cavities where the whole volume of the required complex is less than 2 mL (fibrinogen, antibiotics and thrombin solution). In subse-

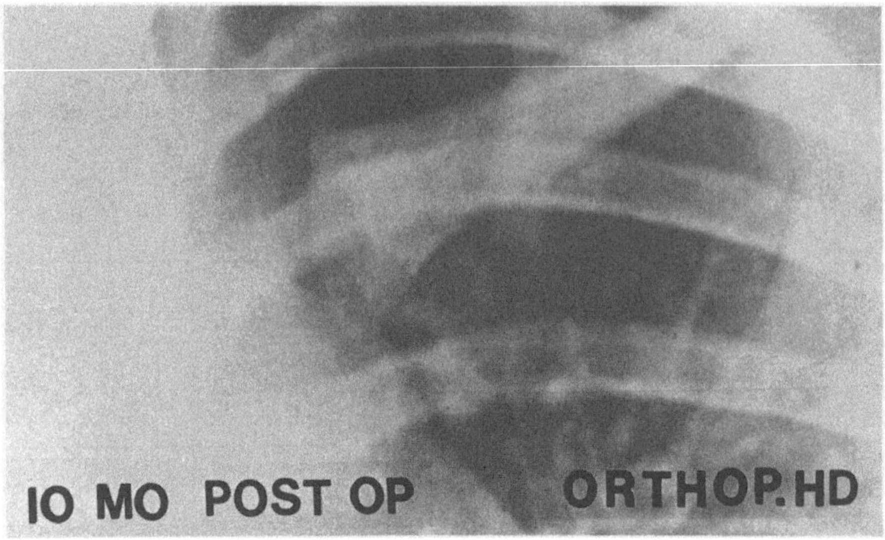

Fig.

quent cases, therefore, we used gentamicin, which is available for clinical trials as gentamicin sulfate powder (500 mg) with an activity of approximately 500 µg/mg. Gentamicin contained in PMMA-beads is locally effective in bone and soft tissue infections. It is sensitive to the most common microbes encountered in orthopedics, has a low rate of resistance development, rarely causes allergic complications, and at low serum concentrations no toxic reactions occur.

Requirements for the application of the fibrin-gentamicin complex are: 1) susceptibility of the microorganism; 2) normal creatinine and urea blood levels which have to be checked preoperatively.

The fibrin-gentamicin complex is prepared during surgery. For example, to achieve 4 mL we use:

- 2 mL highly concentrated human fibrinogen
- 1 mL distilled water containing gentamicin sulfate (8 mg/kg body weight)
- 1 mL thrombin solution (≈500 NIH/mL) and calcium ions (40 mmol/L).

The human fibrinogen is available in cryoprecipitated or lyophilized form. It should be prepared according to the directions and to the required amount. Aprotinin (used to stabilize fibrin-sealing against local fibrinolytic activity) is not used because fibrin in the fibrin-gentamicin complex is a more physiologic carrier for the antibiotic instead of sealing for tissue adhesion. Gentamicin prolongs the coagulation rate; therefore, a high thrombin concentration (≈500 NIH/mL) has to be used. Fibrinogen and gentamicin are premixed and the thrombin solution is added immediately before application. While dissolving, the complex has to fill the entire cavity to avoid a hematoma.

Method of application of the fibrin-gentamicin complex without cancellous bone grafting

A 54-year old woman (Fig. 6) underwent a screw fixation of the distal tibia and fibula (Fig. 6a). A draining sinus developed after removal of the im-

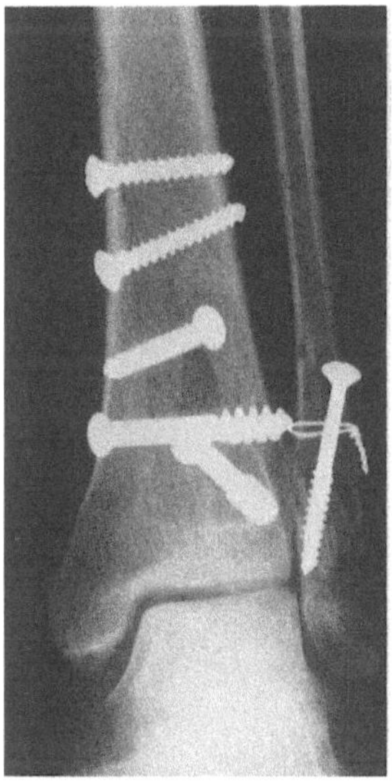

a

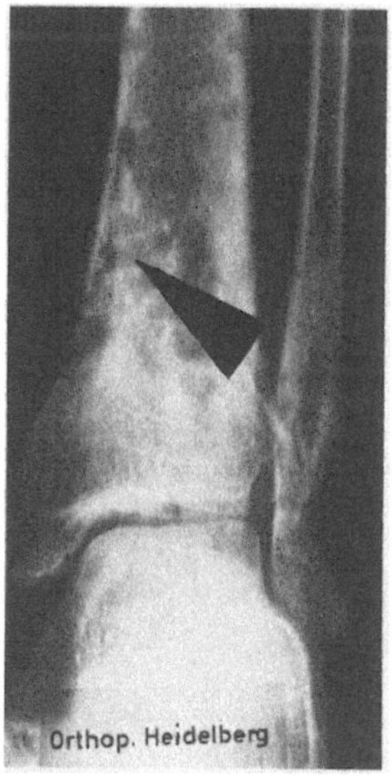

b

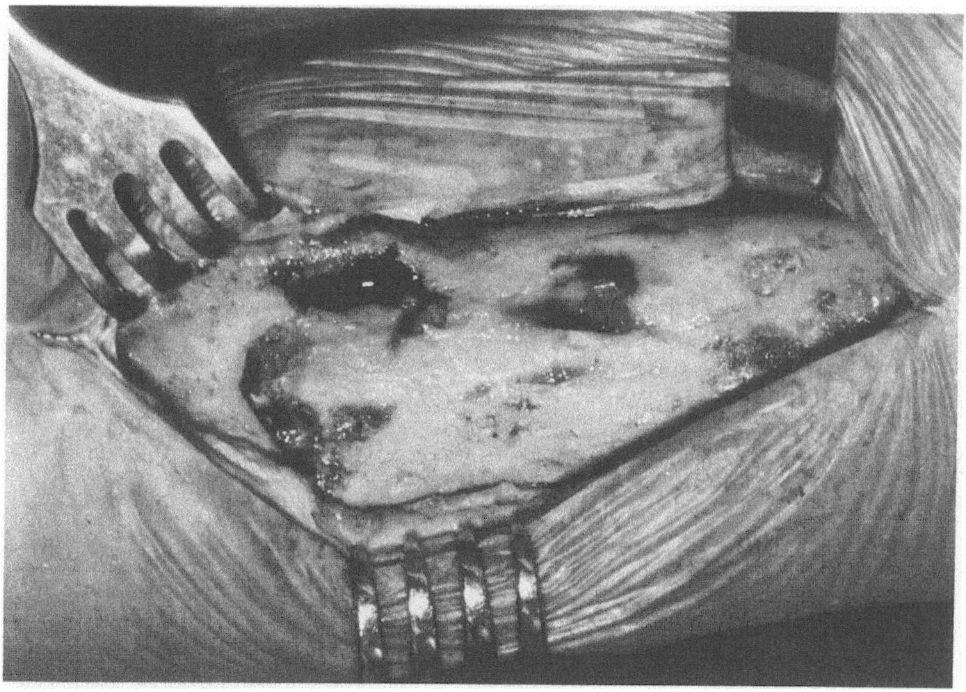

c

Fig. 6. H.R., 54-year old woman. a) Osteosynthesis of the distal tibia and fibula. b) Draining sinus and sequestrum (arrow) after removal of the implants. c) Disulfine-blue staining; sinus and sequestrum. d) Sequestrectomy, curettage and drilling of sclerotic bone. e) The bone cavity filled with the Fibrin-Antibiotic Complex during setting of fibrin. f) Polymerized Fibrin-Antibiotic Complex. Tube drainage, preferably without suction.
g) Roentgenograph 1 year postoperatively. Primary wound healing, no recurrent infection during a 3-year follow-up

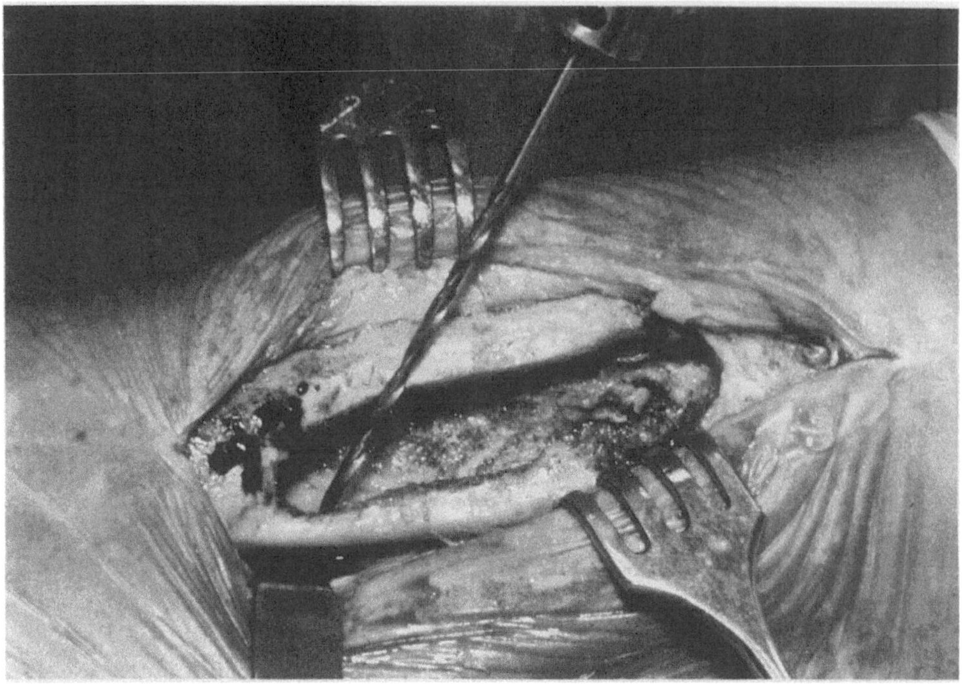

Fig. 6d

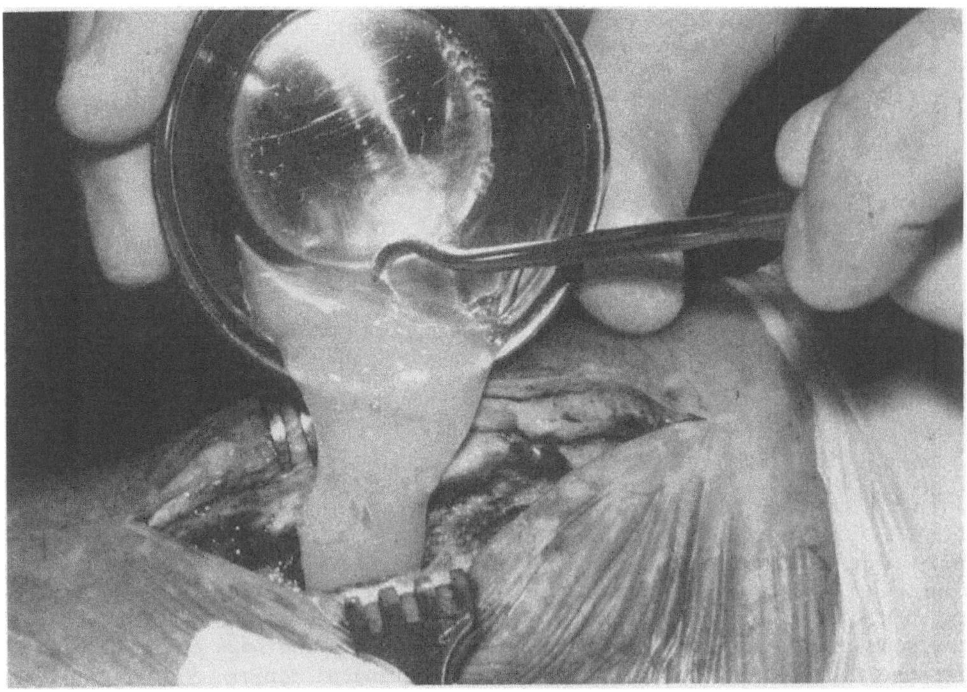

Fig. 6e

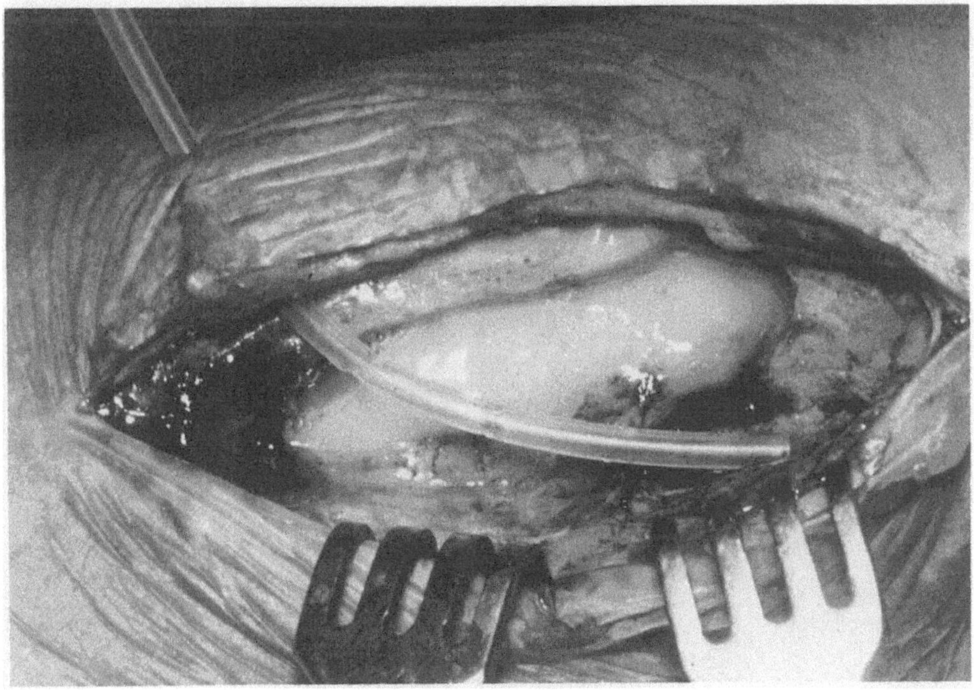

Fig. 6f

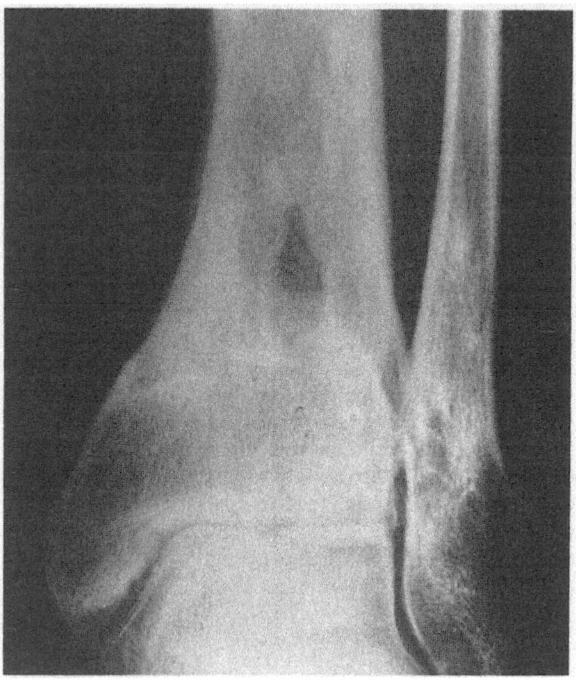

Fig. 6g

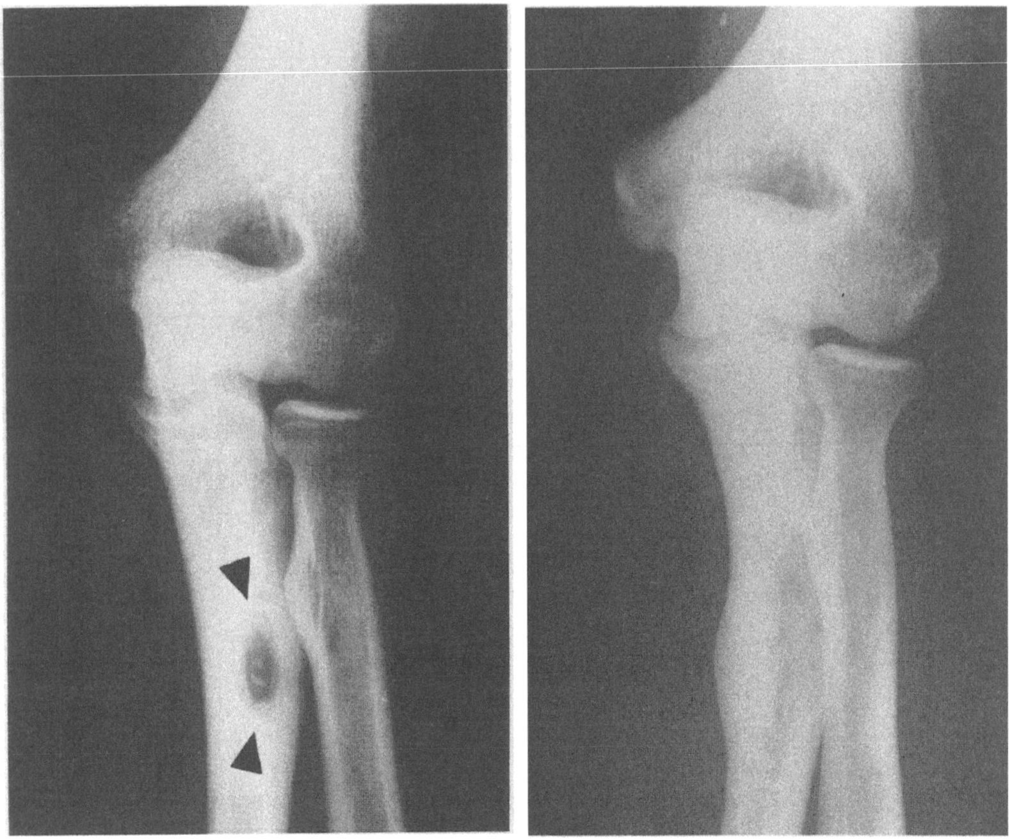

a b

Fig. 7. W.R., 36-year old man. a) Chronic osteomyelitis left ulna with a *S. aureus* draining sinus; third recurrence after surgery. b) Primary wound healing; ten months postoperative remodelling of the bone. c) Debridement and application of Fibrin-Antibiotic Complex. No recurrent infection during a 5-year follow-up

plants (Fig. 6b). The infecting organism was a gentamicin-sensitive *S. aureus*. Creatinine and urea blood levels were normal. A surgical exploration of the infected bone was carried out after intravenous disulfine-blue stain clearly showed the sequestrum (Fig. 6c). Sequestrectomy, curettage, and drilling of sclerotic bone were undertaken to open vascularized bone for surgical debridement (Fig. 6d). Irrigation was done with saline or antiseptic solution. The fibrin-gentamicin complex was mixed, as described above, and the bony cavity filled while the fibrin was settling (Fig. 6e), a process that took a few minutes. Tube drainage (preferably without suction)(Fig. 6f), and primary wound closure were performed to obtain primary healing and to avoid secondary contamination. Primary wound healing followed and the results of the roentgenogram one year postoperatively are shown in Fig. 6g.

A 36-year old man (Fig. 7) was admitted because of chronic osteomyelitis of the left ulna with a *S. aureus* draining sinus. This was his third recurrence (Fig. 7a). Debridement and drilling of sclerotic bone were carried out and irrigation as described above. The Fibrin-Antibiotic Complex was

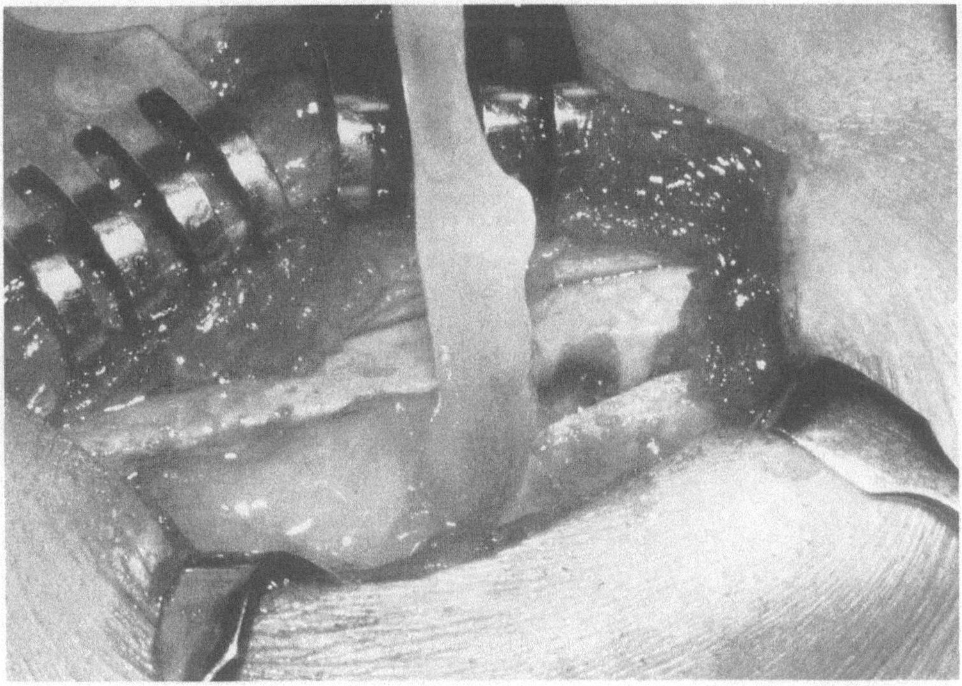

Fig. 7c

applied while the fibrin was settling (Fig. 7c). Primary wound healing resulted, and roentgenograms 10 months postoperatively showed remodelling of the ulna with no signs of recurrent infection (Fig. 7b).

According to the well-established technique of filling infected bone defects after sequestrectomy, saucerization and autologous cancellous bone grafts, we started to combine bone grafting with the fibrin-antibiotic complex. This procedure promised better bone regeneration than fibrin alone. Fresh autologous bone was preferred to allogeneic bone from the bone bank. The surface of the transplanted cancellous bone was coated with antibiotic-impregnated fibrinogen which was coagulated into fibrin by a thrombin solution. The elution of gentamicin provided the as yet unvascularized bone with sufficient bacteriostasis for a few days. The adhesive property of fibrin led to a certain amount of immobilization within the bone grafts.

Method of application of the fibrin-gentamicin complex with cancellous bone grafting

Highly concentrated human fibrinogen is mixed with a gentamicin sulfate solution (8 mg/kg) as described above. The cancellous bone is cut into small pieces and coated with the gentamicin-impregnated fibrinogen. We don't know the exact amount of bone to be mixed with the fibrin complex but we prefer, if available, bone to fibrin as 8:1. Fresh autologous bone is usually taken first from the posterior iliac crest during the same anesthetic procedure. We have had no infection so far at the donor site of the bone graft. Following wound closure of the donor site, the septic wound has to be surgically exposed, foreign bodies and sequesters have to be removed, sclerotic and necrotic bone has to be saucerized, and fragments have

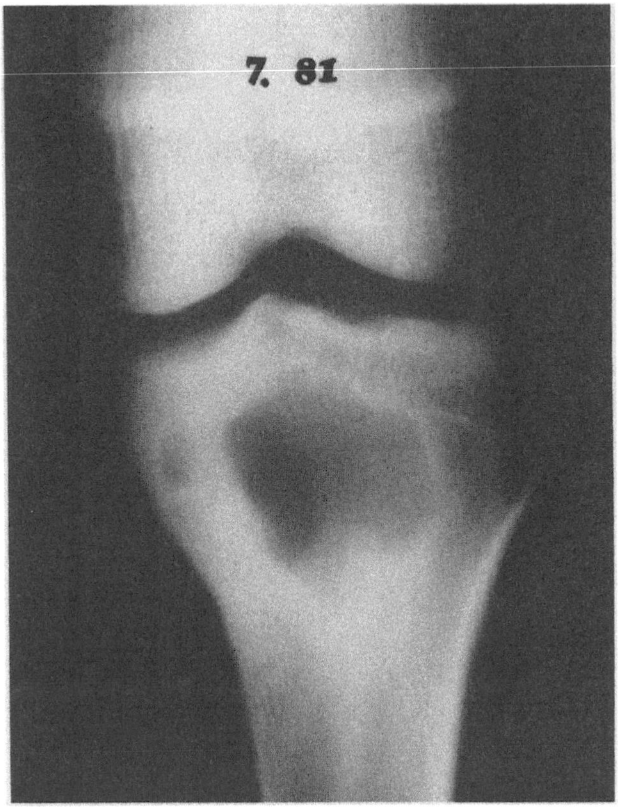

a

Fig. 8. I.B., 26-year old woman. a) Brodie's abscess left proximal tibia. b) Two months postoperatively secondary wound closure with skin graft. c) Debridement and filling of the cavity with cancellous bone mixed with the Fibrin-Antibiotic Complex

to be immobilized, usually by external fixation. Irrigation with saline or antiseptic solution should be performed.

The premixed fibrinogen, gentamicin and cancellous bone is clotted by thrombin solution in a bowl and during fibrin settling filled into the bone defect (Fig. 8c). Tube drainage, preferably without suction, and primary wound closure should be carried out.

A 26-year old woman (Fig. 8) had a Brodie's abscess on the left proximal tibial metaphysis (Fig. 8a) with evidence of *enterobacter* and *pseudomonas* infection sensitive to gentamicin. Curettage and debridement of the abscess and saucerization of the infected cavity were carried out. The defect was filled with cancellous bone mixed with the fibrin-gentamicin complex (Fig. 8c) Two months postoperatively almost complete bone ingrowth was observed (Fig. 8b). Primary closure was not possible and after wound granulation skin grafting had to be performed.

Fig. 9 concerns a 35-year old man with multiple injuries including a fractured right distal femur. A pseudarthrosis (Fig. 9b) was infected with a *S. aureus* draining sinus (Fig. 9a). The infected pseudarthrosis was surgically resected down to bleeding bone. After realignment, an external fixator was applied using the Hoffmann device (Fig. 9c, 9d). Fresh autologous bone grafts from the iliac crest and allogeneic cancellous bank bone were mixed with the fibrin-gentamicin complex and packed into and

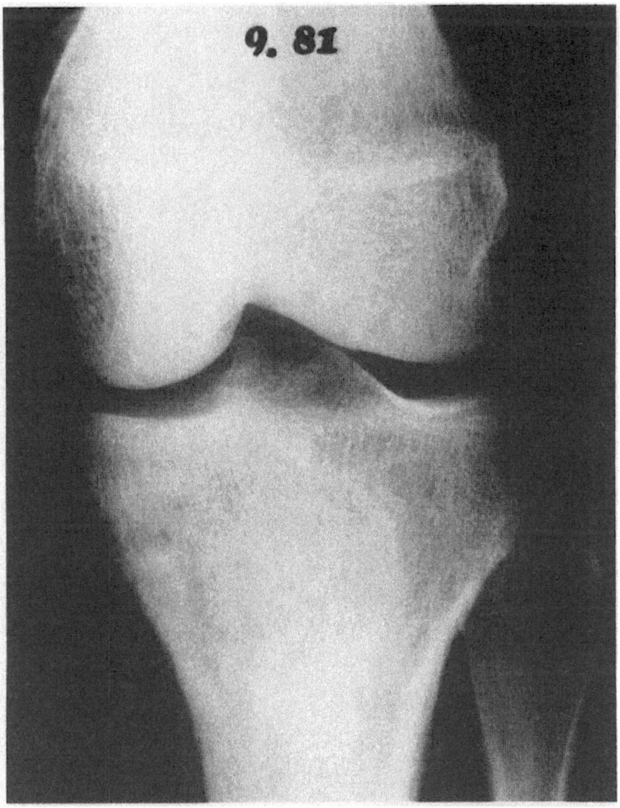

Fig. 8b

Fig. 8c

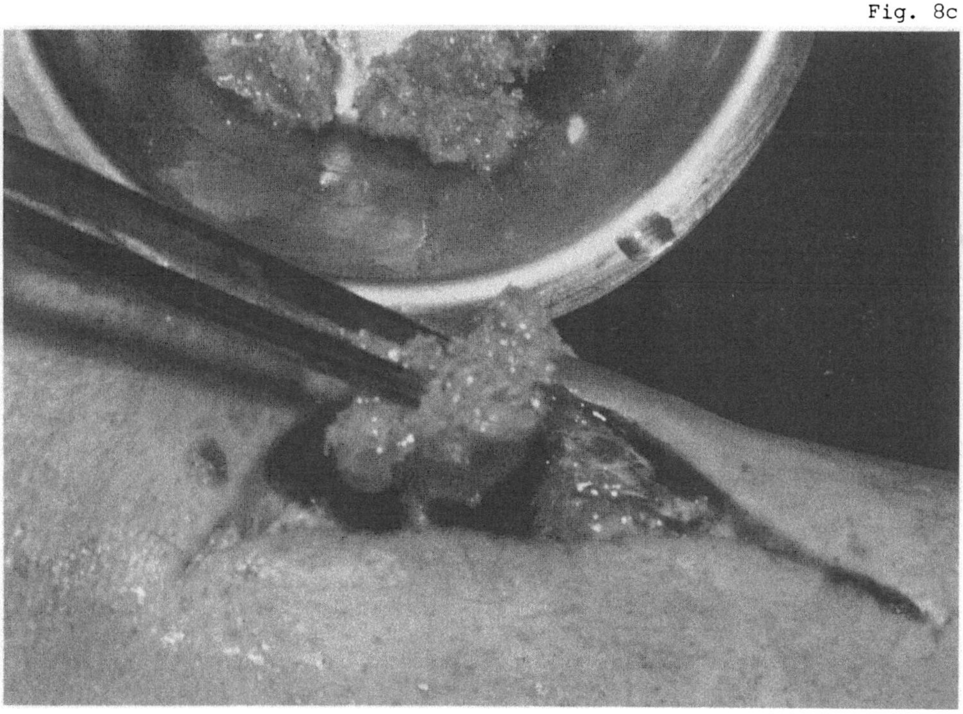

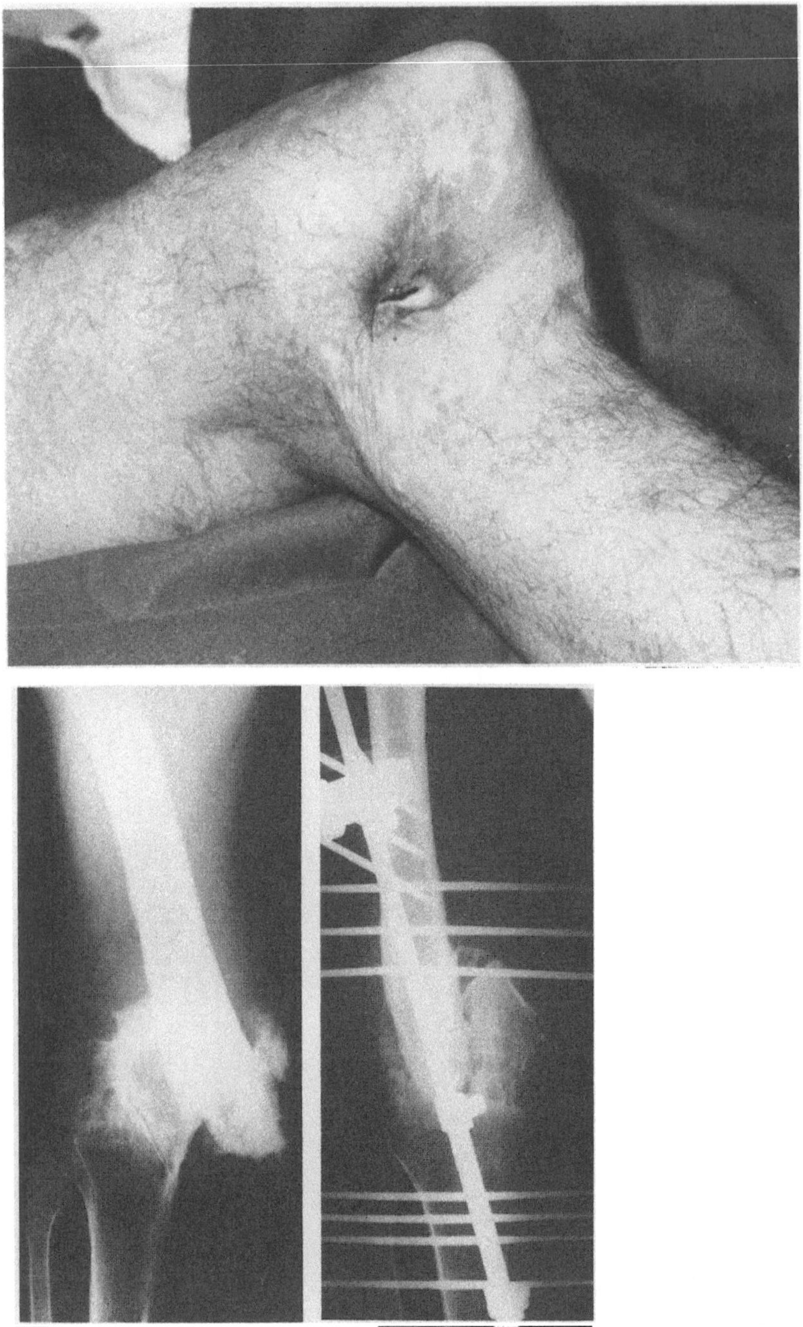

a

b

<u>Fig. 9</u>. W.H., 35-year old man - fracture, distal femur. a) *S. aureus* draining sinus and b) pseudarthrosis. c) December 1981 - debridement, external fixation, autologous and allogeneic cancellous bone grafting with fibrin-antibiotic complex. d) External fixation for 1 year. e) Roentgenograph 2 years postoperatively

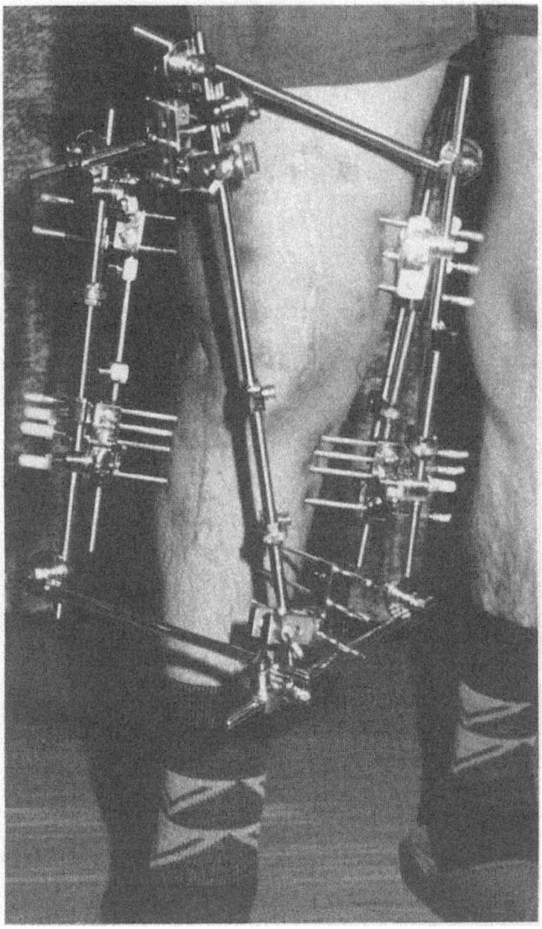

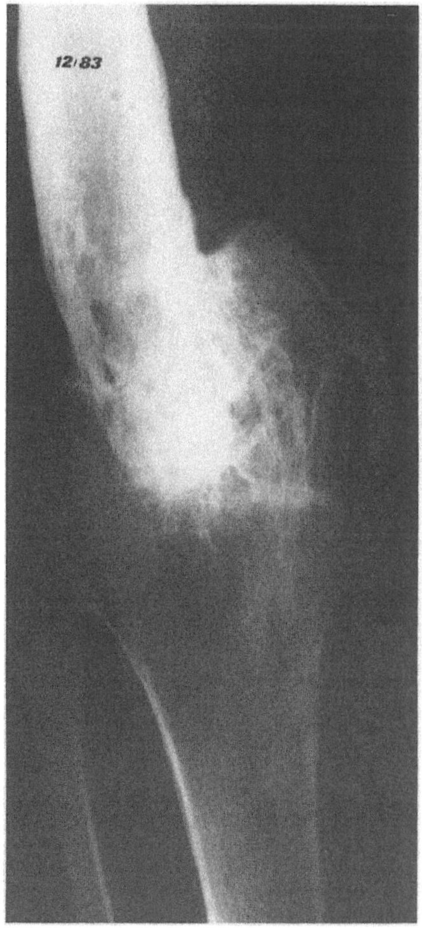

d e

Fig. 9d, e

around the gap in the distal femur (Fig. 9c). The wound was closed primarily with drainage. A cephalosporin was given systemically over a period of four weeks. The external fixation remained for one year. No recurrent infection has occurred so far. The roentgenogram two years postoperatively showed solid bony union (Fig. 9e).

The next case report describes a 20-year old woman (Fig. 10) who had a compound fracture of the left forearm (Fig. 10a) which was plated two weeks after the injury, followed by a deep staphylococcal infection (*S. aureus*). The wound was treated with gentamicin-PMMA beads applied on the radial and ulnar site (Fig. 10b). Due to a persisting deep ulnar infection, the plate was removed and an external fixator applied. We saw the patient for the first time with an insufficient fixation of the infected nonunion of the ulna shaft (Fig. 10c) and with a draining sinus. The causative organism was still *S. aureus*. The external fixator was removed, and one week later autologous cancellous bone was taken from the dorsal iliac crest and, during the same anesthetic procedure, all foreign material (PMMA beads and two screws) and devitalized tissue (sequestrum) were removed from the wound

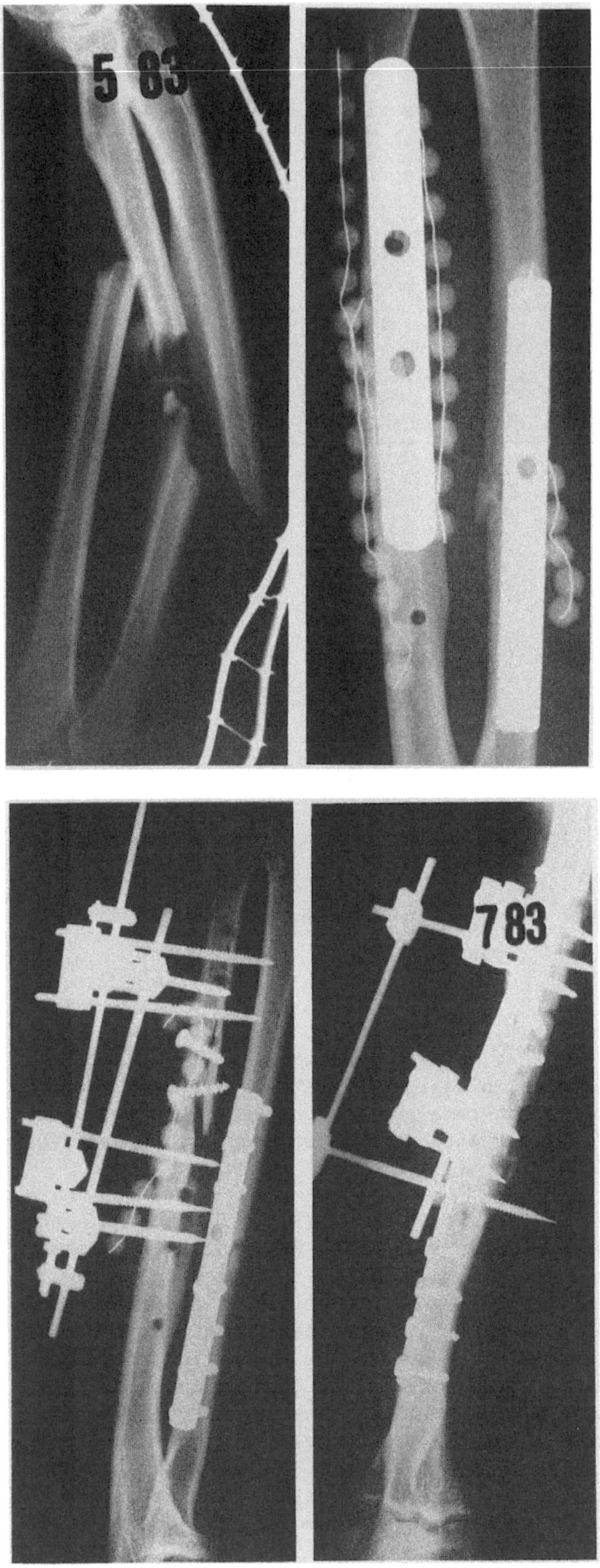

a b c

Fig. 10. M.K., 20-year old woman. a) Fracture left fore arm 5/83. b) Plating followe by deep infection. Gentamici PMMA beads 6/83. c) Persisti infection of ulna. Insuffici external fixation 7/83. d) D bridement. e) and f) Externa fixation and bone grafting w fibrin-gentamicin complex 10 g) Four months postoperative increasing bone remodelling

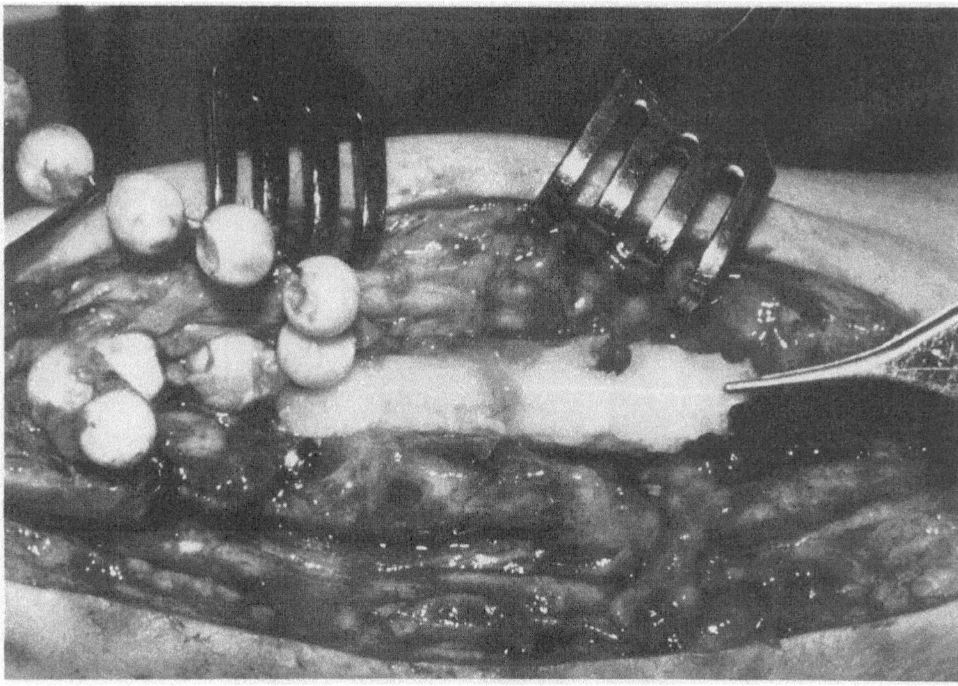

Fig. 10d

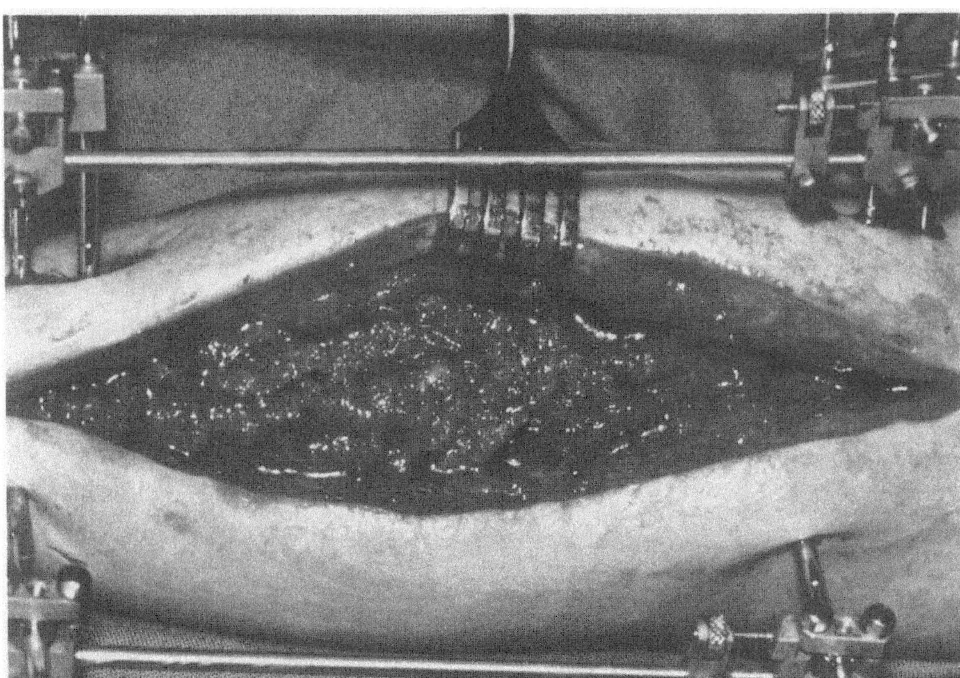

Fig. 10e

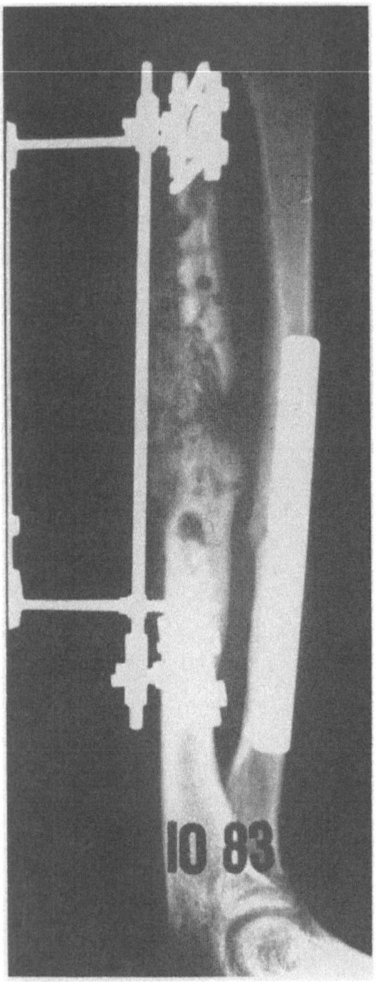

Fig. 10f

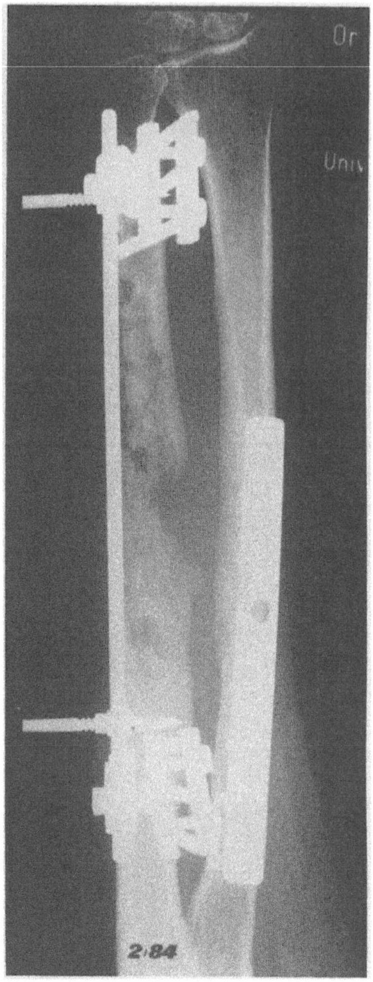

Fig. 10g

(Fig. 10d). The external fixator was reinserted, and the large defect was packed with cancellous bone, impregnated with the fibrin-gentamicin complex (Fig. 10e, 10f). For this procedure, 4 mL of highly concentrated fibrinogen, 1 mL distilled water containing 400 mg gentamicin sulfate and 4 mL thrombin solution were used. The wound was closed with a tube drainage. A cephalosporin was given orally for four weeks. Primary healing was achieved with no recurrent infection. Roentgenograph, four months postoperatively, showed obvious remodelling of the ulna shaft (Fig. 10g).

Results

From April 1979 until December 1983, we treated 69 patients with bone and soft tissue infections with the fibrin-gentamicin complex. Fifty-nine infections healed, 30 primarily and 29 secondarily. Ten patients showed no improvement.

Table II. Bone and soft tissue infections
April 1979 to December 1983 (n = 69)

Results		Number
No recurrent infection		59
primary healing	30	
secondary healing	29	
No improvement		10

Pharmacokinetics

Subsequent to the clinical application of the fibrin-gentamicin complex, serum and urine concentrations of gentamicin were measured (serum: n = 18; urine: n = 17).

Serum level determinations were performed 1, 2, 4, 8, 24 and 48 hours after application of 250 to 500 mg gentamicin sulfate according to body weight. Maximum serum levels were obtained after 2-4 hours. The mean peak values were below 1 µg/mL. After 48 hours, only traces of gentamicin were measurable (<0.05 µg/mL). However, gentamicin could still be measured in three patients after six days (Fig. 11a). Comparing gentamicin serum levels

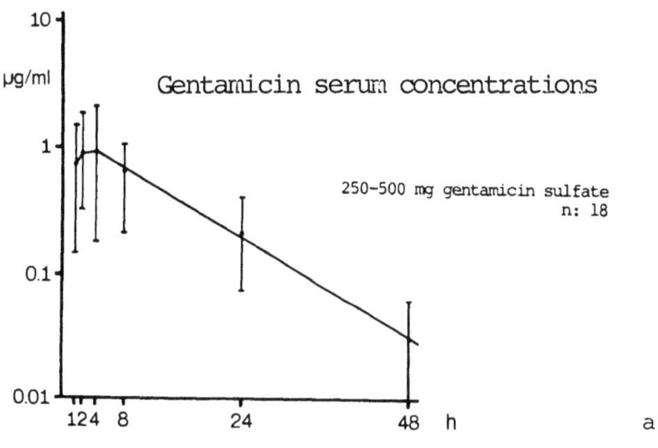

a

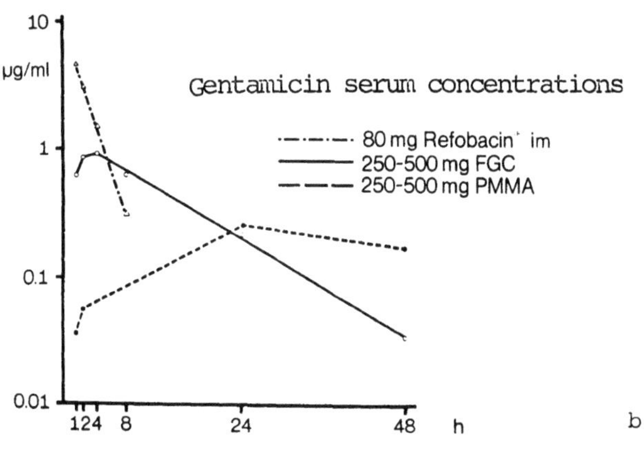

b

Fig. 11. Gentamicin serum concentration: a) after clinical application of the fibrin-gentamicin complex; b) after different techniques of gentamicin application

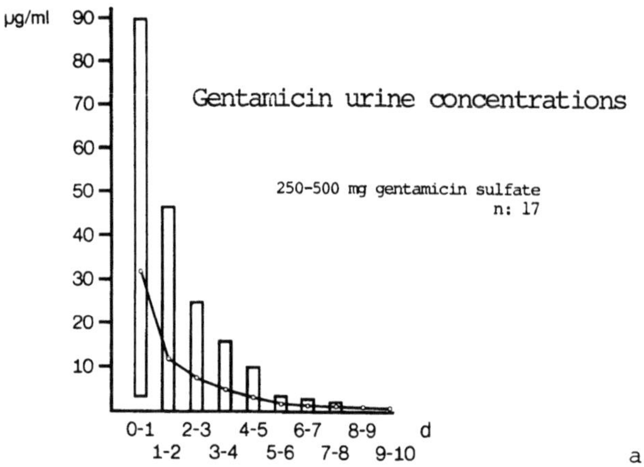

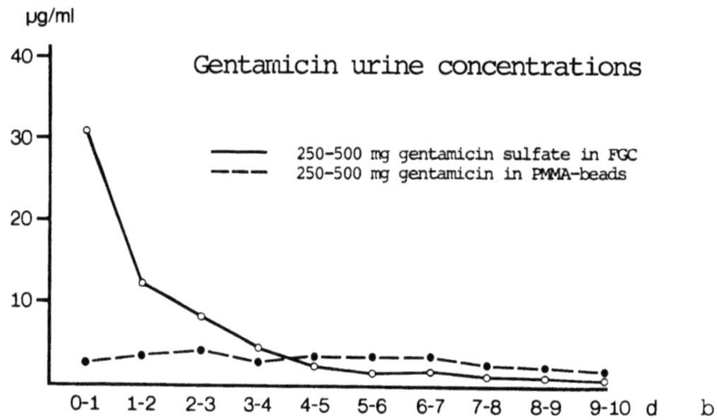

Fig. 12. Gentamicin urine concentration: a) after clinical application of the fibrin gentamicin complex; b) after different techniques of gentamicin application

during treatment with the fibrin-gentamicin complex with values after intramuscular injection of 80 mg of gentamicin and locally applied PMMA beads (250 mg), the elution of gentamicin corresponded to the clinical requirements of a short-term high local antibiotic concentration (Fig. 11b).

Determination of urine levels was performed over seven days following the application of the fibrin-gentamicin complex. During the first three days, the gentamicin levels were high. The mean values ranged from 31 to 8 µg/mL; the peak values from 90 to 24 µg/mL). The mean gentamicin levels decreased to 15 µg/mL within seven days (Fig. 12a). The corresponding values after implantation of PMMA beads, at the fourth day, were below and later slightly above the values measured after application of the fibrin-gentamicin complex (Fig. 12b).

Discussion

The physiologic matrix of the Fibrin-Antibiotic Complex is its main advantage. The replacement of human fibrin in granulation tissue with early capillarization (Böhler et al, 1977; Bösch et al, 1977a, 1977b; Braun et al, 1982e) allows, under high local antibiotic cover, primary reconstructive procedures such as bone grafting and wound closure in septic orthopedic surgery. This means, in most cases, a single surgical procedure compared with suction-irrigation drainage (Willenegger and Roth, 1962) and

PMMA beads (Klemm, 1974, 1977). Bone defects, particularly in poorly vascularized areas, require additional autologous bone grafting. The Fibrin-Antibiotic Complex without bone grafting also showed encouraging results in well vascularized metaphyseal bone defects (Fig. 5c). Our clinical observation in a few patients (Puhl et al, 1982) showed that a thick layer of exogenous fibrin can enhance bone regeneration. This has also been reported by Heine et al (1982). In fibrin-adhered skin grafts, they observed reduced healing when fibrin glue was too thickly applied.

We also recommend the use of fibrin-gentamicin complex for allogeneic cancellous bone grafting in a nonseptic area to provide the not yet vascularized grafts with high local antibiotic coverage.

Like all human plasma derivatives, fibrinogen, theoretically, also carries the same risk of viral hepatitis-B or the non-A non-B type. Plasma donors are carefully selected and we have not encountered a significant incidence of postoperative hepatitis-B in patients in whom fibrin-sealant was used (Panis and Scheele, 1981; Scheele, 1981).

Workability and physiology make human fibrin capable of application. Fast hardening amino acid solutions (Schultheis et al, 1981) or denatured collagen (Burri and Lob, 1982; Götz and Wesch, 1981) are other alternatives as carriers of therapeutic agents in the treatment of chronic osteomyelitis. The denatured pork collagen described by Götz and Wesch (1981) and Burri and Lob (1982) is impregnated with an antiseptic agent. The preliminary results are good but pharmacokinetics and local toxicity are not yet known. The antibiotic-impregnated blood clot (Ecke et al, 1974; Winter, 1951) has been a successful treatment for osteomyelitis. Bösch et al (1982) measured the elution of amicain within the first 24 hours and found that it was twice as fast out of a blood clot as out of the fibrin sealant. They could also show that fibrin is a comparatively poor culture medium for inoculated *S. aureus* and *Pseudomonas aeruginosa*.

Besides gentamicin, different antibiotics have been used clinically in combination with fibrin, such as neomycin sulfate and bacitracin (Goudarzi, 1983) or cefotaxim (Zilch et al, 1982). Neomycin sulfate and bacitracin can cause local allergic reactions and, *in vitro*, cefotaxim has a short half-life and fast elution rate compared with aminoglycosides (Wahlig et al, 1982).

The gentamicin release after clinical application showed maximum serum levels within the first 4 hours. This corresponds to the clinical requirements of a short-term high local gentamicin release. Peak serum values within the first 4 hours were between 2 and 3 µg/mL, far below the margin of toxicity. The fibrin-gentamicin complex can thus contain 8-10 mg gentamicin sulfate per kg body weight. The high gentamicin concentration in serum and urine can be explained by:

1) the different amounts of locally applied gentamicin (250-500 mg);
2) the loss of gentamicin in wound secretions and in the drainage system;
3) the biologic binding of gentamicin with fibrin and transplanted bone grafts; and
4) the different vascularization around the Fibrin-Antibiotic Complex as a criterion for removal of released gentamicin.

Preliminary experimental and clinical results with the fibrin-gentamicin complex for local antibiotic treatment in bone and soft tissue infection are encouraging. It should be considered as supplementary therapy to surgical debridement and immobilization.

Summary

Animal studies and clinical trials in humans are reported to introduce the Fibrin-Antibiotic Complex as effective supplementary therapy for infections encountered in orthopedic surgery. The main advantage of this complex is the physiologic property of fibrin that acts as a carrier for the antibiotic. The replacement of fibrin in granulation tissue allows primary cancellous bone grafting and primary wound closure.

The mixture of human fibrinogen, gentamicin sulfate and thrombin solution is described. Case reports show indications, mode of application, and results of this therapeutic procedure. In this series of 69 patients in whom the Fibrin-Antibiotic Complex was used for a variety of infections, 59 patients had no recurrence of their infections. In 10 patients no improvement could be achieved.

References

1. Badgy, D., Gerendas, M., and Winter, L.: Thrombin-Fibrin-Produkte und ihre therapeutische Anwendung. VEB Fischer Jena 157-171, 1963.

2. Beneke, G., Ecke, H., and Bikfali, A.: Histologische Untersuchungen einiger mit Eigenblut-Antibiotika-Plomben behandelten chronischen Osteomyelitiden. Brun's Beitr.klin.Chir. 209, 430, 1964.

3. Bikfali, A., and Ecke, H.: Behandlung der chronischen Osteomyelitis mit der Eigenblut-Antibiotika-Plombe. Brun's Beitr.klin.Chir. 201, 190, 1960.

4. Bikfali, A., Ecke, H., and Schleifer, D.: Die Eigenblut-Antibiotika-Plombe in der Therapie der chronischen Osteomyelitis - Ergebnisse einer vierjährigen Behandlungsserie. Mschr. Unfallheilk. 66, 257, 1963.

5. Böhler, N., Bösch, P., Sandbach, G., Schlag, G., Eschberger, J., and Schmid, L.: Der Einfluss von homologem Fibrinogen auf die Osteotomieheilung beim Kaninchen. Unfallheilk. 80, 501, 1977.

6. Bösch, P., Braun, F., and Spängler, H.P.: Die Technik der Fibrin-Spongiosaplastik. Arch. orthop.Unfall-Chir. 90, 63, 1977a.

7. Bösch, P., Braun, F., Eschberger, J., Kovac, W., and Spängler, H.P.: Die Beeinflussung der Knochenheilung durch hochkonzentriertes Fibrin - Experimentelle Untersuchungen am Kaninchen. Arch. orthop. Unfall-Chir, 89, 259, 1977b.

8. Bösch, P., Stanek, G., Weber, P., and Arbes, H.: Experimentelle Untersuchungen am Fibrinkleber zur bakteriellen Kontamination und Antibiotikumbeimischung. In, Cotta, H. and Braun, A.: Fibrinkleber in Orthopädie und Traumatologie, Thieme Verlag Stuttgart, 1982, pp 188-190.

9. Braun, A., Schumacher, G., Kratzat, R., Heine, W.-D., and Pasch, B.: Der Fibrin-Antibiotikum-Verbund im Tierexperiment zur lokalen Therapie des staphylococceninfizierten Knochens. Vortrag: 3. Deutsch-österreichisch-schweizerische Unfalltagung Wien, 1979.

10. Braun, A., Schumacher, G., Kratzat, R., Heine, W.-D., Pasch, B., and Fabricius, K.: Der Fibrin-Antibiotikum-Verbund im Tierexperiment. Hefte Unfallheilk. 153, 83, 1981.

11. Braun, A., Kratzat, R., Heine, W.-D., and Pasch, B.: Erste klinische Erfahrungen mit dem Fibrin-Tobramycin-Verbund bei Knocheninfektionen. Hefte Unfallheilk. 157, 66, 1982a.

12. Braun, A., Wahlig, H., and Dingeldein, E.: Freisetzungskinetik von Gentamycin nach klinischer Anwendung des Fibrin-Gentamycin-Verbundes bei der Osteomyelitis. Vortrag: 69 Tagung der Dtsch. Gesellsch. für Orthopädie u. Traumatologie, Mainz, 1982b.

13. Braun, A., Schumacher, G., Kratzat, R., Heine, W.-D. Pasch, B., and Roesler, H.: Der Fibrin-Antibiotikum-Verbund im Tierexperiment. In, Cotta, H. and Braun, A.: Fibrinkleber in Orthopädie und Traumatologie, Thieme Verlag Stuttgart, 1982c, pp 172-177.

14. Braun, A., Güssbacher, A., and Rohe, K.: Experience with the Fibrin-Antibiotic-Complex in bone and soft tissue infection. J. Head Neck Pathol. 3, 75, 1982d.

15. Braun, A., Schumacher, G., and Heine, W.-D.: Fibrinklebung osteochondraler Fragmente im Thierexperiment. In, Cotta, H. and Braun, A.: Fibrinkleber in Orthopädie und Traumatologie, Thieme Verlag Stuttgart, 1982e, pp 110-124.

16. Braun, A., Güssbacher, A., Wahlig, H., and Dingeldein, E.: Der Fibrin-Antibiotikum-Verbund als ergänzende Lokalbehandlung der Osteomyelitis. In, Scheele, J.: Fibrinklebung, Springer Verlag, Berlin-Heidelberg-New York, 1984, pp 205-210

17. Buchholz, H.W. and Engelbrecht, H.: Über die Depotwirkung einiger Antibiotika bei Vermischung mit dem Kunstharz Palacos. Chirurg. 41, 511, 1970.

18. Burri, C. and Henkenmeyer, H.: Autologe Spongiosa bei Osteomyelitis mit Knochen-, Weichteil- und Hautdefekt. Langenbecks Arch. klin. Chir. 329, 1022, 1971.

19. Burri, C.: Posttraumatische Osteitis, 2. Auflage. Verlag Hans Huber, Bern, Stuttgart, Wien, 1979, pp 214-272.

20. Burri, C. and Lob, G.: Trauolin® Gel in der Osteitis-Behandlung. Akt. Traumatol. 12, 159, 1982.

21. Coleman, H.M., Bateman, J.G., Dale, G.M., and Starr, D.E.: Cancellous bone grafts for infected bone defects. A single stage procedures. Surg. Gyn. Obst. 83, 392, 1946.

22. Cotta, H. and Braun, A.: Fibrinkleber in Orthopädie und Traumatologie. Thieme Verlag Stuttgart, 1982.

23. De Grood, M.: Het plomberen van restholten na osteomyelitis met "bone-chips". Nederlandse Tijdskrift for Geneeskunde 91.III. 32, 2192, 1947.

24. Dinges, H.P., Redl, H., and Schlag, G.: Histologische Techniken und tierexperimentelle Modelle zur Untersunchung der Wechselwirkung zwischen Fibrinkleber und Gewebe. In, Cotta, H. and Braun, A.: Fibrinkleber in Orthopädie und Traumatologie, Thieme Verlag Stuttgart, 1982. pp 44-51.

25. Ecke, H.: Behandlung der chronischen Osteomyelitis mit plastischen Operationsverfahren. Chirurg. 33, 123, 1962.

26. Ecke, H., Bernstein, R., and Kyambi, J.: Behandlungsergebnisse nach plastischen Operationsverfahren bei chronischer Osteomyelitis - eine Serie von 19 Jahren. Mschr. Unfallheilk. 77, 36, 1974.

27. Götz, J. and Wesch, G.: Behandlung der chronischen Osteomyelitis mit Taurolin-Gel-Stäben. Z. Orthop. 119, 540, 1981.

28. Goudarzi, Y.M.: Klinische Erfahrungen mit einer Fibrin-Nebacetin-Spongiosaplombe zur Behandlung der chronischen Knocheninfektionen und als lokale Infektionsprophylaxe bei nicht infizierten Knochenherden. Akt. Traumatol. 13, 205, 1983.

29. Hawinger, J., Hammond, D.K., Timmons, S., and Budzynski, A.Z.: Interaction of human fibrinogen with staphylococci: Presence of a binding region on normal and abnormal fibrinogen variants and fibrinogen derivatives. Blood 51, 799, 1978.

30. Heine, W.-D., Edinger, D., and Braun, A.: Wundheilung nach Fibrin-Klebung - Histopathologische Untersuchungen. In, Cotta, H. and Braun, A.: Fibrinkleber in Orthopädie und Traumatologie, Thiem Verlag Stuttgart, 1982, pp 27-34.

31. Heinemann, G.: Beitrag zur Behandlung der chronischen Osteomyelitis. Chirurg. 30, 33, 1959

32. Heiss, F., Ecke, H., Sasse, S., and Bikfali, A.: Tierexperimentelle Untersuchungen zum Wirkungsmechanismus der Eigenblut-Antibiotika-Plombe. Mschr. Unfallheilk. 66, 262, 1963.

33. Hogeman, K.E.: Treatment of infected bone defects with cancellous bone-chip grafts. Acta Chir. Scand. 98, 576, 1949.

34. Klemm, K.: Die Behandlung der posttraumatischen Osteomyelitis mit antibiotikahaltigen Kunststoffkugeln. Vortrag: Symposium Traumatologicum, Brünn, 1974.

35. Klemm, K.: Gentamycin-PMMA-Ketten - eine Alternative zur Spül-Saugdrainage bei Knochen- und Weichteilinfektionen. Langenbecks Arch. Chir. 345, 609, 1977.

36. Kratzat, R., Braun, A., and Schumacher, G.: Erste klinische Erfahrungen mit dem Fibrin-Antibiotikum-Verbund bei der Osteomyelitis. Orthop. Praxis 10, 852, 1981.

37. Kratzat, R., Braun, A., and Schumacher, G.: Erste Erfahrungen mit dem Fibrin-Antibiotikum-Verbund bei Knochen- und Weichteilinfektionen. Akt. Chir. 17, 58, 1982.

38. Marks, K.E., Nelson, C.L., Rock, L., and Lautenschläger, E.P.: Antibiotic-impregnated acrylic bone cement. J. Bone Joint Surg. 58A, 358, 1976.

39. Matras, H., Dinges, H.P., Lassmann, H., and Mamoli, B.: Zur nahtlosen interfaszikulären Nerventransplantation im Tierexperiment. Wien. med. Wschr. 37, 517, 1972.

40. Matti, H.: Über freie Transplantationen von Knochenspongiosa. Langenbecks Arch. klin. Chir. 168, 236, 1932.

41. Mowlem, R.: Cancellous chip bone grafts - Report of 75 cases. Lancet i, 517, 1944.

42. Panis, R. and Scheele, J.: Hepatitisrisiko bei der Fibrinklebung in der HNO-Chirurgie. Laryng.-Rhinol. 60, 367, 1981.

43. Papineau, L.J.: L'excision greffe avec fermeture cutanée retardée délibérée dans l'ostéomyélite chronique. Nouv. Presse Méd. 2, 2753, 1973.

44. Popkirov, S.: Osteoplastische Behandlung der Osteomyelitis. Arch. orthop. Unfall-Chir. 90, 233, 1977.

45. Puhl, W., Böhm, E., Schimpf, K., and Braun, A.: Fibrin zur Blutstillung am spongiösen Knochen bei Hämophilie. In, Cotta, H. and Braun, A.: Fibrinkleber in Orthopädie und Traumatologie, Thieme Verlag Stuttgart, 1982, pp 88-90.

46. Redl, H., Stanek, G., Hirschl, A., and Schlag, G.: Fibrinkleber-Antibiotika-Gemische - Festigkeit und Elutionsverhalten. In, Cotta, H. and Braun, A.: Fibrinkleber in Orthopädie und Traumatologie, Thieme Verlag Stuttgart, 1982, pp 178-181.

47. Redl, H., Stanek, G., Hirschl, A., Seelich, T., and Schlag, G.: Mixtures of fibrin seal and antibiotics: *in vitro* properties (clotting - Crosslinkage - drug release). Biomaterials 4, 29, 1983.

48. Scheele, J.: Hepatitisrisiko der Fibrinklebung in der Allgemeinchirurgie. Med. Welt.32, 783, 1981.

49. Scheele, J. and Pesch , H.-J.: Morphologische Aspekte des Fibrin-Kleberabbaues im Tierexperiment. In, Cotta, H., and Braun, A.: Fibrinkleber in Orthopädie und Traumatologie, Thieme Verlag Stuttgart, 1982, pp 35-43.

50. Spängler,H.P. and Braun, F.: Fibrinklebung in der operativen Medizin. Verlag, Edition Medizin Weinheim - Deerfield Beach, Florida-Basel, 1983.

51. Schumacher, G., Braun, A., Kratzat, R., Fabricius, K., Roesler, H., and Plaue, R.: Zur Antibiotikadiffusion aus dem Fibrin-Gentamycin-Verbund (tierexperimentelle Ergebnisse). In, Parsch, K. and Plaue, R.: Hämatogene Osteomyelitis und posttraumatische Osteitis, Med. Lit. Verlagsgesellschaft mbH, Uelzen, 1982, pp 28-31.

52. Schultheis, K.-H., Schulz, A., and Schiefer, H.-F.: Schnellhärtende Aminosäuren als mögliche Chemotherapeutika-Trägersubstanz zur Behandlung der chronischen Osteomyelitis. Unfallchir. 7, 324, 1981.

53. Ulatowski, L., Thümler, P., Goymann, V., and Meier, M.: Neue Aspekte der Anwendung eines erweiterten Fibrin-Klebesystems (FKS). Orthop. Praxis 10, 795, 1979.

54. Ulatowski, L., Goymann, V., Meier, M., and Thümler, P.: *In vitro*-Ausdiffusion eines Breitbandantibiotikum aus einem Fibrin-Antibiotika-Verbund. Orthop. Praxis 10, 831, 1980.

55. Ulatowski, L., Meier, M., Goymann, V., and Thümler, P.: Zur Wirkung eines Fibrin-Antibiotikum-Verbundes bei Knochen- und Weichteilinfektionen. Fortschr. Med. 99, 864, 1981.

56. Ulatowski, L., Meier, M., Goymann, V., and Thümler, P.: Pharmakokinetik eines Fibrinantibiotikumverbundes. In, Cotta, H. and Braun, A.: Fibrinkleber in Orthopädie und Traumatologie, Thieme Verlag Stuttgart, 1982, pp 196-199.

57. Van Rens, Th.J.G. and Kayser, F.H.: Local antibiotic treatment in osteomyelitis and soft tissue infections. Excerpta Medica, Amsterdam-Oxford-Princeton, 1981.

58. Wahlig, H. and Buchholz, H.W.: Experimentelle und klinische Untersuchungen zur Freisetzung von Gentamycin aus einem Knochenzement. Chirurg. 43, 441, 1972.

59. Wahlig, H., Dingeldein, E., Bergmann, R., and Reuss, K.: Experimentell und pharmakokinetische Untersuchungen mit Gentamycin-PMMA-Kugeln Zbl. Chirurgie 104, 923, 1979.

60. Wahlig, H., Dingeldein, E., Braun, A., and Kratzat, R.: Fibrinkleber und Antibiotika - Untersuchungen zur Freisetzungskinetik. In, Cotta, H. and Braun, A.: Fibrinkleber in Orthopädie und Traumatologie, Thieme Verlag Stuttgart, 1982, pp 182-187.

61. Willenegger, H. and Roth, W.: Die antibakterielle Spüldrainage als Behandlungsprinzip bei chirurgischen Infektionen. Dtsch. med. Wschr. 87, 145, 1962.

62. Winter, L.: Management of chronic osteitis and osteomyelitis with a coagulum of autogenous blood + penicillin + thrombin (on the basis of 56 case results). J. Int. Surg. 1, 510, 1951.

63. Zilch, H., Drehsen, R., Lambiris, E., and Hahn, H.: Diffusionsverhalten von Cefotaxim aus der Fibrin-Antibiotika-Plombe im Tierversuch. In, Cotta, H. and Braun, A.: Fibrinkleber in Orthopädie und Traumatologie, Thieme Verlag Stuttgart, 1982. pp 191-195.

Subject Index

f = figure; t = table

Current Concepts of Diagnosis and Teatment of Bone and Soft Tissue Tumors

Editor: **H.K.Uhthoff**

Associate Editor: **E.Stahl**

1984. 143 figures. XVIII, 436 pages.
ISBN 3-540-12570-1

The prognosis for patients suffering from bone and soft tissue tumors has improved considerably during the last ten years. This success is a result of the increased effectiveness of diagnostic techniques and therapeutic measures made possible by the concerted efforts of pathologists, oncologists, radiologists, and orthopaedic surgeons working as a team to solve one of medicine's more complex problems.

Current Concepts of Diagnosis and Treatment of Bone and Soft Tissue Tumors is designed to foster this effort by keeping all members of the team informed of recent advances in the clinical staging and medicinal and surgical treatment. Written by leading authorities from outstanding medical centers the world over, this book offers access to the expertise and experience necessary for the successful management of these tumors.

Springer-Verlag
Berlin
Heidelberg
New York
Tokyo

MIX
Papier aus verantwortungsvollen Quellen
Paper from responsible sources
FSC® C105338

If you have any concerns about our products,
you can contact us on
ProductSafety@springernature.com

In case Publisher is established outside the EU,
the EU authorized representative is:
Springer Nature Customer Service Center GmbH
Europaplatz 3, 69115 Heidelberg, Germany

Printed by Libri Plureos GmbH
in Hamburg, Germany